KT-562-412

Contents

Introduction   iv

GNVQ Intermediate Health and Social Care: Summary of units   ix

Core skills: Summary of units at level 2   x

Chapter 1   Promoting health and well-being   1

Chapter 2   Influences on health and well-being   70

Chapter 3   Health and social care services   100

Chapter 4   Communication and interpersonal relationships in health and
               social care   129

Chapter 5   Application of science in health and social care   178

Chapter 6   Meeting the needs of individuals in different care settings   225

Chapter 7   Creative activities in care settings   254

Chapter 8   Practical caring skills   282

Appendix: Human development   317

Index   323

Introduction

What is a GNVQ?

A General National Vocational Qualification (GNVQ) is an alternative to A-levels or GCSEs. There are three levels:

- **Foundation GNVQ** – equivalent to four GCSEs at grades D–G, normally one year of full-time study
- **Intermediate GNVQ** – equivalent to four GCSEs at grades A–C, normally one year of full-time study
- **Advanced GNVQ** – equivalent to two A-levels, normally two years of full-time study.

How is a GNVQ structured?

All GNVQ courses are made up of **units**:

- **mandatory vocational units** – those you **must** study
- **optional vocational units** – those you **choose** to study from a selection of possible units
- **mandatory core skills units** in **Communication, Information Technology** and **Application of Number** – generally not studied as separate units, but taught and tested in the activities and assignments on the vocational units.

What is in a unit?

Let us take Unit 1 of the Intermediate GNVQ in Health and Social Care as an example in the diagram below.

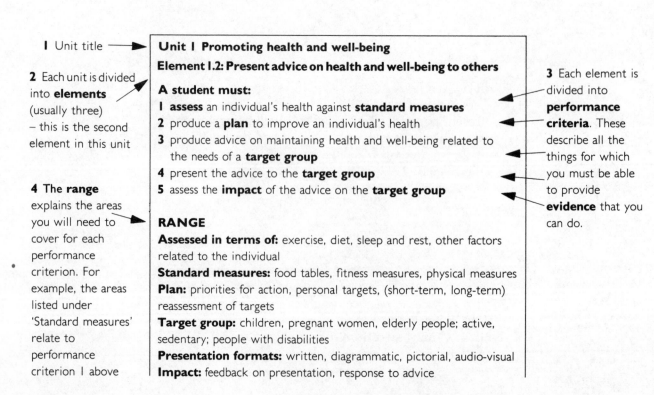

1 Unit title ⟶

2 Each unit is divided into **elements** (usually three) – this is the second element in this unit

4 The range explains the areas you will need to cover for each performance criterion. For example, the areas listed under 'Standard measures' relate to performance criterion 1 above

Unit 1 Promoting health and well-being

Element 1.2: Present advice on health and well-being to others

A student must:
1 **assess** an individual's health against **standard measures**
2 produce a **plan** to improve an individual's health
3 produce advice on maintaining health and well-being related to the needs of a **target group**
4 present the advice to the **target group**
5 assess the **impact** of the advice on the **target group**

RANGE

Assessed in terms of: exercise, diet, sleep and rest, other factors related to the individual

Standard measures: food tables, fitness measures, physical measures

Plan: priorities for action, personal targets, (short-term, long-term) reassessment of targets

Target group: children, pregnant women, elderly people; active, sedentary; people with disabilities

Presentation formats: written, diagrammatic, pictorial, audio-visual

Impact: feedback on presentation, response to advice

3 Each element is divided into **performance criteria**. These describe all the things for which you must be able to provide **evidence** that you can do.

iv

5 The **evidence** ➤ **indicators** describe the **evidence** that you will need to supply to satisfy all the requirements of this element.

EVIDENCE INDICATORS

A plan for improving one person's health and well-being including:
- an assessment of one person's health against standard measures of health and well-being;
- planned improvements to an individual's health; including priorities for action;
- personal targets, and how and when these targets will be reassessed.

A presentation of health promotion advice to one target group using at least two of the presentation formats in the range.

A short report on the impact of the presentation on the target group.

A brief description of the way plans could be adapted and presented to the different groups stated in the range.

What is the Intermediate GNVQ in Health and Social Care?

It is made up of:
- **four mandatory vocational units**
  Unit 1: Promoting health and well-being
  Unit 2: Influences on health and well-being
  Unit 3: Health and social care services
  Unit 4: Communication and interpersonal relationships in health and social care
- **four optional vocational units**, which **differ according to the awarding body offering the GNVQ**. Those for BTEC, and covered in this book, are:
  Unit 5: Application of science in health and social care
  Unit 6: Meeting the needs of individuals in different care settings
  Unit 7: Creative activities in care settings
  Unit 8: Practical caring skills

At Intermediate level you must study the four mandatory vocational units and choose two optional vocational units to study.

What do the units cover?

- **Unit 1: Promoting health and well-being**
  - Personal health
  - Presenting advice on health and well-being to others
  - How to reduce the risk of injury and deal with emergencies
- **Unit 2: Influence on health and well-being**
  - The development of individuals and how they manage change
  - The nature of interpersonal relationships and their influence on health and well-being
  - The interaction of individuals within society and how they may influence health and well-being
- **Unit 3: Health and social care services**
  - The provision of health and social care services
  - How the needs of different client groups are met by health and social care services
  - Jobs in health and social care
- **Unit 4: Communication and interpersonal relationships in health and social care**
  - Developing communication skills

- How interpersonal relationships may be affected by discriminatory behaviour
- Aspects of working with clients
- **Unit 5: Application of science in health and social care**
  - The basic organisation and functions of human body systems
  - Observation and measurement of individuals in care settings
  - The ways science is applied in care contexts
- **Unit 6: Meeting the needs of individuals in different care settings**
  - Methods used to assess individual care needs
  - How individual needs are met in care settings
  - Factors which influence the delivery of care in care settings
- **Unit 7: Creative activities in care settings**
  - The contribution of creative activities to the development of individuals
  - Carrying out creative activities of value to individuals and client groups
  - The contribution of creative activities to care settings
- **Unit 8: Practical caring skills**
  - The function of different care settings
  - The methods for supporting social and life skills
  - Practical skills to support physical needs

How is a GNVQ assessed?

External assessment

Written tests on the four mandatory units are set by either BTEC, RSA or City & Guilds. They are either multiple-choice or short-answer questions. Each test lasts for about one hour and the pass mark is 70 per cent.

Internal assessment

This will take place at your school or college. Your **assessors** will probably be your teachers. Their assessments are checked by **verifiers** (internal and external) to ensure that the assessments agree with national standards.

Assessment is based on showing the assessor what you have achieved. You will need to compile a **portfolio** of relevent **evidence** of your achievements. Your assessor will advise whether you have provided enough evidence to pass a unit, and how to provide any missing evidence.

You may complete the units one by one. There is no time limit on gaining your GNVQ – you can resit external tests and resubmit your portfolio as often as you like to reach the required standard.

What grades are there?

For each unit completed to the national standard, you will obtain a **pass**.

To obtain the GNVQ, you must obtain a pass for each of the required units and written tests, including the core skills. To obtain a **merit** or **distinction** for the complete GNVQ, you must show that you have consistently exhibited skills in the following areas (themes):
- **planning**
- **information-seeking and information-handling**
- **evaluation**
- **quality of outcomes.**

Your tutors will explain these skills.

The award of a final grade for your GNVQ is based on the best third of the evidence for each of the four themes. In order to get a merit or a distinction, you must achieve a third of the evidence in all four themes.

What if I don't agree with an assessment?
You may appeal against an assessment. Every school and college **must** have an appeals procedure to deal with this. You are entitled to a copy of this at the beginning of your course.

Creating your portfolio

A portfolio is a record of your achievements during your course. It will demonstrate to your assessors that you have achieved the relevant skills, knowledge and understanding to gain your GNVQ.

Store your written evidence in an A4 ring-binder divided into sections for each unit you are studying. The portfolio should include forms to be completed by your assessor relating to your evidence.

It will need an **index** as a single piece of evidence may be useful for more than one unit or element. Devise a coding system so that you can cross-reference evidence to more than one unit in the index. The index should include evidence that is not in the ring-binder, such as video or audio tapes, large drawings, maps, etc., which you will need to keep separately.

Types of evidence
- **Performance** or **direct evidence**, for example, reports, assignments (remember to plan carefully how you are going to carry out assignments and projects), an assessor's written report or a written observation (by someone else) of something you have done, such as how you behave in a group, or how you organise other people.
- **Supplementary** or **indirect evidence**, for example, photographs, videos, audio tapes, evidence of written or oral questioning (which will allow you to elaborate on your evidence) and practical tests, references from workplace supervisors.

All evidence should arise from the work you have agreed to complete during discussions with your assessor. How much and what sort of evidence will also be discussed and should form the basis of your **individual action plan** for an activity or assignment. Evidence indicators in the specifications set out what is assessed and what evidence you will need to provide for your portfolio. You do not need to provide any other evidence in your portfolio than that described by the evidence indicators.

Remember
- When planning any piece of work, think carefully about which **vocational** and **core skills** units, elements and performance criteria you can cover. **Remember that a piece of work can provide evidence for more than one element or unit.** For example, a leaflet on healthy eating would be far better produced using a computer, than handwritten.

- Present your portfolio in a professional way.
- The evidence should be **sufficient** (enough), **authentic** (your own work) and **relevant** (test what the performance criteria asks to be tested).
- The assessor and verifiers should find the portfolio easy to read, understand and access. The index should identify what the evidence refers to.
- The documentation should be easy to read.
- You should know exactly what is in your portfolio as you will be asked questions about it by the assessor and the verifiers.

GNVQ Intermediate health and social care: Summary of units and elements

This summary shows how the activities and assignments relate to the units and elements. By keeping a record of your work, many of these exercises will generate useful evidence for your portfolio.

MANDATORY UNITS	Activities	Assignments
1 Promoting health and well-being		
1.1 Investigate personal health	1.1–1.22	A1.1
1.2 Present advice on health and well-being to others	1.23–1.31	A1.2
1.3 Reduce risk of injury and deal with emergencies	1.32–1.35	A1.3
2 Influences on health and well-being		
2.1 Explore the development of individuals and how they manage change	2.1–2.9	A2.1
2.2 Explore the nature of interpersonal relationships and their influence on health and well-being	2.10–2.19	A2.2
2.3 Explore the interaction of individuals within society and how they may influence health and well-being	2.20–2.22	A2.3
3 Health and social care services		
3.1 Investigate the provision of health and social care services	3.1–3.4	A3.1
3.2 Describe how the needs of different client groups are met by health and social care services	3.5–3.10	A3.2
3.3 Investigate jobs in health and social care	3.11–3.12	A3.3
4 Communication and interpersonal relationships in health and social care		
4.1 Develop communication skills	4.1–4.25	
4.2 Explore how interpersonal relationships may be affected by discriminatory behaviour	4.26–4.35	A4.1
4.3 Investigate aspects of working with clients in health and social care	4.36–4.47	
OPTIONAL UNITS		
5 Application of science in health and social care		
5.1 Explain the basic organisation and functions of human body systems	5.1	A5.1
5.2 Investigate observation and measurement of individuals in care settings	5.2–5.6	A5.2
5.3 Investigate the ways science is applied in care contexts	5.7–5.8	A5.3
6 Meeting the needs of individuals in different care settings		
6.1 Examine methods used to assess individual care needs	6.1–6.11	A6.1
6.2 Explore the way individual care needs are met in care settings	6.12–6.19	A6.2
6.3 Investigate factors which influence the delivery of care in different settings	6.20–6.22	A6.3
7 Creative activities in care settings		
7.1 Examine the contribution of creative activities to the development of individuals	7.1–7.4	A7.1
7.2 Carry out creative activity of value to individuals and client groups	7.5	A7.2
7.3 Investigate the contribution of creative activities in care settings	7.6	A7.3
8 Practical caring skills		
8.1 Investigate the function of different care settings	8.1–8.3	A8.1
8.2 Describe methods used to support social and life skills	8.4–8.7	A8.2
8.3 Use the practical skills required to support physical needs	8.8–8.13	A8.3

Core skills: Summary of units at level 2

This summary shows how the activites and assignments provide opportunities to provide evidence of the core skills. When planning a piece of work, think carefully about the core skills you can provide evidence for. For example, use information technology as often as possible when producing written work, leaflets, poster, charts and diagrams.

Core skills	Activities	Assignments
Communication		
2.1 Take part in discussions	1.1, 1.2, 1.8, 1.12, 1.14, 1.23, 1.24, 1.26, 1.30, 1.33, 2.2, 2.7, 2.10, 2.11, 2.12, 2.15, 2.17, 2.18, 2.19, 2.21, 2.22, 3.1, 3.4, 3.10, 3.11, 3.12, 4.1, 4.2, 4.4, 4.6, 4.7, 4.8, 4.10, 4.14, 4.16, 4.17, 4.22, 4.26, 4.36, 4.37, 6.2, 6.8, 6.22, 8.9	A1.1, A3.1, A3.3, A4.1, A7.2, A7.3, A8.3
2.2 Produce written material	1.1, 1.2, 1.6, 1.8, 1.14, 1.15, 1.18, 1.19, 1.20, 1.22, 1.29, 1.33, 1.34, 2.1, 2.9, 2.11, 2.12, 2.13, 2.15, 2.22, 3.8, 3.10, 3.11, 4.2, 4.10, 4.11, 4.12, 4.14, 4.17, 4.22, 4.26, 4.31, 4.33, 5.1, 6.4, 6.8, 6.11, 8.1, 8.8, 8.9, 8.11	A1.1, A1.2, A2.1, A2.3, A3.1, A3.3, A4.1, A5.1, A6.1, A7.1, A7.2, A7.3, A8.1, A8.2, A8.3
2.3 Use images	1.8, 1.20, 1.29, 1.34, 2.19, 3.4, 3.5, 4.12, 4.22, 5.8, 6.16, 8.6	A1.1, A1.2, A5.1, A6.1, A7.1, A8.1, A8.3
2.4 Read and respond to written materials	1.8, 1.9, 1.14, 1.15, 1.26, 1.28, 2.1, 2.2, 2.4, 2.5, 2.6, 2.8, 2.17, 3.5, 3.8, 4.4, 4.22, 4.33, 4.34, 6.8, 7.3	A1.1, A2.2, A2.3, A3.3, A8.3
Information technology		
2.1 Prepare information	1.2, 1.13, 1.20, 1.24, 1.26, 1.34, 5.1, 5.6, 5.8, 8.1, 8.8, 8.11	A1.1, A1.2, A2.1, A2.2, A2.3, A3.1, A3.2, A3.3, A4.1, A5.1, A5.2, A7.3
2.2 Process information	1.2, 1.13, 1.15, 1.20, 1.24, 1.26, 1.34, 4.22, 5.1, 5.6, 5.8, 8.1, 8.8, 8.11	A1.1, A1.2, A2.1, A2.2, A2.3, A3.1, A3.2, A3.3, A4.1, A5.1, A5.2, A7.3
2.3 Present information	1.2, 1.13, 1.15, 1.20, 1.24, 1.26, 1.34, 4.22, 5.1, 5.6, 5.8, 8.1, 8.8, 8.11	A1.1, A1.2, A2.1, A2.2, A2.3, A3.1, A3.2, A3.3, A4.1, A5.1, A5.2, A7.3
2.4 Evaluate the use of information technology	1.2, 1.13, 1.15, 1.20, 1.24, 1.26, 1.34, 4.22	A4.1, A5.1
Application of number		
2.1 Collect and record data	1.1, 1.5, 1.8, 1.11, 1.14, 1.16, 1.24, 1.27, 1.28, 4.22, 5.2, 5.5	A3.2, A4.1, A5.2, A8.1
2.2 Tackle problems	1.8, 1.16, 1.27, 4.22, 5.2, 5.5	A4.1, A5.2
2.3 Interpret and present data	1.5, 1.8, 1.11, 1.13, 1.15, 1.16, 1.19, 1.20, 1.24, 1.27, 1.28, 1.29, 4.22, 5.2, 5.5, 5.6, 5.7	A3.2, A4.1, A5.2, A8.1, A8.2

CHAPTER I

Promoting health and well-being

Element 1.1: Investigate personal health
Element 1.2: Present advice on health and well-being to others
Element 1.3: Reduce risk of injury and deal with emergencies

What is covered in this chapter

- Investigating personal health and well-being
- Diet
- Exercise
- Stress
- Smoking
- Alcohol abuse
- Drug abuse

- Sexual behaviour
- Hygiene
- Advising others on health and well-being
- Accidents
- Dealing with an emergency
- Reducing the risk of injury to others

These are the resources you will need for your Promoting Health and Well-being file:

- your own notes and observations
- your written answers to the activities in this chapter
- evidence of action plans and research you used to carry out the activities, including health promotion material you have collected
- your written answers to the review questions at the end of this chapter
- your completed tasks for Assignments A1.1, A1.2, and A1.3 including your report on the health promotion display and the checklist of your competence in life-saving skills signed by your tutor.

Introduction

Everyone wants to be healthy. Sometimes we take being healthy for granted until for some reason we become ill or find it difficult to cope.

In the last decade there has been unprecedented interest on the part of individuals in their own health care. People want to participate in their own health care and governments are keen to encourage them in order to cut down on increasing health costs. In 1978 the World Health Organisation's Declaration of Alma Ata stated that it was the right and duty of people to participate collectively and as individuals in their own health care.

Information is the first step towards making healthy choices. This chapter identifies health risks associated with certain lifestyles.

Investigating personal health and well-being

Consider how healthy you are. You know how unpleasant it is to feel unwell, but what does being healthy really mean? A person who is in good health is someone whose body is working at maximum efficiency mentally and physically.

Here are some factors which affect your health:
- inheritance
- age
- gender
- climate
- pollution
- environment
- organisms, microbes, parasites
- education
- national services relating to health and welfare.

In addition to these factors, increasing attention is being paid to 'lifestyle' factors. Why do cancer, heart disease and strokes occur particularly in our western society? The quest for finding out is known as *epidemiology*. Epidemiologists are now identifying 'lifestyle' factors, particularly diet and lack of exercise, as causes of health problems. We all have the power to influence our own health and that of our family.

Activity 1.1

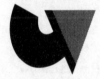

a Write down what you do in a typical week in terms of:
  i) rest
  ii) relaxation
  iii) sleep
  iv) exercise
  v) recreation
  vi) work and study.
Give approximate daily timings for each activity.

b What sort of pattern is there to your week? Is there a balance of different types of activity? Compare your notes with other members of your group.

The effects of lack of exercise

It is often said that the people who would benefit most from exercise feel least like taking it! Certainly lack of exercise contributes to obesity, cardiovascular problems, muscle weakness and stress. You will find more information on exercise in pages 12–17.

Recreation

After work or studying, a complete change is good for you. Do you know what is available in your locality?

Activity 1.2

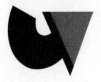

a Make a list of all the recreational activities in which you participate.

b Find out about recreational activities in your local area. Produce a concise booklet which would inform teenagers about activities that are available.

The effects of lack of sleep

When you don't get enough sleep, you are less fun to be with and you may appear dull and lethargic. Different people need different amounts of sleep. Adults average eight hours a night, older people need less and younger people more.

While we sleep our bodies repair themselves. Good sleep is vital for the processes of renewal in the body. A person who is deprived of sleep experiences great difficulty in concentrating and dealing with even simple problems.

There are two types of sleep. We sleep deeply for about two hours then we pass through a stage of lighter sleep, when we dream. During this time our eyes make rapid movements and the brain waves are faster than in ordinary sleep. Both types of sleep are needed. If we are unable to sleep properly, it may indicate that we are worried, depressed, drinking too much or taking insufficient exercise. There is nothing better than natural sleep and people who are experiencing problems might consider some of the following remedies:
- taking more exercise – try walking or jogging
- having a milky drink before bed
- avoiding rich, highly spiced foods
- reading before going to sleep
- trying a mental task like counting sheep
- keeping warm
- cutting down on noise
- not smoking in the bedroom
- having a really comfortable bed.

On some occasions a doctor might prescribe a sleeping tablet as a short-term solution to help a person through a difficult time.

Activity 1.3

Monitor and record your sleep pattern. For a week note how you react if you do not get enough sleep.

Effects of stress

Stress is a condition which can result from many different life activities and events. Some stress can be good for us and can be used positively. But in certain situations it can be detrimental to our mental and physical health. Stress is discussed fully on pages 17–23.

Relaxation

When stress is unavoidable we can try to negate its effects by using relaxation techniques. Here are some examples:

- a regular relaxation period each day
- massage
- muscle control
- breathing exercises
- yoga.

Activity 1.4

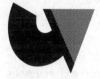

Find out more about the above techniques. Add any other methods of relaxation you know about.

Some aspects of health are difficult to control, for example heredity, environmental hazards and social influences. However there are some risks which we can do something about:

- unhealthy diet
- smoking
- alcohol abuse
- drug abuse
- unsafe sexual behaviour
- lack of exercise
- stress
- poor hygiene precautions
- accidents.

We will look at each of these in detail.

Diet

Does it matter what we eat?

If we want to feel well, stay fit, have good teeth and keep our weight in proportion to our size, then we need to think about the foods that we eat. It is possible to eat nothing but buscuits, chocolates, snack foods and cake for a day or two without feeling too many ill effects. However, if we continued with this type of diet for a longer period we would begin to put on weight, be at greater risk from dental caries and generally feel less fit.

The current recommendations for a healthy diet include:

- eating more fibre
- eating less sugar
- eating less fat.

All of these recommendations could be implemented by simple changes in our daily diet.

Activity 1.5

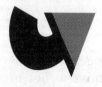

a Keep a record over three days of all that you eat and drink.

b Interview an elderly person and find out what they normally eat and drink.

Write down the differences between the two eating habits. What do you think are the reasons for the differences?

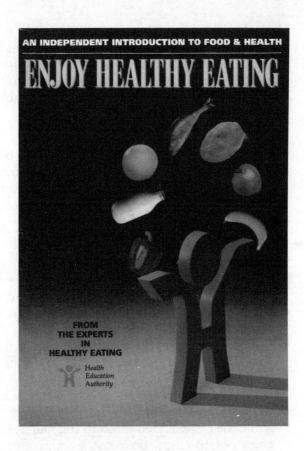

The basic nutrients

The basic nutrients are:
● proteins
● carbohydrates
● fats
● minerals
● vitamins.

Each nutrient has a particular part to play in the body's function. A variety of nutrients from different foods are necessary to keep the body in good working order.

Protein

This is needed for the growth and repair of body tissues. It is found mainly in meat, fish, eggs, milk and cheese. Vegetarians obtain most of their protein from soya products, nuts, cereals, peas, beans and lentils. The protein allowance should be divided up between all the day's meals.

Protein should be eaten with carbohydrates as the body uses proteins to supply energy if it is short of carbohydrates. This is an expensive form of energy and it also deprives the body of its source of nutrients for growth.

Proteins cannot be stored by the body and protein-rich foods can be expensive, but it is important that every member of the family should have a regular supply. In particular, children need a large quantity of protein as their bodies are growing. Adults need a smaller quantity for the repair of tissue.

Carbohydrates

These give us energy. The main carbohydrates are sugar and starches. Cellulose is also a carbohydrate, but it cannot be digested and is used as roughage (dietary fibre). Starches are of vegetable origin and contain other useful nutrients. Sugar, however, has no nutritional value other than warmth and energy, so it is the least useful of fuel foods.

Fats

These also provide energy. Fats and oils are obtained from plants and animals and are a very concentrated form of energy. If we eat more fats and carbohydrates than our body needs they are stored and this can lead to obesity. The main fats in our diet may include butter, margarine, lard, vegetable oils and cream.

Minerals

This is a large group of nutrients but we only need them in very small quantities:
- **iron**, which helps to prevent anaemia. This is found particularly in liver and kidney, dried fruits, eggs, spinach and cocoa.
- **calcium** and **phosphorus**, which give us strong bones and teeth. Main sources are cheese, milk and flour.
- **iodine**, which is necessary for the proper functioning of the thyroid gland. Main sources are fish, water, milk and milk products.
- **sodium**, which is found in all body fluids. It helps in the function of muscles. It is mainly found in salt, cheese, kippers, ham and bacon.
- **potassium**, which is mainly present in body fluids. Like sodium, it is absorbed and excess is excreted through the kidneys. Good sources are milk, cheese, eggs, potato crisps, breakfast cereal, coffee and Marmite.
- **fluorine**, which is found in tea, sea food, toothpaste and water. Fluoride can help to prevent tooth decay.
- **zinc**, which is mainly present in bones. It helps the healing of wounds, and is found in a wide variety of foods, meat and dairy products.

Fluorine, iodine and zinc are known as **trace elements**. Other trace elements include cobalt, chromium and copper.

Vitamins

The four main vitamins which need to be remembered are only available in a limited number of foods. They are divided into two main groups.
- **Vitamins A and D are fat-soluble** and are generally found in fatty foods.
- **Vitamins B and C are water-soluble**, cannot be stored by the body and therefore daily supplies are needed.

Vitamin A

Vitamin A is sometimes known as the *anti-infective vitamin* and can be stored by the body to be used when needed. It is found mainly in dairy products, egg yolk, fatty fish and fish liver oils. A secondary source can also be found in orange, yellow or green plants containing carotene, such as carrots and green cabbage. Vitamin A is used by the body to aid growth in children; it helps our eyes to see in dim light; protects our skin; and keeps the lining of the throat, lungs and stomach moist.

Vitamin B

The vitamin B group contains a number of vitamins, all of which are water-soluble.
- **Vitamin B_1 (thiamine)** is found in brown flour, potatoes, vegetables, meat

and yeast. Its main use is in the release of energy from carbohydrate foods as well as maintaining the nervous system and helping in growth.

- **Vitamin B₂ (riboflavin)** can be found in eggs, cheese, milk, liver and yeast products. It plays a role in the growth of children, keeps the mouth and tongue free from infection and keeps the cornea of the eye clear.
- **Nicotinic acid** (sometimes called **niacin**) is found in bread, cereals, flour, meat and potatoes. Again it is necessary for the growth of children and prevents digestive disorders.

Vitamin C

Vitamin C or ascorbic acid is water-soluble so daily supplies are needed. It is found in citrus fruits, blackcurrants, rose hips, green vegetables and tomatoes. It helps the body resist infection, keeps gums healthy, helps wounds and fractures to heal and ensures a healthy skin. Vitamin C is the vitamin most likely to be lacking in the UK diet. It is very easily lost from food in storage and during cooking. You can only ensure that there is sufficient in the diet by:

- using fruit and vegetables in as fresh a state as possible
- serving fruits and vegetables raw whenever possible
- keeping cooking times to a minimum
- dishing up and serving food immediately
- using the cooking water (stock) which contains dissolved vitamins for making gravy or sauces.

Vitamin D

Vitamin D is often known as the sunshine vitamin and like vitamin A can also be stored by the body. It is found in fish liver oils, margarine, butter, cheese and eggs. It is important in the formation of strong bones and teeth, and promotes growth. This vitamin can also be made by the body itself by the action of sunlight on the skin.

Water

This is not usually regarded as a food, but it is important in the diet. Every part and function of the body depends on water and it is being lost continuously through the skin, lungs, kidneys and bowels. This water must be replaced and is obtained from the liquids that we drink and the food that we eat.

Nutritional deficiences

Everyone has different nutritional needs, and some people can cope with nutritional deficiencies better than others. It has been seen that prisoners of war given exactly the same diet suffered a range of effects, from being hardly affected (apart from weight loss) to blindness and death.

The body is able to adapt to reduced food intake, but too little food over a period of time can lead to ill-health through under-nitrition. In extreme cases, as in developing countries of the world, starvation causes stunting of physical and mental development and wasting. Diseases like scurvy and some forms of anaemia are caused by a deficiency (shortage) of certain nutrients or by the body's inability to absorb those nutrients.

In the UK, we may not necessarily have the problem of starvation, but excessive amounts of food can also cause malnutrition (literally, 'bad eating'), which may lead to conditions of ill-health such as obesity, heart disease or high blood pressure. Too much sugar, for example, may cause tooth decay. In poor countries, diets are often low in fat, while in the West we are advised to reduce our fat intake to prevent heart disease. Adults and children over 5 years are recommended to avoid fat making up more than one third of their total energy or calorie intake.

It is useful to check labels on products and prepared foods just to see the amount of fat or sugar in the product. The greatest amount is listed first. There has been some publicity (and disagreement) about certain fats being connected with particular diseases. It is thought that high intakes of saturated fats (lard, suet, cocoa butter) can increase the cholesterol level in some individuals and so increase the risk of heart disease.

Some nutrients are necessary for good health. The possible effects of deficiencies of these nutrients are mentioned below. Don't forget that people have differing needs.

Carbohydrate deficiency

If a person's carbohydrate intake is too low, their protein intake has to be used for energy and so the 'growth and repair' function of the protein has less effect.

Mineral deficiency

Iron

Deficiency of iron can result in anaemia. A person with anaemia may feel tired, lethargic and be pale. Anaemia can also arise from a shortage of folic acid and vitamin B_{12}. The absorption of iron from food is generally low, but it is increased when the body's stores are low as during menstruation.

Calcium

Calcium is the most abundant mineral in the body. Too little calcium in young children may result in stunted growth and rickets (a condition where the bones develop badly and the legs are often bowed). The condition is rarely seen in the UK today. Among elderly people, the condition may show as osteomalacia. The main cause of such conditions is lack of vitamin D which assists the absorption of calcium.

Phosphorus

Phosphorus is found in many foods and it is difficult to have too little. If too much phosphorus is taken in the first few days of life, this may produce low levels of calcium in the blood and muscular spasms. Phosphorus is found in cows' milk and that is why babies must only have 'modified' milk, special baby milk or breast milk.

Sodium

Sodium and water requirements are closely linked. Too little sodium may result in muscle cramps.

Salt is present naturally in foods and many prepared foods have a high salt content (check the labels). Habitual high salt intake is associated with high blood pressure. Young infants and people with kidney complaints or water retention problems cannot tolerate high salt intakes.

Potassium

Losses of potassium may be large if laxatives or diuretics (medication to reduce water retention) are used or if carbohydrate level is so low that protein is used for energy. In extreme cases deficiency of potassium can result in heart failure.

Fluorine

Fluorine is found in tea, sea food, toothpaste and water. Fluorine or fluoride level in water varies in different parts of the country. Fluorine can help to prevent tooth decay. Take care, however, because an excess of fluoride can cause the teeth to become mottled.

Iodine

A shortage of iodine causes the thyroid gland to swell and this condition is known as goitre.

Zinc

If a diet is too high in fibre, the zinc in food may not be absorbed and this may affect growth and repair.

More knowledge is needed about the trace elements (fluorine, iodine and zinc). The effects of deficiencies of them isn't fully known, neither is it known how one may affect another.

Vitamin deficiency

In general terms, a shortage of vitamins can lead to a reduced resistance to disease and feeling unwell. An excess of certain vitamins can also be harmful. The more specific deficiencies are:

- **vitamin A** – poor vision and, in extreme cases, blindness. An excess of vitamin A is poisonous
- **vitamin B_1 (thiamin)** – depression, tiredness and, in cases of severe lack, diseases of the nervous system. Also beri-beri in rice-eating communities
- **vitamin B_2 (riboflavin)** – rarely deficient, occasionally sores in the mouth. Can be destroyed by sunlight, so avoid leaving milk on a sunny doorstep
- **nicotinic acid (niacin)** – pellegra in famine areas, a condition where the skin becomes dark and scaly when exposed to light
- **vitamin C** – bleeding from small blood vessels, gums, wounds heal more slowly. Scurvy from prolonged lack. There is no scientific evidence that a lack of vitamin C means more colds.
- **vitamin D** – rickets (see Calcium deficiency, page 8).

The nutritional needs of different client groups

People have different dietary needs at different times in their lives.

Young children

Young children have a great need for protein, thiamin and calcium as they grow, particularly at around 7–8 years of age. Some children may find it difficult to eat well for a variety of reasons.

Activity 1.6

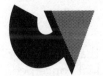

Make a list of factors which might affect a child's eating pattern.

Adolescents

Adolescents also have high nutritional needs. They may find it difficult to eat balanced meals because they are busy or because they may not care for food prepared by their parents and considered to be nourishing. They may miss meals because of demands on their time.

This is also a time when they may be aware of their body shape and feel they need to lose or gain weight. Adolescence is a vulnerable time for eating disorders such as anorexia and bulimia. Sometimes young people are influenced by media images of what they should eat, what they should drink and how they should appear. Emotionally, adolescence can be a turbulent time and eating can be seen as an escape or a comfort at a time of possible exam pressure, career dilemma, parental tension and relationship worries. Apart from all that, some people do enjoy their adolescent years!

Adults
Adults may be concerned about time and costs in connection with food. This is particularly the case if they work and have family responsibilities and/or if they are on a low income.

Sometimes people fail to eat well because they are anxious or stressed about matters which are important to them, such as relationships, family and work or lack of work. The reverse situation can also happen when people overeat, possibly because they feel it doesn't matter about weight as they grow older or possibly because they are overwrought or overworked. There are many reasons why people overeat or become overweight. You might like to discuss some of these reasons in class. Think about decreased mobility and the calorie levels of alcoholic drinks.

Pregnant women and breast-feeding mothers
This group of women need high quantities of protein, iron, calcium, folic acid (a B-group vitamin) and vitamins C and D. Sometimes the minerals and vitamins are prescribed by the GP, but a good nutritional intake is also required.

Elderly people
Elderly people may have fewer energy requirements because of decreased mobility and a smaller appetite. There are also social reasons why elderly people may not eat well, for example:
● They may live alone and it may seem pointless to cook for one.
● They may be on a fixed income and find it difficult to afford the food they would like to eat.
● They may find it hard to shop and many pre-packed goods may be too much for them.
● They may find it physically difficult to cook.

Activity 1.7

What might you suggest in each of the cases listed above?

Disabled people
Disabled people are no more likely to be nutritionally deficient than any other group. It depends on the nature of the disability and the individual concerned. Where mobility is restricted, weight gain may be a problem, in which case a reduced calorie intake may be necessary. If you need to plan or cook meals for children or people with disabilities, then you will need to check their dietary requirements with them or with their carers.

Diabetics

Diabetics have a metabolic disorder which reduces the body's ability to control the amount of glucose in the blood. Diabetics need to avoid the rapid rises in blood glucose which result from eating large amounts or readily-adsorbed carbohydrate. Their total carbohydrate intake needs to be controlled. Asian diabetics live well, with 60 per cent of their diet as carbohydrate coming from rice or chapatis, whereas traditional low carbohydrate diets may be high in fat which can lead to heart disease.

Planning meals

What's for tea? What would you like for your supper? When did you last eat a *proper* meal?

Many factors influence what we eat: habit, age, class, income, available money, taste, family background, amount of time we have, who we are with, whether we play sport, etc.

A balanced meal is said to be one with adequate amounts of carbohydrate, protein, minerals, vitamins and fibre, but low in sugar, fat and salt.

There is no point in knowing about nutrients if we do not put that knowledge into practice. Before you plan to eat you should consider these questions:
● What pattern of eating suits my way of living?
● What foods are available and what can I afford?
● Is there anyone in my family who has special dietary needs?
● How do I ensure that I obtain the necessary nutrients?

The nutrient triangle

Most of us prepare meals without really thinking about their nutritional value. We think more about the likes and dislikes of the people who will be eating the meal. While we want to avoid food being wasted, it is important to include foods in each meal that satisfy our dietary needs. No matter what race or culture we belong to, it is possible to provide meals that are healthy and satisfy the family's likes and dislikes.

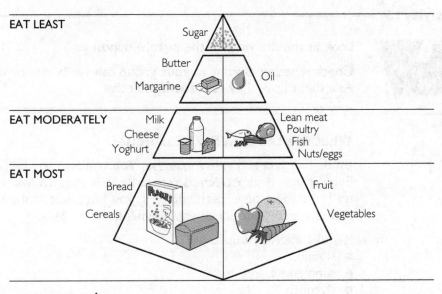

The nutrient triangle

If you divide the main nutrients into three groups then the triangle that they form can be used to check whether the meal you are planning is balanced or not.

Remember that too many energy foods can cause obesity and that fruit and vegetables should be used to supply the bulk of fibre in our diet.

Energy requirements

Different people need different amounts of food each day. The amount needed depends on age, sex, size and activity level. People with high energy needs, such as children, manual workers and teenagers, will need more energy than less-active people. Sedentary people may need to cut down on energy foods.

Activity 1.8

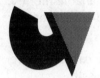

a Plan two days' meals for yourself and a friend. How have you ensured that you are getting the right amounts of nutrients?

b Plan two days' meals for someone with particular dietary needs. (He or she could be elderly/vegetarian/of a different cultural background.) How have you ensured that his or her dietary needs are being met?

Exercise

For some people, the mere mention of the word 'exercise' makes them shrink away. This reaction may be the result of unhappy experiences of exercise and particularly competitive sport. Exercise is an extremely individual matter. People can select from a whole range of exercise patterns and sports to find something which suits their level and their lifestyle.

Activity 1.9

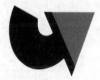

Look at the drawings in the picture opposite.

Check whether anyone in your group can verify one or more of these points. Ask them how they feel about exercise.

What are the benefits of exercise?

If you try, you will enjoy exercise. You will also feel better for it – eventually! Even if you have exercised regularly, it is easy to lose the habit if you give up for a short time, particularly if you have just embarked on a new course and changed your social environment.

Regular exercise improves:
● stamina
● suppleness
● strength.

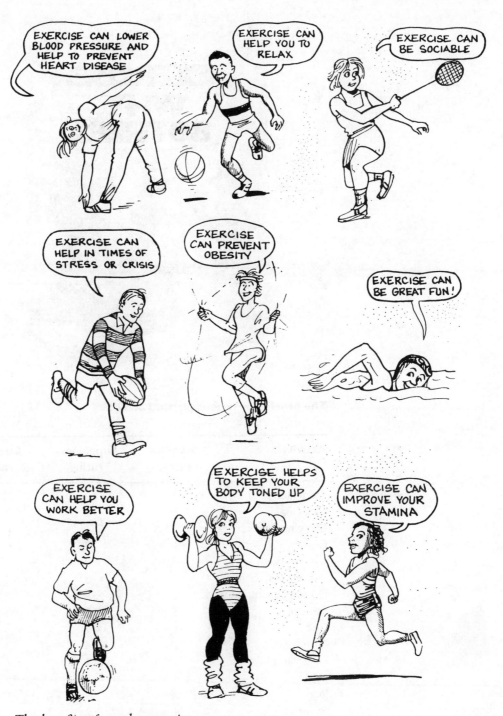

The benefits of regular exercise

The table on page 14 illustrates the benefits from various physical activities. Bear in mind, however, that the actual benefits will depend on how vigorously the activity is carried out.

Regular exercise

If you exercise vigorously but spasmodically, you are shocking your body into action and your muscles are jolted into performance. On the other hand,

13

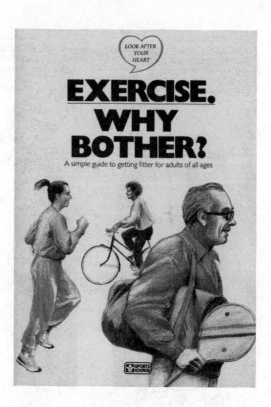

The benefits of various physical activities

Activity	Stamina rating	Suppleness rating	Strength rating
Badminton	2	3	2
Canoeing	3	2	3
Climbing stairs	3	1	2
Cricket	1	2	1
Cycling (hard)	4	2	3
Dancing (ballroom)	1	3	1
Dancing (disco)	3	4	1
Football	3	3	3
Golf	1	2	1
Gymnastics	2	4	3
Hillwalking	3	1	2
Jogging	4	2	2
Judo	2	4	2
Rowing	4	2	4
Sailing	1	2	2
Squash	3	3	2
Swimming (hard)	4	4	4
Tennis	2	3	2
Walking (briskly)	2	1	1
Weightlifting	1	1	4
Yoga	1	4	1

Key: 1 – no real effect   2 – beneficial effect
3 – very good effect   4 – excellent effect

if you exercise gradually at first and then build up regularly, your body becomes accustomed to the pressure. Limbs become more flexible and your heart and lungs increase their capacity to supply the body with its extra demands for oxygen.

You are less likely to maintain an exercise plan if it is not suited to your lifestyle.

It is far better to set yourself realistic targets which you know you can fit into your routine – such as running a couple of miles before tea or before dark, twice a week – than a time-consuming or expensive sport. It is better for your self-esteem to keep to a regular exercise pattern than to start and then trail off.

Exercise routines

Exercise routines can be divided into two types:

- **Aerobic** – exercise which works your heart, lungs and blood system, such as running, fast swimming and fast cycling.
- **Anaerobic** – exercise which concentrates on stretching and flexing the muscles, such as yoga and general stretch work.

A good exercise programme will combine the two types of exercise depending on individual needs.

Whichever activity you choose, try to build up gradually. To gain and maintain a fitness level you ought to aim for three, 20-minute sessions per week. Exercise which is boring, gruelling or difficult to fit in which your lifestyle will be a problem to maintain. Choose something you feel happy with and which is not too disruptive of your routine at work and home. You may encourage friends and family to join you.

Another point concerning anaerobic work is that some people of average flexibility try to work at levels which are beyond them and injury results.

Try to:

- warm up thoroughly
- avoid jerky movements
- avoid exercises which leave the back unsupported like the 'bridge' (**a** in the illustration below)
- take care doing double-leg raises (**b**) or exercises which involve lifting the leg high to a fixed point (**c**)
- be cautious doing sit-ups with straight legs (**d**).

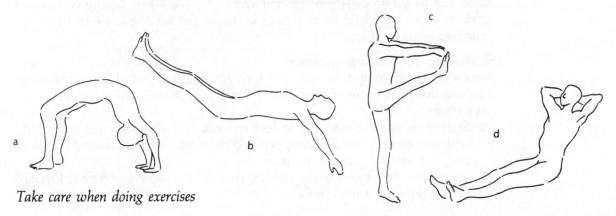

Take care when doing exercises

Questions to consider before exercise
- Can you afford the cost of the exercise?
- Are you fit or do you need a medical check-up?
- Do you have suitable clothes?
- Do you have suitable footwear?
- Is the weather suitable and safe for the exercise?
- Do you have enough time to warm up before and cool down after?
- Have you eaten enough and sufficiently early so that the food is digested?

Monitoring exercise

You will find it encouraging to monitor your progress in terms of how fit you are getting during the training programme.

Pulse rate
Taking your pulse is one way of monitoring your fitness. The slower your pulse the fitter you are getting.

To check your pulse, press the artery on the inside of your wrist with your first three fingers. Count how many beats you can feel in 10 seconds and then multiply by six; alternatively count the number of beats you can feel in 60 seconds. The average pulse rate is about 70 beats per minute.

Now that you can check your pulse try a few exercises to monitor your fitness level:
- Walk up and down a flight of steps, say 15 to 20 in total. On the whole, if you are more than mildly breathless and your pulse is higher than average then you may be unfit.
- Run on the spot for about three minutes. If your pulse is over 90 and you are midly breathless then you are fairly unfit.
- Using a firm bench or the second step of a stair, step up and down briskly. Aim for about two steps up and down every six seconds for about three minutes. If you are very breathless and your pulse rate is about 90 then you are pretty unfit.
- Jog gently for about one mile. This should take about 10 minutes. If you are not breathless then you are fairly fit.

Useful exercises for carers

Caring can be a hectic and stressful occupation. You are often on your feet for long hours. There is a temptation when you are very busy to rush your meals and to slump down in the first chair you see when you have finished work. A more beneficial habit would be to lie flat on the floor or bed with your feet slightly raised.

Stretching and flexing exercises
Remember to warm up thoroughly before you begin any stretching or flexing. You can do this by running on the spot for two minutes or skipping if you have room.
1 Start with some head rolls to loosen neck and shoulder muscles. Stand with feet apart, shoulders dropped and then roll the head around six times one way and six times the other.
2 Turn head three times to the left and three to the right. Drop head forward – chin on chest three times.

3 Hunch right shoulder to ear and drop three times. Same for left and then both together.

4 Strong abdominal muscles are important – this exercise helps:
- lie flat on the floor
- raise knees
- feet flat on the floor
- slowly lift up through a rounded spine so that hands go just above the knees.

Try four of these at first and then hug your knees to your chest. Then try a further four. Try to work towards six continual raises. Go slowly. Do *not* jerk. Breathe in as you go down and out as you come up.

5 Still on the floor, raise yourself onto your elbows and cycle your legs forward. Work towards 12 pedals and then hug your knees in.

6 For back strength. Lie on your tummy. Raise one leg straight behind you and hold for a count of two. Then raise the other leg and hold for a count of two. Finally, raise both legs for a count of two. Eventually try to work to holding both legs to a count of four.

7 For general flexibility try side bends. Stand legs apart with hands on hips. Bend eight times to the right and eight times to the left.

8 Same as 7 but this time with hands behind the head.

9 Same position, but slide your right arm down the right leg. Repeat for the left.

10 Body bender. Stand with feet apart. Raise your arms above your head and then swoop round in a big circle around your own body. First clockwise and then anti-clockwise.

11 Lie on your side with both legs stretched out. Raise the top leg eight times. Then swing the leg in front and behind the body eight times. Change legs.

12 Relaxation position. Lie flat on tummy, arms stretched out in front, and head facing down. Draw the knees up and you should feel a good stretch in the spine. Arch and then drop the back like a cat three times.

Stress

Most people are aware that too much stress can endanger your health, but too little stress can also be bad for you. People who have few demands made on them or who have little stimulation may find themselves feeling very tired without doing very much or wanting to do very much. Some people thrive on stress, but others find even a minimal disruption difficult to cope with.

What is stress?

Stress is a response. It is the imbalance between an individual and the demands made of that individual. The term *stressor* is used to describe the demand. This could be a noise, a task or a thought which makes the demand that produces a stress response in the individual.

An extreme and sudden stress produces a physical reaction. For example, if you think a child is about to run out in front of a car:
- Your eyes and ears receive an alarm signal.
- Your brain registers the child is in danger and sends messages out along the nerves.

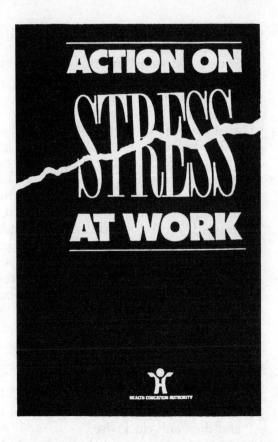

- Your muscles contract in readiness for action.
- The strength of your heart beat increases so blood is pumped more quickly to where it is most needed, i.e. your muscles.
- Chemicals in the brain set off a number of hormonal changes in your body. Adrenalin is produced.
- Your hearing becomes more sensitive.
- Your skin goes pale because the blood has to go elsewhere.
- Your breathing gets faster.
- Your blood pressure rises, carrying oxygen more quickly to the heart, muscles and brain.
- Your sweating increases.
- You may be left feeling faint because the fear causes you to breathe too fast, leading to less blood in the brain.

Interestingly, a similar physical reaction may be felt if somebody you feel quite strongly about actually enters the room where you are.

Reactions to stress

People may react differently to stress or have different reactions at different times. There are three types of reaction. For example, if you are engrossed in a piece of work and some friends call round, you might take a:

- **fight response** – you throw down your pen, open the door muttering irritably that you are busy. This sort of person tends to be the conscientious type, who works hard and finds it difficult to relax. Sometimes a person may suppress the fight response so that they appear to be calm and in control, but in fact they are seething within.

- **flight response** – you might think to yourself that you might as well take a break and put the kettle on. This sort of person is trying to escape from stressful situations. Such a person tends to be more cautious, may withdraw from stressful situations and pass up opportunities for advancement.
- **flow response** – neither fighting nor running away, this is an attempt to go with whatever the current trend happens to be. This sort of person usually stays fairly cool, and may be viewed as erratic and having no fixed values, but is very tolerant.

No one response is better than another. Overuse of one particular response, however, may lead to a fixed, rigid pattern and eventually to a stressed state.

Obviously, the responses outlined here are broad stereotypes, and many people fall between these categories, or may vary from one type to another.

Activity 1.10

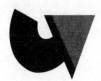

Think of something which might cause you stress in the next week and try to monitor your own response to it.

Did you fight or run away? Why? On reflection, do you think that was the best reaction to the situation?

Causes of stress

Stress is a highly individual matter. Different things cause stress in different people. Noisy or hazardous environments, relationships or work may all be stressful. Experts acknowledge that major life changes are generally stressful. The quiz in Activity 1.11 gives crisis ratings for various life events.

Activity 1.11

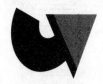

Life changes and stress

Look at the list of life events on p. 20. If any of the events have happened to you in the last two years, make a note of the numbers and then add up your score.

The higher your score, the more stressful the past two years have been for you.

Stress at work

The people who experience stress at work are not always top managers. Shift work can be stressful too. Many jobs may involve working with physical and chemical hazards. Safety measures may make it difficult to have working relationships; for example, it is difficult to have any sort of converstion if you have to wear ear muffs or indeed if factory or construction site noise levels are high.

Another cause of stress at work is relationships. Sometimes seniors may exert unreasonable pressure to achieve tasks in unreasonable deadlines.

Life event (in the last two years)	Crisis unit	Score
Death of spouse or partner	100	_____
Divorce	73	_____
Marital separation	65	_____
Jail term	63	_____
Death of close family member	63	_____
Personal injury or illness	53	_____
Marriage	50	_____
Fired at work	47	_____
Made redundant	45	_____
Martial reconciliation	45	_____
Retirement	45	_____
Pregnancy	40	_____
Change of health of family member	39	_____
Sex difficulties	39	_____
Gain of new family member	39	_____
Business readjustment	39	_____
Change in financial state	38	_____
Death of close friend	37	_____
Change to a different line of work	36	_____
Change in number of arguments with spouse or partner	35	_____
Mortgage over £10 000	31	_____
Foreclosure of mortgage or loan	30	_____
Change in responsibilities at work	29	_____
Son or daughter leaving home	29	_____
Trouble with in-laws	29	_____
Outstanding personal achievement	28	_____
Wife or female partner begins or stops work	26	_____
Begin or end school	26	_____
Change in living conditions	25	_____
Revision of personal habits	24	_____
Trouble with boss at work	23	_____
Change in work hours or conditions	23	_____
Change in residence	20	_____
Change in school	20	_____
Change in recreation	19	_____
Change in religious activities	19	_____
Change in social activities	18	_____
Mortgage or loan less than £10 000	17	_____
Change in sleeping habits	16	_____
Change in number of family get-togethers	15	_____
Change in eating habits	15	_____
Holiday	15	_____
Minor violation of the law	11	_____

Below are listed some of the factors people find stressful about work and which may be very difficult to cope with:

- **Money worries** Your income is low. You cannot earn more. Your job is not secure.
- **Relationships** You do not get on well with some or all of your colleagues. You are forced to work with people you do not like.
- **Poor working conditions** You have to put up with noise, vibration, poor lighting, heat, cold, poor ventilation, danger from physical or chemical hazards, fear of accidents, dirt and grime, long hours of overtime and shift work.
- **Poor administration and company policy** You get a lot of bother from inefficient administration.
- **Work load** You have too much responsibility or work to handle or not enough work or responsibility
- **Prospects** There is no hope of promotion or advancement.
- **Recognition** No one appreciates what you do.
- **Satisfaction** The job is boring and you have too much time on your hands or so demanding you have no time left for yourself.
- **Goals** You do not feel you can ever achieve or finish anything because the demands are constantly changing.

Signs of stress in the workplace
- High turnover of staff
- High absenteeism
- High illness rates
- High strike rates
- High accident rates

If a job has satisfaction and meaning to those who do it, and if there is pride in the work, then the turnover rates, absenteeism, illness, strike and accident rates are all low. Studies in Sweden have shown that where workers can arrange their own schedules in consultation with a supervisor rather than doing the same job over and over again, there is far greater interest and satisfaction in the work. Control and variety can also lead to higher standards of work.

The symptoms and results of stress

Extreme stress can cause ill-health, but remember that people have differing stress tolerances and that stress can be prevented and managed.

Physical symptoms
These can include any of the following:
- tension in the muscular system, in the back of the neck or lower back (may result in headaches)
- nausea (feeling sick)
- tension in the jaw – grinding teeth
- diaphram and pelvic muscles become tense
- throat muscles change leading to changes in voice or nervous laughter
- if the muscle tension is severe, this can lead to blinking, nervous tics, trembling and shaking
- raised blood pressure
- disorders of the glandular system including excessive sweating, dry throat and difficulty in swallowing

- heart and lungs are affected resulting in rapid pulse rates, a pounding heart and rapid, shallow breathing
- the nervous system is affected, resulting in dizziness, fainting spells, weakness, lethargy and difficulty in sleeping, too much sleep or disturbed sleep.

Psychological symptoms

These can include any of the following:

- inability to concentrate
- general irritability
- being over-exact
- sense of mild fear or panic
- inability to enjoy yourself
- inattention to hygiene or dress

- general dullness and flatness
- emotional and social withdrawal
- poor work performance
- difficulty in communicating
- loss of sex drive.

Stress management

What can be done to reduce stress? There are many aspects of stress management, but the first is to be aware of your own stresses and reactions to them.

Activity 1.12

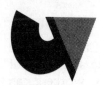

In pairs, work through the interview questions below. One person should be the interviewer and the other the interviewee (the person being asked the questions). You could then swop places if you have time.

Interview questions

1 Think about something that happened to you that was a very stressful experience for you. Tell me about it.

2 Was this experience something you knew was going to happen or was it a surprise to you?

3 What did you feel when this happened and what did you do?

4 Can you remember doing anything that made you feel any better or less anxious?

5 Did you turn to anyone else for help? What happened?

6 If you had to face this experience again would you do anything different the second time? Could you have done anything to prevent this experience happening or that would have made it less stressful for you?

7 Did you learn anything about yourself as a result of the experience?

8 What factors do you generally find stressful?

9 What helps you to cope with these factors?

Stress management techniques
The key to managing stress is to consider three important areas. These are:
- physical fitness
- good diet
- time management.

The first two are connected with your physical well-being. Time management is being aware of how you spend your time. Can you alter your life to relieve certain pressures at busy times? Being organised about your time avoids leaving things to the last minute. There are certain aspects of stress management:
- assertiveness – saying 'No' without feeling guilty
- meditation
- relaxation
- massage
- emotional release, such as tears or talking
- self-talk and positive thinking – telling yourself to treat each situation as positively as possible
- communication skills, for example, talking through your problems with a friend or counsellor
- support systems – using friends and family or more formal guidance and counselling systems.

Activity 1.13

a Consider the above list of stress management techniques. See which ones might suit you.

b Choose one technique and research it further.

c As a class, discuss a possible design and format for a booklet entitled 'Dealing with Stress'.

d The individual pieces of research could be collated and presented in the form of bar charts using a computer.

Some tips for stress survival
- Do one thing at a time.
- Find a quiet nook at home to be by yourself.
- Do not rush.
- Eat well and enjoy your food.
- Listen, do not interrupt.
- Plan a treat for yourself.

Smoking

Most smokers admit that they wish that they had never started to smoke, not least because of the health risks that they face. In fact 100 000 deaths each year are caused by smoking. Particular problems include:
- **Lung cancer** There are 40 000 cases of lung cancer diagnosed in Britain each year. Ninety per cent of these cases are caused by smoking and 90 per cent of these people are dead within two years.

Lung cancer occurs when the lethal cocktail of chemicals in cigarette smoke attacks the genetic material in the lung cells. This causes changes that make the cells multiply wildly so that they collect together. Masses of cells build up and the lungs cannot work.

- **Throat and mouth cancer**   Smokers are four times more at risk from these cancers even if they do not inhale.
- **Bronchitis**   This is a serious inflammation of the tubes leading to the lungs. The tubes become blocked by a jelly-like mucus and then the damaged tissue is easily infected by bacteria. Bronchitis can also affect non-smokers, but it is more common and worse in smokers.
- **Emphysema**   This is caused by the destruction of the feathery branches deep in the lungs. People suffering from the condition are initially short of breath, but eventually so dependent on oxygen supplies that they can hardly move outside their own home. Nine out of ten cases of emphysema are caused by smoking.
- **Hardening of the arteries**   Another condition associated with heavy smoking is the 'furring up' of the arteries. This makes it extremely painful to walk and can lead to amputation of limbs.

  Arteries are the tubes that carry blood from the heart. The tubes become 'furred up' when fatty deposits, caused by factors such as smoking and high blood cholesterol, collect. These fatty deposits are called *atheroma*. The presence of atheroma makes it harder to pump blood through the tubes and limits the amount of oxygen that can be carried around the body. The narrowing of the heart's own arteries can result in severe chest pain. A heart attack occurs when one of the arteries is completely blocked by a blood clot and this can kill.
- **Heart disease**   The specific ways in which smoking promotes heart disease are not certain. Nicotine may be involved because it makes the heart beat faster and therefore the heart's requirement for oxygen is greater. It also makes the blood stickier and harder to pump

  Smokers also take in carbon monoxide which reduces the oxygen-carrying capacity of a smoker's blood by as much as 15 per cent. In an attempt to compensate for this loss, the body produces extra haemoglobin which means that the blood becomes more likely to clot. Carbon monoxide also contributes to the hardening of the arteries.

  So, smoking goads the heart to beat faster while making the blood harder to pump, more likely to clot and less likely to carry oxygen.
- **Post-operative complications**   Because of the extra pressure smokers place on the heart they run greater risks during and after surgery.
- **Cervical cancer**   Woman smokers run twice the risk of cervical cancer than women non-smokers.
- **Miscarriage**   Pregnant women, even those smoking less than 20 cigarettes per day, are 20 per cent more likely to miscarry. Premature births and stillbirths are also more common amongst smokers than non-smokers. The same is true for infertility.
- **Gum disease**   Smokers are more likely to have gum disease and consequently dental problems.

Passive smoking

The health risks from smoking are undoubtedly heavy. The risks of ill-health, however, are also run by other people in terms of *passive smoking*. People who live or work in smoky atmospheres without smoking themselves are termed

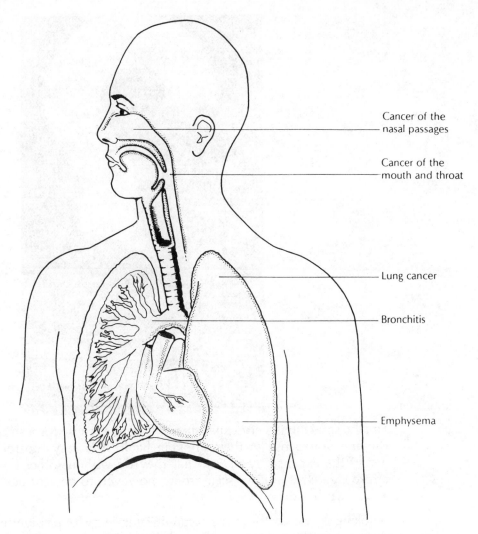

Cancer of the
nasal passages

Cancer of the
mouth and throat

Lung cancer

Bronchitis

Emphysema

Problems caused by smoking

passive smokers. They are vulnerable to the same diseases, as explained above, but to a lesser extent. It is very difficult to estimate the risk of passive smoking, but two studies of children with parents who both smoked estimated that the children breathed in the equivalent amount of smoke as that associated with actively smoking 80–150 cigarettes per year.

Passive smoking can also aggravate asthma and other bronchial conditions.

Stopping smoking

It is difficult to stop, but if you do then within one year the health risks you run are 50 per cent above non-smokers. After five years of non-smoking you have little more risk of heart disease than a life-long non-smoker.

Another reason for giving up smoking is that it has become an anti-social habit. More and more venues are becoming completely smoke-free or have special smoke-free zones. People generally feel smoking leaves unpleasant smells on clothes, hair and breath. It is no longer considered sophisticated or attractive to smoke.

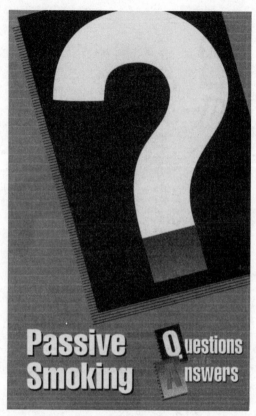

Finally, smoking is very expensive. It is hard exercise for a smoker to calculate the annual expense of their smoking habit. It is easy too for the smoker to justify the expense by saying that they do without other things in order to afford cigarettes. It does seem ironic, however, to pay for possible damage to your own health.

Smoking is also costly to the community in terms of passive smoking, nursing care and working days lost through ill-health caused by smoking. About half the fires dealt with by the fire brigade are caused by smoking. In 1985, the fire at Bradford Football Ground, in which 56 people died, was caused by a discarded cigarette. Similarly, in the tragic Kings Cross fire, the dirt and debris in the escalator shafts were ignited by a cigarette.

How to stop
If you are young and only smoke occasionally, it is worth noting that many heavy smokers started with an occasional, social smoke, once a week perhaps, but the habit became established and very difficult to break.

As smoking is an addiction rather than just a habit, the smoker must really want to stop. It needs a lot of willpower to stop as the smoker will probably feel the effects of withdrawing from the nicotine.

Some people switch to low-tar cigarettes and these do cause less damage. It is difficult, however, for heavy smokers to adjust to the change and some may smoke more because they find the low-tar cigarettes are less satisfying. In some areas, Health Promotion Councils offer group therapy sessions to support people as they give up.

Few people manage to reduce their level of smoking so low that they stop entirely. The temptation is to creep back up gradually. On the other hand, to 'cold turkey' and stop suddenly is very difficult because of the effects of nicotine withdrawal.

In Britain there are 10 million ex-smokers. It is not easy, but it can be done!

Activity 1.14

a Discuss the following issues:
   i) Is the government doing enough to discourage smoking? (At present there is a partial ban on advertising tobacco products, Government Health Warnings are being displayed and it is illegal for cigarettes to be sold to those under 16 years of age.)
   ii) Is it true to say that people have a right to enjoy themselves how they wish?
   iii) More than half the world's tobacco is grown by poor developing nations who desperately need the cash that the tobacco crops bring. Thousands of people in these countries are employed in making and selling tobacco. Is it right that every job in the tobacco manufacturing industry should equal the deaths of five smokers in the Western world each year?

b Within your own group, ask the smokers how they started and what advice they would give to anyone who is tempted to smoke.

Summarise your discussions in your file.

Alcohol abuse

Unlike smoking, drinking alcohol is still very socially acceptable. Indeed it is expected that we will drink on certain occasions. To refuse alcohol may seem embarrassing. You may think that people will consider you odd or cranky if you refuse even a mildly-alcoholic drink. It is often overlooked that alcohol is in fact a drug. It is a legal, socially-accepted drug, but one which can cause much personal and social damage. In fact, there are more deaths through excessive drinking than through heroin abuse.

What is alcohol?

Alcohol is formed by the fermentation action of yeasts on various fruits or cereals. The resulting liquid, with various additions, may be drunk as wines or beers. The alcohol may be further concentrated by distilling or boiling off to produce spirits, such as whisky, gin or vodka. Different drinks contain different amounts of alcohol.

Ten grams of pure alcohol, the amount contained in half a pint of beer, is regarded as one unit. This unit measure is the equivalent of one glass of wine or a pub measure of spirits. The table on page 28 lists the unit levels of various alcoholic drinks, but it is important to note that:
- Wines vary a great deal in strength and it is better to check the label than assume a particular unit level.
- There is also a range of strengths in beers from fairly light beers and lagers, at two units per pint, through to stronger ones, such as *Guinness* and *Stella Artois*, which contain three units per pint. Some beers are even stronger.

Unit levels of various alcoholic drinks

Drink	Units
1 bottle of spirits	30.0
1 bottle of table wine	10.0–18.0 or 7.0–12.0
1 bottle of sherry/martini/port	14.0
1 can of special lager	4.0
1 bottle of special lager	2.5
1 can of beer	1.5
1 pint of cider	2.0–4.0
1 pint of beer	2.0–3.0
1 glass of wine	1.0–2.0
1 glass of sherry/martini/port	1.0
1 measure ($\frac{1}{6}$ gill) of spirits	1.0

Alcohol levels

Current advice is that men ought to consume no more than 21 units per week and women no more than 14.

When the police stop drivers suspected of 'driving whilst under the influence of drink', they measure the **B**lood **A**lcohol **C**oncentration – **BAC**. This is the concentration of alcohol in the body's system. It is difficult to state precisely how much alcohol needs to be consumed in order for a person to be above the legal limit because people have different tolerance levels in relation to alcohol. As a broad rule, one unit of alcohol or half a pint of beer is equivalent to a BAC of 15 mg (milligrams) per 100 ml (millilitres) BAC. The legal limit for driving is 80 mg per 100 ml BAC, so an averaged-sized man would be around the legal limit for driving if he has drunk five units or 2.5 pints of ordinary beer (or its equivalent). A smaller man or a woman may be above the BAC legal limit by drinking five units of alcohol.

Alcohol concentration in the body
The factors which affect alcohol concentration in the body are:
- the amount of alcohol consumed
- the size of the drinker
- the sex of the drinker (women have proportionately less body fluid than men and are therefore less able to absorb alcohol)
- the rate at which drinks are consumed
- the amount of food in the stomach.

Almost all of the alcohol in a pint of beer is absorbed after one hour if it is drunk on an empty stomach. If there is food in the stomach the alcohol is absorbed more slowly.

Most of the alcohol consumed is removed from the body by the liver. A little is eliminated through breathing and urine. On average, one pint of ordinary beer takes about two hours to filter out of the body.

Activity 1.15

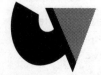

Read the case study opposite concerning Alicia Robson and then plot the graph outlined.

Alicia Robson runs a small boutique. The boutique was a thriving concern but high interest rates have meant that recent months have been more difficult. On Friday evening she arranges a promotion for the boutique to coincide with some new garments arriving from France. It is a cheese and wine celebration. So:

- On Friday evening Alicia drinks five glasses of wine very rapidly. **5 units**
- On Saturday at lunchtime Alicia meets her boyfriend for a pub lunch. She has half a pint of cider, one sherry and some sandwiches. **2 units**
- On Saturday evening Alicia goes to a dinner dance. She drinks two gins and four glasses of wine. **6 units**

Plot the level of Alicia's BAC on a graph like the one below.

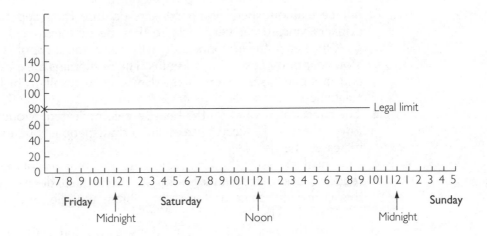

Remember:

- One unit of alcohol = 15 mg/100 ml BAC.
- Five units is very near the legal limit.
- Two units of alcohol takes about two hours to filter through the body (rough guide only).

a Roughly how long would it take for Alicia to eliminate the alcohol from the cheese and wine celebration on Friday evening?

b When is Alicia's BAC at its highest?

c What arrangements might Alicia consider concerning her journeys home on Friday and Saturday nights?

How excessive alcohol consumption affects the body

- Many people turn to drink in times of **stress**. Alcohol is a *depressant* drug which can act as a tranquilliser if amounts below the recommended units are taken. If excess alcohol is taken, however, the nervous system is initially 'weighed down' by the depressant nature of the drug, and then when the effects wear off the nervous system rebounds like a coiled spring. This 'rebound' produces feelings of nervousness, tension and restlessness.

- **Stomach disorders** like gastritis are also common amongst many drinkers. Gastritis is the result of alcohol stripping parts of the stomach of its mucous lining, producing pain and eventually diarrhoea. Peptic ulcers are also associated with prolonged heavy drinking.
- In the short term, alcohol may have a positive effect on **sleep** patterns. In the long term, however, alcohol increases anxiety, depression and therefore insomnia.
- Alcohol also has the effect of suppressing the body's own **immune system** making heavy drinkers more vulnerable to infection and disease.
- Alcohol stimulates **insulin production** in the pancreas. Insulin reduces sugar levels in the blood and can lead to very low blood sugar counts. Thus the person feels drowsy, weak, trembly and may faint.
- Alcohol can simultaneously **increase weight** and **cause malnutrition**. Alcohol provides calories – one gin and tonic is 150 calories and a pint of beer 300 – but it does *not* provide nutrition. So you can become quite fat but be malnourished. Some drinkers do lose their appetite and excessive drinkers tend to eat very little so they become extremely thin.

  A further point in connection with food and alcohol is that alcohol can stop your body absorbing vitamins. The B-vitamins are especially vulnerable and in some cases severe brain damage can result from the deficiency of thiamine (B_1).
- The effects of alcohol on the **heart** are complicated. Moderate drinking can lower the risk of heart disease in certain people, but excessive drinking increases the risk.
- Continual excessive drinking may cause inflammation of the **brain**, gradually reducing brain size and resulting in intellectual deterioration. (Note that this is not the same as temporary 'brain muddle' after occasional heavy bouts of drinking.)
- One of the best known conditions associated with heavy drinking is **cirrhosis** of the liver. Cirrhosis means that the liver is at first enlarged by the continual work that it has to do in dealing with the alcohol. Subsequently, it becomes inflamed and packed with fat. Eventually it becomes scarred and shrunken so that it can no longer function.

  A fatty liver can generally become healthy with a nutritious diet and avoiding all alcohol. Alcoholic hepatitis leads to cirrhosis in about 50 per cent of cases, but in itself is not quite as serious as cirrhosis. Cirrhosis kills about 10 per cent of people who have been problem drinkers for ten years or more.
- When you have a drink, you experience a warm glow and that signifies that many of the cells in your body are bathed in ethyl alcohol. If this happens often enough and with sufficient quantities of alcohol, then changes take place in some cells. At times, these changes can be malignant, so heavy drinkers are at a higher than average risk of **cancers** of the throat and liver.
- Some heavy drinkers suffer from **delirium tremens**. This is a dangerous state of alcohol withdrawal which causes violent tremors, hallucinations, rambling speech and hyperactivity. It usually takes place three to four days after very heavy drinking has stopped. Between 15 and 30 per cent of people with the so-called DTs die. There are several, less severe levels of withdrawal which come as soon as heavy drinking stops.

  Some heavy drinkers actually suffer alcohol-induced, epileptic-type fits.

- It is ironic that media images of drink often portray it as an *aphrodisiac* (increasing sexual desire). In fact, heavy drinking **reduces sexual function** in both men and women. **Impotence** in heavy drinkers is not uncommon.

Activity 1.16

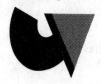

Calorie count on popular drinks	
Drink	**Calories**
1 pint of beer	300
1 glass of wine	80
1 whisky	90
1 vodka and orange	130

a Compare the calorie levels above to those of fruit juices, tea, coffee, slimline tonics and bitter lemon.

b If 10 000 extra calories can produce three pounds of fat, how much weight would you gain drinking 2.5 pints of beer each day for a fortnight?

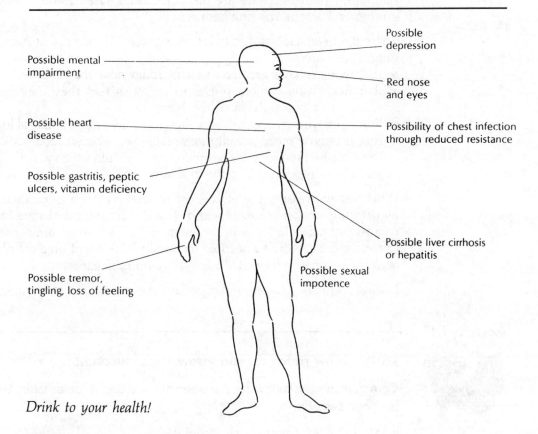

Possible mental impairment

Possible heart disease

Possible gastritis, peptic ulcers, vitamin deficiency

Possible tremor, tingling, loss of feeling

Possible depression

Red nose and eyes

Possibility of chest infection through reduced resistance

Possible liver cirrhosis or hepatitis

Possible sexual impotence

Drink to your health!

The effects of alcohol abuse

- Alcohol is a factor in many road deaths.
- Alcohol is a factor in many criminal offences.
- Alcohol is a factor in much family violence.

It is impossible to record the amount of misery, pain and unhappiness that heavy drinking causes in families.

Alcohol and driving

In connection with road traffic accidents, research shows that even after only two pints of beer, some people's judgement and co-ordination can be less reliable. After five pints there may be a loss of self-control, more aggression, less balance and blurred vision.

The idea of testing drivers to check alcohol levels was first introduced in 1962, but there was no maximum level fixed at that time. In 1967, the 80 mg/100 ml limit was introduced and the police had the power to stop drivers. In May 1983, a cheaper, quicker way of measuring BAC, with instant computerised print-out was initiated.

If the results are positive, then the driver is taken to the police station for further tests. In court, the lowest level reading is the one used. If the driver is found guilty then he or she may be disqualified from driving for a year and the licence is endorsed.

Female drinking patterns

During the mid 1960s and 1970s, male alcoholism doubled, but female alcoholism trebled! There are also increasing rates among women of drunk driving and arrests for drunkenness.

There has been a lot of discussion about why women are drinking more. Some suggestions are:
● that women have greater social freedom now than before
● that women have more pressures today in that they may be expected to work inside and outside of the home
● that more women do work and, therefore, have more financial independence
● that it is now more socially acceptable for women to drink
● that drinks favoured by women, such as gin, sherry and liqueurs, have actually gone down in price in real terms.

Whatever the reason, the effects are serious. Women can damage their livers by drinking smaller amounts and over a shorter period of time than their male counterparts. Similarly, women are more at risk from brain damage, certain cancers and ulcers. They become physically dependent on alcohol more quickly than men, so they show withdrawal symptoms earlier.

During pregnancy, drinking is especially dangerous as it can damage the foetus.

Activity 1.17 ──

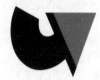

Quiz – How much do you know about alcohol?

Comment on the following statements – are they true of false? Give reasons for your decision.

a Alcohol warms you up on a cold day.

b Alcohol makes you sleep well.

c Alcohol causes as much damage in society as heroin.

d Alcohol provides important dietary requirements.

e Alcohol is OK taken with mild tranquillisers.

f The effects of alcohol are temporary.

g Women get drunk more easily than men.

h Alcohol is a stimulant.

i Only the liver can remove alcohol from the bloodstream.

j The best advice to pregnant women is to abstain from alcohol completely.

k It takes about four hours for your body to eliminate two pints of beer.

l Drinking spirits is more dangerous than drinking beer.

Compare your answers with others in your group.

Activity 1.18

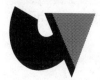

Controlling alcohol consumption

Make a list of the reasons why you think people drink. Think about why you drink yourself. Then look at the list of reasons below and comment on them in the light of what you have read in this chapter.

- It helps me relax.
- It helps me to feel confident.
- It helps me pull myself together.
- It helps me sleep.
- I like to be sociable.
- I enjoy the taste.
- I find it refreshing.
- I drink out of habit.
- I drink to forget my worries.
- I drink when I am under pressure at work.

Activity 1.19

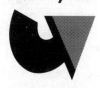

Keeping a drink diary

If you are worried about how much you drink or even how much you spend on drink, a useful monitoring exercise is to keep a drink diary.

Record your alcohol consumption every day for about 12 weeks. It may help to use the headings below so that you can see if any particular patterns emerge.

Date	Time	Hours spent	Place	Money spent	Units consumed	Other activities	With whom	Consequences/ how you felt
Sun 4/11/9-	12.30– 1.30 p.m.	1.5	'Hammer & Pincers' pub		2.5	Darts	George and Alex	Quite relaxed; good chat about football
5/11/9-	7 p.m.– 10.30 p.m.	3.5	West End		10	None	Nobody	Had awful day at work; drank to console myself; felt very rough Tues a.m.
9/11/9-	8 p.m.	1.5	'Hammer & Pincers' pub		2	Cards	George and Alex	Good – enjoyed myself

Once you have kept your diary ask yourself:

a Did you drink more than you intended to in each case?

b Do you sometimes regret how much you drank the day before?

c Does your drinking ever cause trouble?

Very heavy drinkers are sometimes encouraged to draw up 'troublesome' and 'trouble-free' drink diaries. Obviously, factors like who you are drinking with, how much money and time you spend and whether drinking is the sole activity, all affect consumption levels. Below is a list of steps which you may consider if you are trying to reduce your alcohol intake or if you are working with people who are trying to cut down.

How to cut down

- Tell people you are cutting down, but be careful as some may see this as provocation and aim to make you drink.
- Start drinking later than you do at present.
- Take smaller sips.
- Put your glass down between sips.
- Occupy yourself, either with an activity or by conversation.
- Do not take spirits and lager or beer together; you take in alcohol much faster that way.
- Dilute spirits with water or a mixer.
- Eat a meal before you drink.
- Learn to refuse drinks.
- Know *exactly* how much you have drunk.
- Have some 'rest days' when you do not drink at all.
- Learn to relax without drinking – see the section on Stress on pages 17–23.

Obviously, if people have serious problems then professional help must be sought. People may need help for underlying problems such as bereavement, marital strains or pressures from work. Some psychiatric hospitals run group therapy sessions at alcohol treatment units. In severe cases, people may need to be admitted to hospital for de-toxification or 'drying out'. This does not cure alcoholism, but helps to arrest the physical damage incurred by it.

Drug abuse

The definition of illegal drugs

Drug misuse means those forms of drug-taking which meet with social disapproval. This includes possession, for non-medical use, of illegal drugs under the Misuse of Drugs Act 1972. Cannabis, LSD, opiates, amphetamines and solvents are all illegal drugs.

Numbers of young people involved with drugs

A survey carried out in 1986 by *New Society* found that 17 per cent of secondary school pupils used cannabis; 6 per cent solvents and 2 per cent heroin. Asian pupils registered the lowest number for the question asking whether they had ever tried drugs. Some schools were particularly high, for

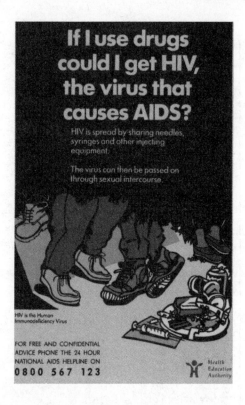

example one boys' school in Glasgow where 20 per cent of pupils were involved with solvent misuse.

Studies indicate that problematic drug-taking is worse in the cities and in areas of high unemployment and social deprivation. Official statistics demonstrate an overall increase in the number of drug addicts. If drug addicts inject they run a strong risk of contracting AIDS (Acquired Immune Deficiency Syndrome, see page 39).

Why people misuse drugs

People take illegal drugs for all sorts of reasons from curiosity to searching for some form of escape. Studies indicate four main reasons why people take drugs:
- a mixture of curiosity and pleasure seeking
- encouragement from peers
- to relieve stress or solve problems, but mostly as a gesture of rebellion rather than deep anxiety
- availability – if drugs are around at a party or concert there is often pressure to take them.

Help available for drug users

The majority of drug users do not come into contact with health service personnel unless the toxic effects of the drugs do evident damage or because a relative is worried about them.

People who work with drug users have found that multi-disciplinary teams obtain the most effective results. This means drawing staff from health, probation, social services and voluntary organisations together to work in teams. They can then work with the individual as a total person discussing

Illegal drug uses and effects

Drug	Nicknames	Use	Effect
Cannabis	Dope, Pot, Blow, Weed, Smoke, Tea, Puff.	Smoked in the form of 'joints' (hand-rolled cigarettes).	Loss of sense of time, relaxes and also heightens appreciation of music and colour.
LSD (Lysergic Acid Diethylamide)	Acid, Flash, Sugar, Paper mushrooms.	Tablet form or impregnated onto sheets of paper. Sometimes taken on a sugar cube or set in gelatine.	Main damage is psychological.
Cocaine	Coke, Charlie Girl, Lady, Toot, Happy, Dust, Candy.	Can be mixed with flour, baking powder and water, and even cooked. Can also be smoked.	Strong psychological dependence, nausea, restlessness and insomnia.
Barbiturates	Barbs, Goof balls.	Tablet form.	Psychological dependence; sudden withdrawal can be fatal.
Heroin	Junk, Horse, Dragon, Henry.	Injected or smoked.	Range of physical effects. Higher doses can produce sedation, stupor and coma.
Amphetamines	Speed, Whizz, Wake-ups.	Tablet form or injected.	Stimulates the central nervous system. Long-term use can affect the heart.

and co-ordinating their broad approach. It is in this way that the psychological, social, emotional and economic needs of the user are taken into account.

The table opposite shows some common illegal drugs, how they are used and the effects they have both short- and long-term.

'Everyday' drugs

The drugs described above are illegal and potentially very dangerous. It is interesting to note, however, that tea, coffee and cocoa all contain active chemicals, caffeine, theophylline and theobromine, which are absorbed into the bloodstream. The structure of these chemicals is similar to that of adrenaline, the body's own stimulant.

People who drink more than two cups of coffee or four cups of tea per day will have levels of chemicals in their bloodstream which will keep their 'rate of arousal' at a higher than normal level. Maintaining an artificially high level of arousal will reduce your ability to cope with any additional stress, and will keep your body and mind in perpetual tension. When tea and coffee are reduced you may well feel lethargic and slow for a few days. You may even develop a 'coffee withdrawal' headache. The table below shows a list of caffeine indicators. The recommended adult intake of coffee is two cups per day and for tea, four cups. Have you tried herbal teas, many of which contain none of the active chemicals mentioned above?

Amounts of caffeine in different food and drink

Food or drink	Amount of caffeine it contains
1 cup of instant coffee	90 mg
1 cup of filter coffee	200 mg
1 cup of tea (depending on how long you allow it to brew)	40–70 mg
1 can of coca-cola	40 mg
1 150 g bar of plain chocolate	100 mg
1 150 g bar of milk chocolate	30 mg

Solvents

Several hundred substances can be used for solvent abuse: glue, paint, petrol and lighter fuel are just a few. The solvent vapours act as a depressant and hallucinations can be experienced when solvents are inhaled.

Accidental death or injury can happen because the 'sniffer' (solvent user) is 'drunk', especially if they are sniffing in an unsafe environment, such as on a roof or near a canal bank. Sniffing to the point of becoming unconscious risks death through choking on vomit. Very long-term use might cause brain damage. The after-effects of poor concentration, fatigue and forgetfulness can become habitual and affect whole lifestyles and opportunities.

It is an offence for shopkeepers to sell potentially dangerous solvents to people under 18 years of age.

Activity 1.20

a Find out what help is available within your own community for people involved with drugs.

b Organise a display warning people of the dangers of illegal drug taking. You could:

- Check out suitable places to mount the display, for example in the college reception area or library.
- Contact the Health Promotion Unit of your local health authority for posters and pamphlets.
- Research your own information from as many sources as you can, for example, magazines, books, journals and videos, and use the computer to word-process and present them well.
- Capitalise on the artistic talent within the group. There are bound to be some eye-catching methods of presentation. Make sure all work is correct, neat, straight and well-mounted.

Record your contribution to the display in your file.

Sexual behaviour

Some infections can be transmitted as a result of unsafe sexual behaviour. This is sometimes known as **sexual infection** or **sexually transmitted disease** (STD).

People may feel embarrassed if they have a sexually transmitted infection, but in fact apart from the common cold STDs are the most common type of infection. The main STDs are:

- syphilis
- gonorrhoea
- non-specific urethritis
- trichomonas
- thrush
- genital herpes
- genital warts
- hepatitis
- pubic lice
- HIV.

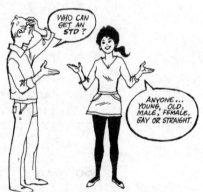

Avoiding STDs

Sexual activity is most appropriate within a secure, loving relationship where partners have respect for each other.

- Don't take risks.
- Take precautions.

STDs are no respectors of persons.

Preventing STDs

- Know and understand about 'safe sex'.
- Restrict the number of sexual partners.
- Use condoms.
- Practise good personal hygiene.

Activity 1.21

a Find out the signs, symptoms and treatment of two different STDs. Be prepared to present your information to the rest of your group.

b Collect leaflets and fact sheets about STDs from your local Health Promotion Unit. Keep them in your file for reference.

c Find out and note the addresses of your local Genito-Urinary Medicine Clinic and/or STD Clinic.

d Find out about and make a note of any 'helplines' available for people who are worried about STDs.

AIDS

AIDS stands for Acquired Immune Deficiency Syndrome:
- **Acquired** – it is caught from someone or something
- **Immune Deficiency** – you have an immune deficiency when your body cannot defend itself against certain illnesses
- **Syndrome** – the particular pattern of illnesses you can get as a result.

AIDS is a disease which results from contracting HIV (Human Immune Deficiency Virus).

Numbers of victims

By the end of 1991, AIDS had resulted in over 3391 deaths in Britain since the first case was recorded in 1981. At the end of 1991, 5451 cases of AIDS were recorded and over 950 of these are or were heterosexual men and women. The disturbing aspect of AIDS, however, is that the number of AIDS cases is doubling every ten months and at least 30 000 people are thought to be virus carriers (i.e. potential AIDS victims). Experts fear that there may be an epidemic; AIDS could be the greatest public health problem of the century.

Groups at risk

The main groups at risk are:
- sexual partners of AIDS sufferers or virus carriers
- homosexuals and bi-sexuals
- drug addicts
- sufferers of a blood clotting disorder called *haemophilia*
- babies born to AIDS sufferers or virus carriers
- prostitutes (both male and female).

However, all sexually-active people are at risk if they have several partners and do not protect themselves.

How the virus is spread

The virus is found in its most concentrated form in the blood and sperm and so any form of sex that involves penetration into the body can spread the disease. Thus all types of *unprotected intercourse*, that is intercourse without using condoms, can spread the virus. The risk can be reduced but not eliminated if condoms are used.

Needles and syringes shared by drug addicts can cause blood infection. This means that the virus can be passed from one addict to another via the same needle or syringe.

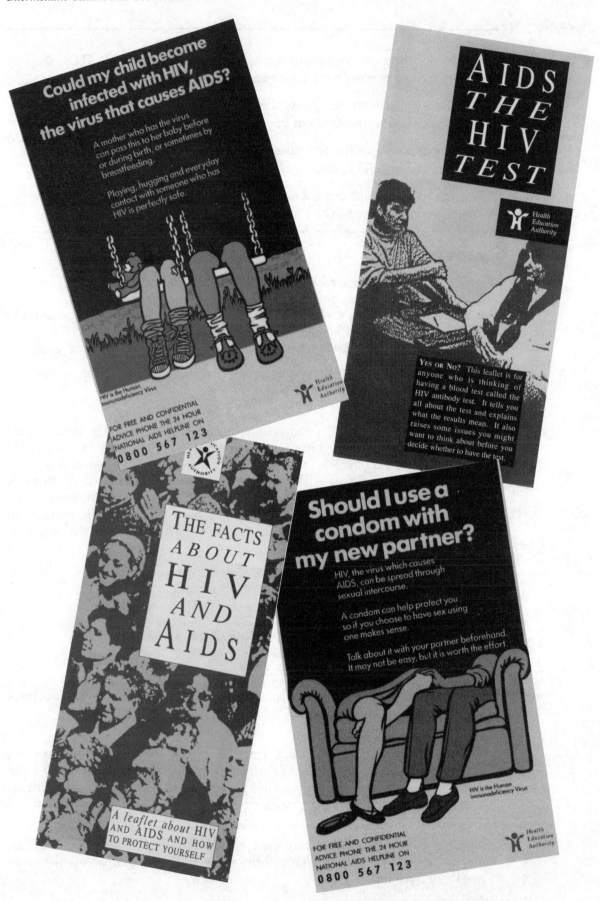

Some haemophiliacs have been infected by contaminated doses of a blood product called *Factor 8* which is now heat-treated to destroy the virus. A few people have been infected through ordinary blood transfusions.

People can actually be 'carriers' of the virus (they are called *HIV positive*), without showing signs of the AIDS condition itself. They can knowingly or unknowingly infect other people. The carriers can be healthy for years.

The effects of AIDS

Those who demonstrate signs of the AIDS condition may be ill for nine months to six years. About 50 per cent die within a year of diagnosis. Once a diagnosis of AIDS is made it obviously has many far-reaching implications, practically, socially and medically, for the individual. First, AIDS sufferers may be refused insurance and mortgages. Secondly, other people may feel that they may also contract the virus and be uncertain about relating to the sufferer. Finally, there is no cure at present for the disease.

Help available

GU (Genito Urinary) clinics:
- can give general advice about AIDS
- can give the HIV antibody test (the test that shows if you are HIV positive and so have the virus that could develop into AIDS)
- offer special advice and counselling from people who have the virus or AIDS itself.

The advice and treatment is free and confidential. You do not need a letter from your doctor. At some clinics you can just turn up but it is best to phone first to check. The number will be in the telephone directory. If you have difficulty, then phone your nearest main hospital.

The Terrence Higgins Trust, based in London:
- offers help and counselling to people with the virus or AIDS itself, and their friends or relatives
- gives detailed information on what is 'safe sex' and what is 'risky sex'
- gives advice and information to people thinking about having the HIV antibody test. Your own doctor can advise and arrange for you to have the test.

Hygiene

Personal hygiene

Some bits of us are not that nice! No one would want to be anything less than fresh and squeaky clean in any situation, but it is especially important to pay attention to personal hygiene if you are working closely with people.

Activity 1.22

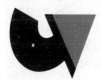

Write out your own rules for maintaining your personal hygiene. What daily routines do you have and what other regular routines are important to your general appearance and well-being?

Skin

Remember that the skin has pores which need to be kept clean as the body rids itself of grease and sweat. If skin is left unwashed, then the smell is obvious and the growth of germs is encouraged. Summer weather, hectic sports and certain clothing can necessitate frequent baths or showers. When sweat is trapped in the folds of the skin this needs extra care. Most people try to prevent stale odours by using deodorants. Check what the difference is between a deodorant and an anti-perspirant next time you purchase one.

Consider reasons why people may not perform personal hygiene routines:

- Practically it may be difficult for them if they are living in poor housing which may be cold, damp and a disincentive to keeping clean. Laundry may be more difficult for such people. Some may 'cut corners' financially and not bother with deodorants or tooth brushes.
- Adolescents may feel self-conscious about using a deodorant or taking a shower after games at school. Ironically, because of body changes and hormones working overtime, they need showers more than ever.
- Young children may have difficult situations at home so their personal care routines are not taught or encouraged. There are many reasons why they may arrive at school unkempt or unwashed.
- Sometimes when people are depressed to the point of mental illness, they neglect themselves and lose interest in how they look or appear to others.
- People who live rough because they are homeless have obvious difficulties. Hostels for homeless people provide washing facilities and often clean clothing. Some hostels insist that people take advantage of the provision others offer and leave it to the client.

Activity 1.23

Imagine you are a community nurse. You visit an elderly lady who has mobility problems. You can smell the fact that she hasn't had a bath for some time. You suggest tactfully that you could help her to take a bath. She refuses. You have a good relationship with the lady so you try to persuade her a little more. You mention how much better she will feel once she has taken the bath. She still refuses. Discuss with your group what you should do and why.

Hair

Most people know how often their hair needs washing and conditioning. Some people need to wash their hair more frequently than others because their skin and scalp are naturally more oily. Factors like taking exercise, cooking or being in a smoky environment also affects how often the hair needs washing.

A small percentage of the school population have head lice at any one time. Most people have had head lice at some point in their lives even if they don't care to admit it. Some people are more prone than others, so watch out! If you discover you have caught head lice, ask your chemist for the latest preparation to clear head lice and follow the manufacturer's instructions carefully. Allow the time stated for the preparation to work thoroughly otherwise the remaining eggs from the lice will breed and you will be re-infested. Regular brushing and combing helps to disturb the nasty creatures. Now you can stop scratching!

Teeth
Clean teeth means healthy teeth and less chance of bad breath.

It is far better for your teeth if you eat to your satisfaction at meal times and then avoid eating between meals. Every time you eat, the plaque or harmful substance starts to build up and everything has to work hard to combat the plaque, like the saliva in your mouth. If you are constantly eating then the plaque wins the battle and decay results. Sugar is particularly hard on teeth, so boiled sweets which last a long time may be nice at the time but too many could cause pain later. Raisins flip off the teeth quite well and chocolate melts away, but this is not to say that such foods are harmless to teeth. Watch out also for drinks like coke and diet coke which are bad for teeth, and foods which contain other forms of sugars, such as dextrose. Apples were once regarded as better for teeth than sweet foods. Apples are sweet, but they also contain a type of acid which the mouth can find difficult to deal with. Use a fluoride toothpaste, dental floss and chew a disclosing tablet occasionally to check your own brushing. See your dentist at least twice a year. You need to brush extremely well if you wear a brace.

If you are working with young children encourage them to eat wisely. Think about ways to avoid sugar. It's harder to think of rewards other than sweets but it is better in the end. Don't let children drink sweetened drinks last thing at night after they have cleaned their teeth or put anything sweet on dummies.

First teeth are precious and the child should be shown how to use a soft toothbrush using 'round and round' movements rather than hard up and down movements which may cause the gums to recede. Carers or parents should brush the baby's gums before first teeth appear and then gently brush the new teeth as they come through.

If you work with the elderly then once again clean mouths prevent gum disease and bad breath. Some elderly people will have dentures which need removing and cleansing in special preparations.

Nails
Clean and short is probably the best habit for health and social care work and general appearance.

Feet
You will probably be on your feet a lot, so keeping them fresh, clean and comfortable is positive.

Keep toe nails short and remove hard skin, but anything more major like athlete's foot, bunions or corns should be seen by a doctor or a chiropodist.

It's tempting to squeeze your feet into fashionable shoes at times but this can cause deformities later. Children's feet are particularly vulnerable in this way and it is best to have their feet measured and shoes properly fitted.

The need for professional care for feet increases with age. Some elderly people may need to see a chiropodist regularly.

Indoors/outdoors
Pressures of work and studying often mean that we can be stuck inside for long periods of time in hunched positions over desks. It can be really beneficial to take some exercise outdoors on a regular basis. It is healthy to take some fresh air and stretch out the limbs with a walk or a run if energy permits.

Similarly with clients, to build some outdoor excursion into a day makes a difference to the outlook, appetite and sleep patterns. If the weather is very warm then care needs to be taken about sunburn which can happen very quickly on unprotected skin with very young or elderly clients.

Community health and hygiene

Nowadays we expect:
- good quality housing
- good town planning
- clean, wholesome water
- clear air
- effective sewage disposal
- effective refuse disposal
- clean cities and towns
- unspoiled country and coastal areas
- clean milk
- clean, safe food
- high levels of vaccination to prevent outbreaks of infectious diseases.

Some problems caused by poor community health and hygiene

Problem		Possible effects
Poor housing	• Old – in need of modernisation • Inappropriate for user group • Over-crowded • Lacking in adequate sanitary facilities • Damp	Stress Increased accident rate Infections Respiratory problems
Poor quality water	• Dirty – untreated • Contaminated with micro-organisms • Excess levels of chemicals, e.g. nitrates	Gastric upsets Dysentery Hepatitis Typhoid Cholera
Inadequate sewage treatment	• Poor drainage • Old drains which need replacing • Untreated sewage getting into water supply • Untreated sewage in areas where people bathe	Water-borne infections, such as gastro-enteritis, dysentery, hepatitis, typhoid, polio, cholera
Inadequate refuse disposal	• Poor facilities for collecting rubbish • Lack of proper refuse disposal sites	Infestations of: • rats and mice, causing food poisoning (and possibly Weils Disease, a rare jaundice spread in rats' urine) • flies, causing gastro-enteritis, dysentery, typhoid, cholera

Activity 1.24

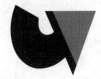

Divide into small groups. Each group should study one or more services relating to public health and hygiene, such as water, sewage or housing.

In your town or area:

a Find out all you can about the services. Collect leaflets and information.

b Note how the service is provided, for example by the local authority, a private company or contracted out to private organisation.

c Find out what the costs of the service are to individuals.

d Carry out and analyse a small survey to establish levels of public satisfaction with the service.

e Present your findings to the rest of your group.

Keep a note in your file of *your* contribution to this work.

Advising others on health and well-being

People do not readily respond to preaching and lecturing on health matters so it is necessary to plan **health promotion** campaigns carefully.

Aims of health promotion programmes

● Empowerment of individuals so that they can make informed choices.
● To bring about changes in behaviour.
● To provide knowledge, and increase awareness, of health promotion issues.

Assessing needs against standard measures

Before embarking on a fitness programme, an individual will usually have their personal fitness assessed against standard measures. The checks made to assess physical fitness will include:
● height
● weight
● blood pressure
● pulse
● muscular strength
● body measurements (chest, waist, hips, thighs, calves, biceps)
● lung efficiency
● aerobic capacity.

Activity 1.25

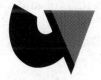

a Visit a fitness centre in your locality and find out what assessments are made on individuals before they start a fitness programme.

b Obtain copies of assessment sheets.

c If possible take part in a personal fitness assessment.

Health messages are usually targeted so that they reach certain groups. Examples of target groups include:

- children
- adolescents
- pregnant women
- active people
- sedentary people
- people with disabilities
- elderly people.

More precisely the following groups could be targeted:

- smokers
- drinkers
- drug users
- glue sniffers
- obese people.

Health promotion information can be presented in a variety of different ways, including:

- leaflets
- models
- posters
- videos
- advertisements
- bill boards
- displays
- games
- role-play activities
- slides
- magazine articles.

You may have noticed particular posters on TV adverts which give very clear health messages. Make a note in your portfolio of any which have particularly caught your attention.

Activity 1.26

a Within your group, discuss the advantages and disadvantages of each method of presentation of health promotion material. Present the findings of the group in the form of a chart.

b Choose one aspect of health promotion which interests you. Collect as many leaflets on this topic as you can. Rate the leaflets in order of effectiveness. Explain your ratings.

Accidents

Living is a hazardous activity!

- Hazards or dangers are all around us.
- At different stages in our lives we are more vulnerable to certain hazards. The old and young are most vulnerable.
- It is important that we can recognise potential hazards.
- More accidents occur at times of peak activity in the day.
- Seasonal factors affect number of accidents.
- Accidents don't just happen. They are usually the result of human, environmental or material factors.

Accidents in the home

Every year thousands of people are injured in the home. The most common types of accident are:

- falls from stairs, ladders, buildings
- bites – from animals or insects
- cuts
- blows – being struck by an object or by a person
- burns, scalds
- foreign bodies
- inhaling poisons
- swallowing poisons
- suffocation
- choking
- electric current.

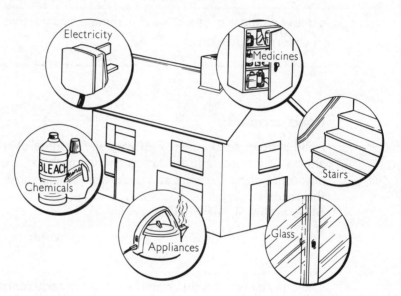

Some hazards in the home

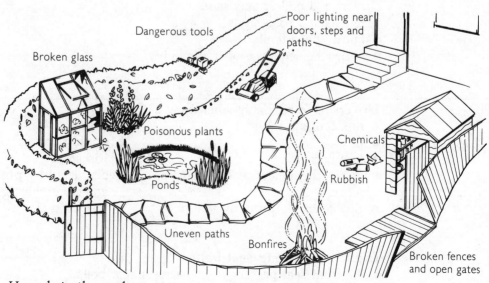

Hazards in the garden

Poisonous plants

Berries and flowers look attractive and can be a danger to children who may put them in their mouths.

Activity 1.27

a i) Draw a plan of a house.
  ii) Divide it into: Kitchen, Lounge/Dining room, Stairs, Bedrooms, Bathroom/toilet.
  iii) On your drawing, note the potential hazards in each room.

b If possible look up *Home Accidents Surveillance System 1988 Data UK*.
  i) How many home accidents occur per annum?
  ii) Which are the most common types of accident?

c How would a prospective childminder ensure that her house was safe or children in her care?

Road accidents

Road accidents have increased with the volume of traffic using our roads. The effects of an accident are far-reaching involving the victim, their family and innocent people. Drivers and pedestrians must show responsible behaviour on the roads:
● Be aware of potential dangers.
● Consider other people.
● Be polite.

The most dangerous times on the roads are early morning, evening and between 11.00 p.m. and midnight.

Drivers and pedestrians should:
● understand road signs
● know speed limits
● know the sequence of traffic lights.

Drivers have accidents when they are:
● not concentrating
● ill
● in a hurry
● under the influence of drugs or alcohol
● unable to see properly
● angry
● driving dangerously, i.e. too fast, too close
● distracted by other passengers and when they ignore fog, ice and wet road signs.

The law regarding seat belts
● All front seat passengers must wear seat belts.
● All rear seat passengers must wear seat belts where fitted.

- All children under 14 must use a seat belt, child seat or harness where fitted and available.
- A child under 1 year of age in the front passenger seat of a car must use an approved child restraint.

Activity 1.28

a Find out whether there are any exceptions to wearing seat belts.

b Find out the best type of car safety device for the following:
  i) a baby weighing up to 10 kg
  ii) a child between 4 and 9 years, weighing between 118 and 136 kg
  iii) an older child, 10 years and above.

Ways of reducing pedestrian accidents
- Pedestrians must behave responsibly.
- Drivers must be aware of the dangers of speed and carelessness.
- Children, parents, teachers and drivers can all co-operate to cut down accidents involving children.

Ways of reducing accidents involving children
- Introduction of traffic calming measures
- Educating children once they can understand
- Teaching by rote
- Teaching the Green Cross Code

Cycling hazards
The bicycle is potentially dangerous and is frequently used by inexperienced, untrained riders on busy roads. Serious injuries following cycling accidents include:
- head injuries
- fractured limbs
- severe lacerations and grazes.

Ways of reducing cycling accidents
- Children should attend cycling proficiency schemes.
- Children under 9 years of age should not ride on the road.
- Crash helmets should always be worn.
- The bicycle should be in good condition and well maintained to BSI standards.
- Off-the-road provision and recognition of cyclists' needs by local authorities.

Playground accidents

Although playgrounds are designed for enjoyment many accidents do occur within them. The most common causes are:
- poor design and layout
- over-exuberance by children.

Not surprisingly most playground accidents occur in the summer months.

Equipment most commonly implicated in playground accidents includes:
- swings
- climbing frames

- slides
- see-saws
- roundabouts.

Landing on hard surfaces causes many injuries. What can be done?
- Playgrounds should be close to housing to allow safe local play.
- Equipment should be safe and well-maintained, with no sharp protuberances.
- Moving apparatus, e.g. swings, should be sited away from static play areas.
- There should be smaller play areas for under 5s.
- Surfaces should be made of rubber, tree bark or sand, not concrete or tarmac.
- There should be adequate adult supervision.

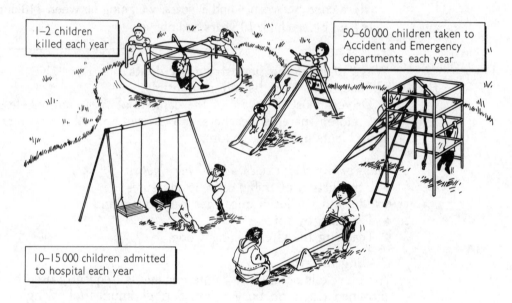

1–2 children killed each year

50–60 000 children taken to Accident and Emergency departments each year

10–15 000 children admitted to hospital each year

Activity 1.29

Visit a playground in your area. Make notes on the following points:

a Monitor usage of the playground over a morning or afternoon. Note how many children use it and what age groups.

b How much supervision is there?

c What type of equipment is in use?

d Comment on the appropriateness and quality of the equipment.

e Do you think any improvements could be made?

Other local hazards

Overhead power lines
Electrocution and death can occur if people come in contact with cables.
- Children should never play near, or climb, pylons, towers or poles.
- Never fly kites or model planes near power lines.

- Never climb trees which overhang power lines.
- Never throw stones or wires over power lines.

Derelict buildings and building sites
Dangers include:
- unsafe buildings
- building equipment
- broken glass
- sharp metal
- asbestos
- lead
- dumped waste
- rats and mice.

Railways
Dangers include:
- falling onto the line
- electrocution
- level crossings.

Parents need to make their children aware of potential dangers and keep them under constant surveillance until they are old enough to be responsible for their own actions.

Water dangers
- Sea
- Ponds
- Lakes
- Rivers
- Swimming pools
- Canals
- Baths

Never leave small children unsupervised. Parents should teach children to swim and be safe in water as soon as possible. Instructions regarding water safety require constant reinforcement for all age groups. Tragedies occur every year – around 60 children drown every year.
- Most drownings occur in the summer.
- Drowning can occur where there is water of any kind – in the home: a bucket, a jacuzzi or a paddling pool.
- The majority of cases of small babies drowning are due to being left in the bath at home.
- In the UK most incidents of children drowning occur in rivers and canals.
- Public swimming baths have a good safety record. Trained attendants are present.

Ways of preventing drowning
- Awareness of avoidance of local dangers
- Fencing-off of ponds and pools
- Learning to swim
- Obeying instructions
- Not swimming alone
- Learning resuscitation techniques
- Never leaving babies, small children and frail elderly people alone in the bath
- Being aware of the hazards of water sports

Dealing with an emergency

On occasions during your work with various groups of people you may be faced with a 'health emergency'. An emergency is an unforeseen thing or event needing prompt action. You can prepare yourself for this kind of situation by taking a basic first aid course. The information contained in this section will serve as a reminder and reinforce the practical skills you learn.

If you are employed you may be able to take a full (Health and Safety Executive (HSE) approved) first aid qualification which would enable you to take on the responsibilities of 'first aider'. Your employer will advise you about this. You will find that courses are run by your local college, St John Ambulance Association or the British Red Cross Society.

Priorities in an emergency

Stay calm!
1 Quickly assess the situation.
2 Ensure safety for yourself, the casualty and other helpers.
3 Identify the condition.
4 Get help.
   Only move the casualty if he or she is in risk of further danger.
5 Give essential treatment, the three main priorities are problems with:
   ● Airway – **A**. See page 58.
   ● Breathing – **B**. See page 57.
   ● Circulation – **C**. See page 58.
   Other priorities are:
   ● Severe bleeding – see page 62.
   ● Unconsciousness – see page 57.
6 Be attentive to the emotional needs of the casualty by showing understanding and giving reassurance.

Summoning help

Things to know in advance:
● the procedure following an incident in your particular work place or placement
● who the qualified first aiders are
● where colleagues, especially those who are qualified first aiders, are likely to be at any given time
● location of any medical facilities or equipment in the establishment
● location of the telephone and how to make emergency calls
● location of emergency numbers, doctor, nurse, relatives.

Activity 1.30

In your group discuss the anxieties and needs of a seriously injured casualty. Make a note of the outcomes of your discussion in your file.

Information to give when calling the emergency services:

- service required (ambulance, fire, police)
- your telephone number
- name of establishment
- exact address
- exact location in building, e.g. front entrance, back entrance
- type of incident, number of casualties
- precise nature of the emergency, e.g.
    90-year-old person totally collapsed
    unconscious
    difficulty in breathing
    feeble pulse
    time incident occurred.

Your responsibility as first aider ends when more qualified help arrives, such as a paramedic or a doctor.

Protecting yourself

- Make sure that you are familiar with safety and fire procedures in your workplace/placement.
- Always sign the fire book when you arrive and again when you leave.
- Check the fire drill, emergency exits and arrangements for evacuating the building should a fire occur.
- Be sure that you know the rules for safe moving and handling (pages 220–1).
- Use protective clothing and equipment provided whenever you are in contact with blood and other body fluids.

Activity 1.31

Write a report on the fire safety provision and first aid facilities at the school or college you attend.

Reducing the risk of injury to others

Some simple hygiene measures

- **Wounds and cuts**   Allow free bleeding and wash.
- **Bites and puncture wounds**   As above, and always seek medical aid.
- **Splashes in mouth and eyes**   Irrigate with water for ten minutes.
- **Cuts and grazes**   Cover with waterproof dressings.
- **Blood and body fluids**   Wash hands with soap and water after contact. Spills should be cleaned up as soon as possible using a chlorine-based product, e.g. *Titan Sanitizer*. Always wear latex gloves and an apron. Wash the gloves before removing and place gloves, apron and any soiled paper towels in a yellow plastic bag and seal.
- **Clothes and dishes**   Normal washing in hot water and detergent is safe.
- Incinerate or double bag any contaminated waste.
- **Needles and blades** or other sharp objects should be placed in a special 'Sharps' container.

Hygiene, HIV and Hepatitis B
Additional information from Health and Safety Code of Practice C7:
The Hepatitis B Virus and Human Immunodeficiency Virus (HIV) may be present in blood and body fluids.

Hepatitis B and HIV are spread in the following ways:
● blood to blood contact
● sexual transmission
● mother to foetus.

Remember:
● Normal social contact carries no risk.
● No case of infection has yet been reported from any part of the world as a result of giving mouth-to-mouth resuscitation.
● Good hygiene prevents the spread of infection (see above).

Provision for first aid in the workplace

First aid is the immediate care given to a casualty to save life and improve or maintain his or her condition.

Provision for first aid in the workplace is set out in the Health and Safety (First Aid) Regulations 1981. These regulations state that:
● Employers must ensure that adequate and appropriate equipment and facilities are provided for employees/students/residents.
● Employers may also wish to make provision for others visiting the premises e.g. customers, contract workers.
● Different work activities involve different hazards and therefore different first aid provision is required.

How many first aiders?
This depends on the types of hazard present in the workplace. In a bank, for example, one first aider for every 50 workers is recommended. In a more dangerous workplace, more first aiders are required.

First aiders must have undertaken training and obtained a HSE-approved qualification.

Appointed persons
The Regulations state that there should be 'appointed persons', who are authorised to take charge in the absence of a trained first aider, or where a first aider is not required, such as in a small non-hazardous work area. Appointed persons should undergo emergency first aid training.

Advice and training to deal with specific hazards can be obtained from your local Employment Medical Advisory Service (see page 56).

The first aid room
The first aid room should contain:
● a sink – hot, cold and drinking water, and disposable cups
● soap and paper towels
● a smoothed-topped working surface
● a suitable store for first aid materials
● a suitable refuse container with disposable plastic bag
● a couch with waterproof surface, clean pillows and blankets
● clean protective garments for first aiders, e.g. aprons and gloves

- a chair
- a bowl
- any special first aid equipment
- a first aid record book.

The room should have easy access and a toilet nearby. It should be heated, well-ventilated and properly maintained. It should be clearly identified as a first aid room. There should be a notice on the door of the first aid room clearly displaying the names and locations of the nearest first aiders.

Activity 1.32

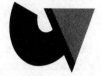

Find out the address of your local HSE office. Find out and write an account of the kind of work which is carried out there.

The first aid box

A first aid box should be made of a material that will protect the contents from damp and dust. It should be clearly identified as a first aid box.

First aid boxes and kits should contain a sufficient quantity of suitable first aid materials and nothing else. **First aid kits** may be provided for particular situations and should be stocked accordingly. An antidote or equipment needed to deal with a specific hazard may be kept near the hazard area or in the first aid box.

Sufficient quantities of each, individually wrapped item should always be available. The Regulations recommend:

Item	First aid box	First aid travelling kit
First aid guidance card	1	1
Individually wrapped sterile adhesive dressings in various sizes	20	6
Sterile unmedicated dressings with bandage attached:		
medium	6	
large	3	
extra large	3	1
eye pads	2	
Triangular bandages	6	
Safety pins	6	2
Individually-wrapped moist cleaning wipes	10	6

Where tap water is not available for eye irrigation, sterile water or sterile normal saline (0.9%) in sealed, disposable containers should be provided – at least 900 ml in three 300 ml containers.

Where soap and water are not available, individually wrapped cleansing wipes (not impregnated with alcohol) may be used. Disposable drying materials should be provided.

Do not use antiseptic lotions or creams or give any medication. It is advisable to keep blankets, scissors, cotton wool and extra triangular bandages nearby.

The contents of the first aid box should be replenished as soon as possible after use.

In the event of a serious incident the Regulations state that you should:
- treat any injuries
- deal with the immediate emergency
- make premises/machinery safe
- do not destroy evidence required by inspector during investigation
- record injuries in accident book.

Riddor (Reporting of Injuries, Diseases and Dangerous Occurrences Regulations 1985)

Failure to comply with Riddor is a criminal offence. The Regulations require immediate notification by phone if anybody dies or is seriously injured in an accident at work or if there is a dangerous occurrence. A written report must be sent within 7 days to confirm above, and:
- if anyone is off work for more than 3 days as a result of an accident at work
- to report occupational diseases suffered by workers
- to report certain events involving flammable gas in domestic and other premises.

EMAS (Employment Medical Advisory Service)

EMAS is the medical division of the Health and Safety Executive. It investigates and gives free advice about health at work. You should contact your local HSE Office or HSE Inspector if you have any queries about health and safety at your place of work. They can supply further information on the Health and Safety at Work Act 1988, Regulations and Approved Codes of Practice and First Aid.

Initial examination and immediate treatment of casualties

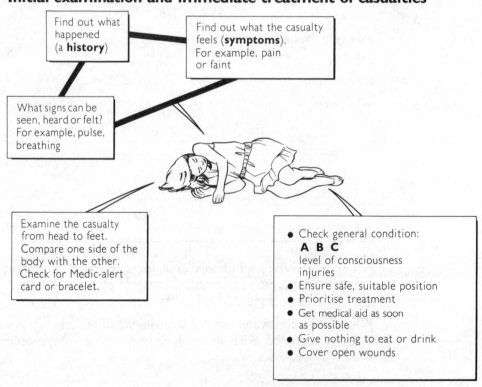

Find out what happened (a **history**)

Find out what the casualty feels (**symptoms**). For example, pain or faint

What signs can be seen, heard or felt? For example, pulse, breathing

Examine the casualty from head to feet. Compare one side of the body with the other. Check for Medic-alert card or bracelet.

- Check general condition:
  A B C
  level of consciousness
  injuries
- Ensure safe, suitable position
- Prioritise treatment
- Get medical aid as soon as possible
- Give nothing to eat or drink
- Cover open wounds

Activity 1.33

a Write a checklist of observations you would make on a casualty who has had a serious accident.

b In groups of two or three, role-play an examination of a casualty.

c Find out about and make a list of the different types of medical card and medi-alert bracelets which are in use.

Major life-threatening situations

Some things you need to know before you can be an effective helper:

● **Check to see in the casualty is conscious**. See if you can make the person respond to you. Touch them, speak to them, call their name, if possible. Note any responses they make and any changes in levels of responsiveness.

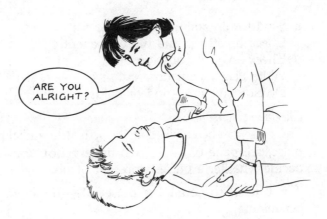

ARE YOU ALRIGHT?

● **Check to see if the casualty is breathing**. Do this by looking to see if the chest is rising and falling and by putting your ear close to the casualty's face and listening for sounds of breathing. Feel expired air on the side of your cheek. Look also for signs of blueness round the lips and the nail beds.

Unconsciousness

You find someone who is unconscious, they do not respond when you speak, they do not move, they are breathing and the heart is beating. What do you do?

Assuming that you do not suspect a spinal injury, you must turn this person onto their side to prevent inhalation of saliva or vomit and to prevent the tongue falling back and obstructing the air passages.

The safe position used for unconscious people is called the **recovery position**.

How to turn a person from his back to the safety of the recovery position
● Kneel beside the casualty.
● Remove glasses, etc.
● The arm which is nearest to you should be placed at right angles to the casualty's body with the elbow bent and the palm uppermost.
● The arm which is furthest away from you should be brought across the chest so that the palm rests against the near cheek.

- Grasp the far thigh of the casualty and pull the knee up, keeping the foot flat against the ground.
- With the casualty's hand still pressed to his cheek, pull the thigh to roll him towards you onto his side.
- Tilt head back to keep the airway open. It may be necessary to adjust the hand under the cheek.
- The hip and knee of the upper leg are bent at right angles.

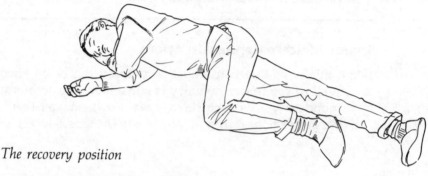

The recovery position

- Send for an ambulance.
  Check breathing and pulse frequently.
  Check level of consciousness.
  Write down your observations.
  Do not give any food or fluids.

Checking for a pulse

The pulse can be checked at the wrist (the radial pulse) or the neck (the carotid pulse, see page 61). Use two fingers, **not** your thumb, feel for 5 seconds to decide whether a pulse is present or not.

If you need to count the pulse rate, the average adult rate is 60–80 beats per minute.

Obstructed airway

- The neck should be extended so that the tongue does not obstruct the airway. To do this, lift the chin forward using the finger and thumb of one hand. At the same time, press the forehead backwards with the heel of the other hand.
- If the person does not breathe, there may be an obstruction. Try to remove this using finger sweeps.

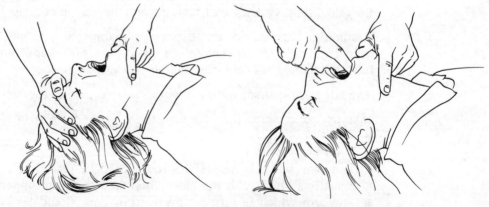

Opening the airway   *Finger sweeps*

● If it is not possible to remove the obstruction and the casualty is conscious you should give firm blows to the person's back and tell the person to cough.

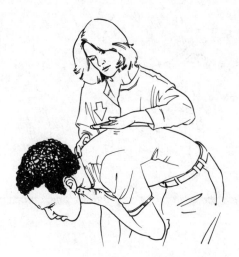

Back blows

   If this does not work, lean the person over a chair and give back blows.
● If all the above fail, give abdominal thrusts. To do this stand behind the person, put your arms round him/her. Grasp your hands together below the person's breast bone and pull them upwards.
● To remove obstructions from unconscious people, the same manoeuvre is carried out but the person is lying in the position shown below right.

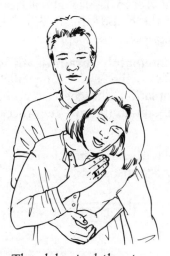

The abdominal thrust

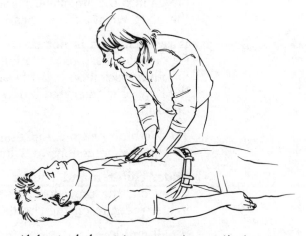

Abdominal thrust in unconscious patient

A child or baby who is choking
An obstruction in the airway of a child or baby is usually caused by food or a small toy.

Place the child or baby face down and apply back blows (see the diagrams on page 60). If back blows are unsuccessful, abdominal thrusts *may* be used. Your tutor will show you the correct way to do this.

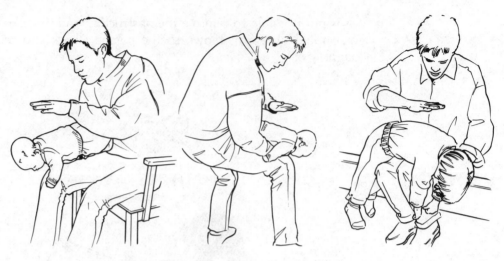

Back blows for choking babies and children

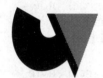

Activity 1.34

Design a poster giving precise instructions about what to do if someone chokes.

Cardiopulmonary resuscitation (CPR)

A person who is not breathing (respiratory arrest) will rapidly become unconscious. When breathing stops, the heart will stop beating within 3 to 4 minutes (cardiac arrest). When we try to resuscitate a casualty, oxygen is blown into the lungs and passes to the blood stream. Blood is pumped round the body when external heart compressions are applied.

If resuscitation is not started immediately, brain death will occur.
Cardiopulmonary resuscitation (CPR) is the use of lung inflations (mouth-to-mouth resuscitation or artificial ventilation) and chest compressions to restore the flow of oxygenated blood to the brain (follow the procedure in the chart opposite).

To combine heart compressions with lung inflations:

15 chest compressions to 2 lung inflations.

Older children and youths

Carry out the procedure described in the chart but slightly faster and use lighter pressure on the chest.

Small children

1 Check and clear mouth.
2 Check breathing.
3 Seal lips round child's nose **and** mouth.
4 Give two small gentle inflations.
5 Check pulse. The brachial artery can be used in babies.
6 If pulse absent, commence chest compressions at a rate of 100 per minute. Compress the breastbone to a depth of 2.5 to 3.5 cm, using one hand just below the centre of the breast bone (centre of the chest, between the nipples).

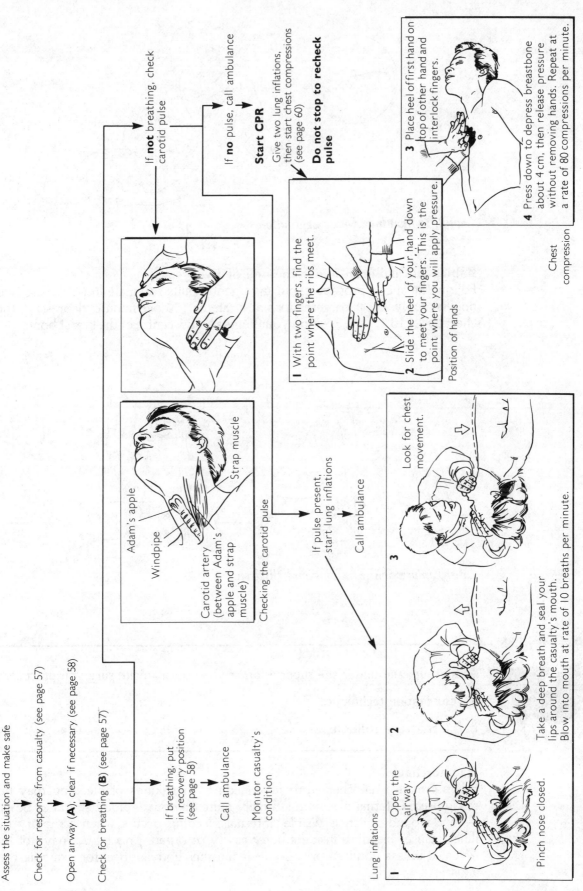

Assess the situation and make safe

Check for response from casualty (see page 57)

Open airway (**A**), clear if necessary (see page 58)

Check for breathing (**B**) (see page 57)

If breathing, put in recovery position (see page 58)

Call ambulance

Monitor casualty's condition

If **not** breathing, check carotid pulse

If **no** pulse, call ambulance

Start CPR

Give two lung inflations, then start chest compressions (see page 60)

Do not stop to recheck pulse

Adam's apple

Windpipe

Strap muscle

Carotid artery (between Adam's apple and strap muscle)

Checking the carotid pulse

If pulse present, start lung inflations

Call ambulance

1 With two fingers, find the point where the ribs meet.

2 Slide the heel of your hand down to meet your fingers. This is the point where you will apply pressure.

Position of hands

3 Place heel of first hand on top of other hand and interlock fingers.

4 Press down to depress breastbone about 4 cm, then release pressure without removing hands. Repeat at a rate of 80 compressions per minute.

Chest compression

Lung inflations

1 Open the airway.

Pinch nose closed.

2 Take a deep breath and seal your lips around the casualty's mouth. Blow into mouth at rate of 10 breaths per minute.

3 Look for chest movement.

CPR: the procedure for adults

61

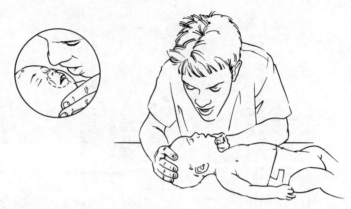

Mouth-to-mouth-and-nose ventilation

Babies and children under the age of two years
Follow the above procedure, but give gentle puffs to inflate lungs. Using two fingers, apply, chest compressions at a rate of 100 per minute, depressing the chest by 1.5 to 2.5 cm. Position your fingers below centre of the breast bone.

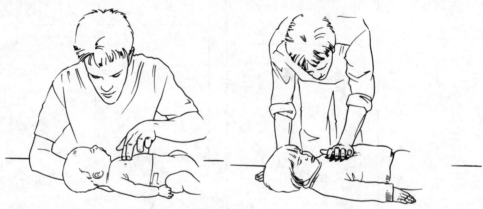

Chest compression in infants and children

Activity 1.35 ―――――――――――――――――――――――――――――――――――――

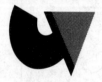

As a group, and under the supervision of your tutor, make sure you practise:

a resuscitation techniques

b the recovery position.

Haemorrhage
Haemorrhage is another word for bleeding. Two kinds of bleeding may be recognised. External bleeding is usually quite obvious – blood spurts or flows from a wound which is visible. Internal bleeding occurs when an injury or illness causes bleeding inside a body cavity or organ. This blood may not be revealed unless vomited or passed via another body orifice, for example the anus.

Why does bleeding occur?
External bleeding can be the result of cuts, blows, tears, grazes and puncture wounds.

Internal bleeding can result from broken bones, blows, crush injuries, stab wounds and certain medical conditions such as a perforated stomach ulcer.

In both instances, the signs and symptoms experienced by the casualty will vary according to the severity of the injury or medical condition.

The average blood volume for adults is 6 litres. When external bleeding occurs, it can look rather dramatic, but remember that a healthy adult can donate 0.5 litres of blood without showing any adverse effects.

Signs that severe bleeding is taking place
- Face and lips become pale
- Skin feels cold and clammy
- Faintness and dizziness
- Pulse is rapid, weak and feeble
- Thirst
- Shallow breathing
- Gasping for air

Internal bleeding: What to do

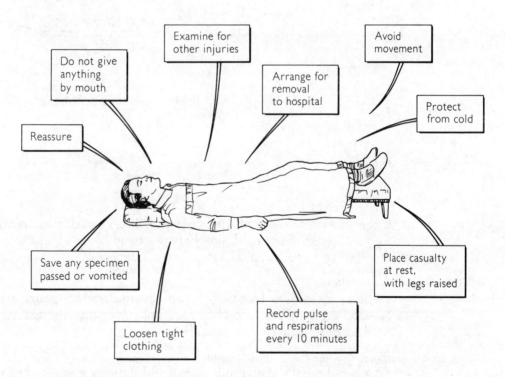

Do not give anything by mouth

Examine for other injuries

Avoid movement

Arrange for removal to hospital

Protect from cold

Reassure

Save any specimen passed or vomited

Place casualty at rest, with legs raised

Loosen tight clothing

Record pulse and respirations every 10 minutes

External bleeding: What to do
- Always wash your hands before dealing with wounds.
- Wear protective clothing when dealing with blood or body fluids.
- Wash your hands after all first aid procedures (see page 53).

Minor wounds
- Lightly rinse the wound with running water until it is clean.

- Clean the surrounding area with soap and water – always wipe away from the wound, using each swab once only.
- Apply a sterile dressing if necessary.

Wounds where there is heavy bleeding
- Pick out any easily removable foreign bodies.
- Cover wound with a sterile dressing and apply pressure.
- Add extra padding if necessary.
- Lay casualty down.
- Raise the injured part, unless a broken bone is suspected.
- If blood soaks through the dressings which you have applied, add more on top of the originals.
- Arrange for immediate transfer to hospital.

Sometimes it may be advisable to use a pressure point to control severe bleeding. Pressure points are areas where large blood vessels (arteries) can be compressed against an underlying bone to prevent the further flow of blood. Pressure should be applied to the appropriate point between the heart and the wound for up to 15 minutes at a time.

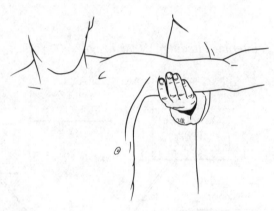

The brachial pressure point

Foreign bodies
If the foreign body is on the surface of the wound, rinse off. Never remove if embedded in the wound, simply protect and cover lightly with an emergency dressing and seek medical aid.

Amputations
Treat as for severe bleeding. Wrap severed part in gauze soaked in saline. Place in a plastic bag and keep cool but never directly against ice. Label and send to hospital with the casualty.

Blood leaking from the ear canal
This is potentially dangerous as it could indicate a severe head injury. It may occur after falls, for example from play equipment.
- Place a dressing or pad gently over the affected ear.
- Place casualty in recovery position, if unconscious.
- Lay the casualty down, head slightly raised and inclined to the injured side.
- Arrange for immediate transfer to hospital.
- Observe and record breathing, pulse and level of consciousness.

Do not plug the ear.

Nose bleeds
- Ask casualty to sit down with head bent slightly forward.
- Ask casualty to breathe through his/her mouth.
- Pinch the soft part of nose for 10 minutes.
- Loosen clothing around neck.
- Warn the casualty not to blow nose for several hours.
- If bleeding does not stop within a short time or recurs, advise casualty to seek medical advice.

Never plug the nose.

Bleeding from a tooth socket following dental extraction
- Place a pad of gauze firmly on the socket – the teeth should not meet.
- Instruct casualty to bite on the pad for 10 to 20 minutes.
- If bleeding does not stop, seek medical or dental advice.

Never give mouth washes as this prevents clotting, and never attempt to plug the tooth socket.

Cuts to the tongue or inside of cheeks
- Apply pressure using a clean dressing between thumb and finger.
- Seek medical advice if bleeding continues.

Bleeding from varicose veins
You may have seen protruding veins on legs of older people. If these veins are knocked they may bleed profusely. If the bleeding is not controlled, it may be fatal.
- Lay the person down, raising the affected leg as high as possible.
- Apply direct pressure using a sterile dressing.
- Loosen any constrictions, such as garters.
- Apply padding and bandage firmly.
- Raise and support leg.
- Transfer to hospital immediately.

Advising casualties about tetanus innoculation
With any wound there is a risk of infection from the tetanus germ. Deep wounds with soil or dirt in them are particularly dangerous. Always ask casualties if their tetanus protection is up-to-date and advise them to seek medical advice if it is not or if they are in any doubt.

Shock
Shock is a medical condition which may accompany a variety of injuries particularly those associated with blood and fluid loss as in haemorrhage, burns and scalds.

Some causes of shock
- Fluid loss due to severe bleeding, severe burns, diarrhoea, vomiting and sweating
- Heart attack
- Electric shock
- Pain

Signs and symptoms of shock
- Skin – pale, cold, clammy
- Pulse – fast, weak

- Breathing – rapid, shallow
- Casualty may feel – sick, dizzy, faint, anxious, thirsty
- Casualty may become unconscious.
- Heart and breathing may stop.

Shock: What to do

1 Put casualty in a suitable position for injury/condition:
   - minor injuries – sit down
   - unconscious – recovery position (see page 58)
   - chest injury – sit up, lean to injured side
   - heart conditions – 'W' position or lie flat
   - otherwise – lie flat, raise feet if possible.
2 Deal with cause.
3 Loosen tight clothing at neck, chest and waist.
4 Cover with blanket or coat. Do not overheat.
5 Reassure.
6 Give medical aid.
7 Observe condition.

Do not move unnecessarily, give food or drink, or allow casualty to smoke.

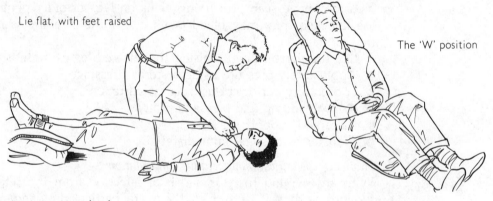

Lie flat, with feet raised

The 'W' position

Positions for shock

Review questions

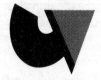

1 List five factors which affect the health of an individual.

2 What do you understand by the word 'lifestyle'?

3 How long, on average, do adults sleep at night?

4 List three benefits of taking regular exercise.

5 Suggest three strategies for coping with stress.

6 List four health problems associated with smoking tobacco.

7 List five ways in which excessive drinking of alcohol affects the body.

8 How could a person try to decrease their alcohol consumption?

9 List three reasons why people misuse drugs.

10 What help is available for drug users?

11 How is HIV spread?

12 Why do accidents occur?

13 Give three recommendations for maintaining a healthy diet.

14 When assessing an accident situation, the first consideration is for the _____ of the casualty and yourself.

15 What is the average adult pulse rate per minute?

16 Name two points in the body where the pulse can easily be counted.

17 Describe the immediate first aid treatment for a casualty who is not breathing.

18 When the heart has stopped beating _____ _____ (___) should be commenced.

19 In cardiac and respiratory arrest the ratio of heart compressions to lung inflations is __ heart compressions to __ lung inflations.

20 Explain how you would treat a severe bleed of the forearm.

Assignment A1.1
Investigate personal health and well-being

Teenscene

How my lifestyle ruined my health
3 true life stories from young people
Ali, Jane and Kevin tell their stories to you

Complete the stories using the information in this chapter on lifestyle and health, for example drug-taking, smoking, solvent abuse, etc.

Assignment A1.2
Present advice about health and well-being

In this assignment you are going to prepare a health promotion display for specific client groups. You should divide into groups of three or four to do this. There are several tasks to complete as part of your action planning.

1 In your groups, decide first on the target group you wish to prepare the display for. You will have to take into account the experience within the group, perhaps from placement or voluntary work. It is good to prepare a display for a group with whom you have had contact and know something about. You may decide to present the display to your contemporaries in your class on a topic which may affect adolescents.

   If the small groups within your class prepare displays for children, adolescents, adults and elders then you will have covered all the client groups mentioned in the range statement.

2 First think about how to research the possible factors affecting the lifestyle of your chosen group. You will need to look at books on general human development and Chapter 2 of this book. You may be able to find newspaper articles, magazine features, health journals and videos. It would be helpful if you could divide these tasks amongst yourselves and agree a time to share the information.

3 Once you have some background information about your client group, you should decide on a likely health promotion topic. Research the topic you decide on – again using similar sources, including establishments connected with the subject, possibly a Health Education Centre. Again, divide the tasks so that you can compete the research more efficiently.

4 When you have gained all the information you can in the time, think about the best methods of display. You will need to present some factual material in an attractive or shocking way to make people take notice. Charts and graphs could be produced on the computer and you may have someone in the group who is good at art!

   Collecting artifacts can also make a stimulating display, for example for Dental Health and Childcare – toothbrushes, kept first teeth or a can of cola are all eye-catching.

5 Once this display is set up you should be prepared to give a short talk to the rest of the group to explain what you have done and why. If your display is for children, for example, then it would be appropriate to treat the group as children using clear language for the designated age group. If you can present the display to real children then this is even better.

6 Write a brief report on the impact of the display.

7 After the period of the display, make sure you dismantle and return any borrowed items. Hand in your background notes, action planning and evaluation of your work for assessment.

Assignment A1.3
Reduce risk of injury and deal with emergencies

1 a Choose an individual, for example a baby, a child, an old person or a teenager. Produce a list of the types of hazard to which the individual is likely to be exposed on a day-to-day basis.

b Prepare an action plan to eliminate potential hazards. The plan should be in a form or style which is readily understood by the particular individual or their carer.

2 **Practical test on health emergencies**
Your tutor will arrange a practical/oral test to assess your life-saving skills. Criteria for assessment will include:
- assessment of the situation
- examination of a casualty
- checks on airway, breathing and circulation
- demonstration of CPR using a manikin and answering questions
- demonstration of recovery position and answering questions
- demonstration of control of bleeding and answering questions on blood loss and shock.

CHAPTER 2
Influences on health and well-being

Element 2.1: Explore the development of individuals and how they manage change

Element 2.2: Explore the nature of interpersonal relationships and their influence on health and well-being

Element 2.3: Explore the interaction of individuals within society and how they may influence health and well-being

What is covered in this chapter

- The development of the individual
- Self-concept
- The impact of changes caused by major events
- Interpersonal relationships and their influence on health and well-being
- The influence of social factors on health and well-being

These are the resources you will need for your Influences on Health and Well-being file:

- your written answers to the activities in this chapter
- your written answers to the review questions at the end of this chapter
- your completed for Assignments A2.1, A2.2 and A2.3.

Introduction

Have you ever thought about why you are the way you are – why *you* are *you*? What has influenced your well-being or otherwise? Can you help being like your parents? Can you work through or avoid some of the factors you don't like about your parents for yourself? Would it matter, in terms of health, which side of the city you were born in or at which end of the country? Is good health simply a matter of looking after yourself or are there other factors which come in to play? Such questions and others are tackled in this chapter.

The development of the individual

Individuals are so complicated that it is helpful to think of *aspects* of an individual's development to assist study. The four aspects usually considered are:

- **physical factors**, such as a person's height, weight, diet, exercise pattern, eye sight, hearing, etc.

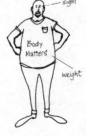
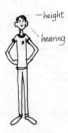

- **intellectual factors**, such as how a person's mind works, whether they absorb or understand information easily or quickly. Also, educational issues and language development.

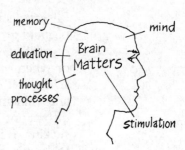

- **emotional factors**, such as how an individual *feels* about him/herself, about their roles and other people.

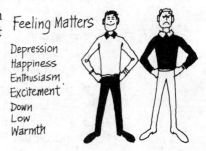

- **social factors**, such as how a person responds in groups and with other individuals.

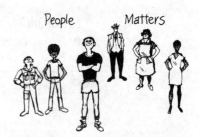

Although these four factors may be studied separately, they are in fact all related. Generally people in good physical health also feel positive and relate well to others. As their personal feelings are good, they probably tackle educational issues confidently and become successful. Conversely, if someone has a lot of illness, it is quite easy to become emotionally low and be less enthusiastic about work and relating to other people. Factors are inter-related – so that if you are physically hungry, it is difficult to concentrate on your assignment!

The physical aspects of development are described in the Appendix.

Nature nurture
It is impossible to say how far we are the way we are because of what we have inherited genetically or because of what we have learned. Is a child intelligent because of his/her genetic make up or because of a stimulating, encouraging home? Is he or she born intelligent or made intelligent? There is no definite answer to this question.

Characteristics of development in different stages of life

As individuals we are changing and developing throughout our lives. Everyone develops at different rates so that when comparisons are made between babies, allowances are made for individuality. If, however, a child or baby was assessed to be considerably behind his or her contemporaries then other investigations would need to be carried out.

Research shows that the development process is made up of alternating periods of rapid growth (often accompanied by disruption in life – 'hassle') and periods of relative calm, or consolidation. There are times when the changes pile up or when one central change affects the entire system, such as when we start school. Often these changes in role are accompanied by big changes in language and thinking so that a child starting school, for example, may seem a bit distant until he or she adjusts. They may even revert to old habits, such as thumb sucking. Relationships need a new pattern and it is best to keep other changes to a minimum at such times. Familiar foods, leisure patterns, rooms and decoration all help to gain consolidation in the period of transition or change.

Summary of the stages of human development

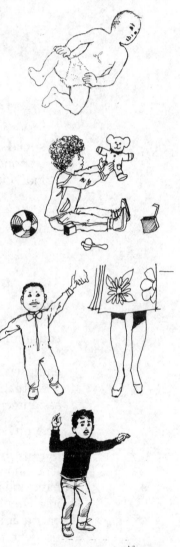

0–2 months
- Child mainly behaves in an instinctive, reflexive way – cries for food or if in pain.
- Begins to smile, may show interest in the world around.
- Probably no clear cut attachment to a single individual.

2–8 months
- Child now coos and babbles.
- May show preference for one adult over another, vision improves, can sit up and reach for things.

8–18 months
- Child learns to crawl and walk.
- Can use a series of actions to gain what he or she wants.
- Speaks words and half sentences.
- Will show attachment to other care givers and shows an interest in other children.

18 months–2 years
- More complex language.
- Transition time – possible disruption of sleeping and eating patterns.

2–6 years
- Motor skills are refined.
- Co-ordination improves so that games of bat and ball become fun.
- In terms of thinking, the child can use words or images to stand for things, develops a gender awareness, can put things into groups and can take other people's perspectives into account.

- Strong attachments to primary care givers, especially if under stress (child always calls for Mummy or Daddy if frightened or under pressure).
- Play choice may begin to be with the same gender and be for traditionally gender-related toys – little boys may want trains, etc.
- Early friendships formed, evidence of sharing, generosity and aggression.
- Explores further from own base – growing independence.

6–12 years

- Physical growth steady until puberty. Girls may see the beginning of puberty.
- Gross motor skills improve – mountain bike for Christmas!
- In terms of thinking, 'child' can subtract, order, add up, etc. Can perform tasks in the mind, for example, reading and mental arithmetic.

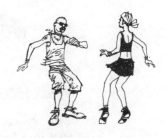

- Friends or peers become important, usually same gender. Individual friendships become more important. Attachments to parents less obvious, but still very much needed. Continues to absorb gender roles.

12–18 years: Adolescence

- Puberty is completed in this period. Increase in physical strength and speed.
- Most adolescents can reason morally – what is right and wrong, and why.
- Need to seek out future career, as well as interest in opposite gender.
- A lot of conflict as peer pressure mounts, possibly against parental influence.
- Questioning of taught values, roles, ideas, mood swings, depression, elation.

18–22 years

- No significant physical changes.
- In relationships, idea of giving and taking is consolidated – mature response.
- Understanding that identity is a complex product of past experiences and background.
- Intimate relationships, possibly new self-concept through work, religious and political views may be worked through.

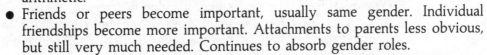

22–40

- Physically most people function at the maximum before the end of this stage, similarly with mental performance.
- Socially – possible marriage, parenthood, work peak.

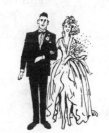

40–65

- Physically and mentally possibly some loss of abilities.
- May be demands from children and ageing parents.
- Marriage may be reassessed, friendships may increase in importance.
- Mid-life physical and emotional upheavals will occur in the early part of this stage.

65–

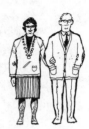

- Further decline physically and mentally.
- May experience loss of social contacts and gradual withdrawing or 'disengagement', cutting off from wider issues.
- Retirement. Readjustment to post-retirement phase.
- Family may be more significant in terms of mutual help.

Self-concept

What is self-concept?

Self-concept means the image you have of yourself. How you see yourself. Some people have a very realistic concept of who they are and what they are capable of. Most of us have an *ideal* self-concept – someone who we would like to be or be like. It helps in terms of being content if your ideal concept isn't too far from your actual self-concept. It is useful to try to understand something of your own identity or self-concept in caring because it will affect what you say and do in relation to others. Chapter 4 also explores this area.

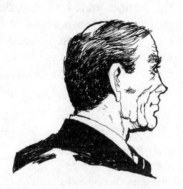
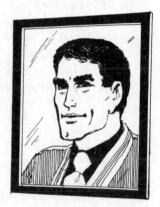

What influences self-concept?

Our self-concept is formed by how people behave towards us and then our response to them. It is a two-way process. We have an image of who we are, and we choose our friends because they are similar to us and like the things we do. In return, they reinforce aspects of our personality that are like them.

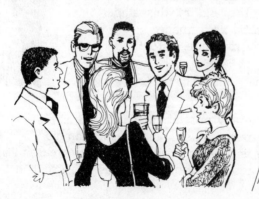
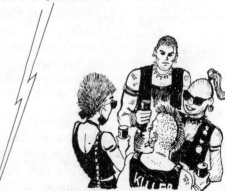

They confirm what we are 'Birds of a feather flock together, not out of luxury but out of necessity'.

A major influence on our self-concept are our primary carers or parents. They help to form our values, attitudes, patterns of behaviour and roles. They are one of the main agents of **socialisation**.

What is socialisation?

Socialisation is **not** socialising – you may do that at discos. Socialisation is a sociological term which is more significant than just socialising – it affects every individual.

Socialisation is the process whereby we become members of society. We are born with instincts to eat, to rest, etc., but we are **taught** manners, how to dress, language, etc. We absorb our cultural patterns through our parents, friends, education, media and work.

Socialisation starts when we are born and only ends when we die. We are continually being socialised by the new situations we meet in our lives.

Look at Activity 4.32 and remind yourself of how your parents have affected your own development. Page 85 also deals with family relationships and how they affect the individual.

Activity 2.1

a Read the case study below and then write down whether you think James has a positive or a negative self-concept. This is also a judgement on the level of his **self-esteem** or how he rates himself. Write down also *why* you think his self-concept is positive or not, giving specific reasons.

> James is 11 years old. He has just finished junior school. He is a tall, healthy-looking boy with blonde hair and pale blue eyes. He has a perfect set of evenly-spaced, white teeth which are displayed by his frequent grins and smiles. He is old for his school year – his birthday is in September so throughout his school life so far he has been physically and educationally ahead. He is good at sport and plays for the school football team and county tennis. His parents support him totally. They help him with any school work he has in the evenings and transport him to his many sporting events. His mother takes particular pride in buying his attractive, up-to-the-minute clothes and makes sure his tennis outfits are always immaculately laundered.
>
> At school his favourite subject is mathematics. His teacher says he is better than she is at maths, but he is also pretty good at English, science, geography and history. He is often so far ahead that he helps the others and they think he is really good.
>
> Each year a prize is awarded in the school to the girl and boy who have made the most contribution to the school. The staff of the school vote for who they think should gain the prize: James won the prize.

b When you have considered the first question, think about the following and write down your answers.

  i) How many friends do you think James will have?

  ii) How do friendships and popularity affect self-concept? How do you feel if you know you are liked?

  iii) How will James face the transition to his new secondary school? What attitude will he have?

  iv) Educationally, how do you rate his chances in the long term?

  v) If you feel you are good at a particular subject does this affect your motivation to work at that subject?

  vi) If you are good at one subject, what sort of attitude might you have towards other subjects?

  vii) What sort of relationship do you think James has with his teacher in the junior school? How will this affect his self-concept?

  viii) At home James is very much loved and his parents are proud to have such a son. What difference does this make to James? (Think about what James might lose if he was badly behaved for some reason – would it be worth James risking the loss of his parents' affection?)

  ix) When questions are asked in class, James often puts his hand up and gives a correct answer. Would it matter very much to him if he gave a wrong answer in terms of embarrassment or loss of self-esteem?

  x) How do you think James' physical capacity in terms of his height and sporting prowess affect his self-concept?

'You can be my friend, you can be in our gang'
Research shows that it is only when children become less egocentric – that is, concerned with self – at the age of about 6, that they develop stronger friendships. Once children are 7 or 8 they are in roles which unfortunately are extremely difficult to break. At this age it is extremely important for children to be accepted by their friends or 'the group'. Being accepted by the group doesn't necessarily mean that the child is popular. Some children rejected by the group do have friends. Sometimes the child who is popular at playgroup remains popular right through school. Similarly if a child has a reputation as a 'cry baby' or a 'trouble maker', he or she may find it hard to shake off that label.

Activity 2.2

As a class, discuss the following questions. Summarise your discussions for your file.

a How do children gain reputations?

b How significant are the things we say about children in terms of:
  i) how these comments make them feel about themselves?
  ii) how others perceive a particular child?

c What are the possible long-term implications of 'labelling' children?

Using the notes from your discussion see if you can work out the meaning of a term used by psychologists in relation to adults and children about a wide range of issues from education to criminal behaviour. The term is **self-fulfilling prophecy**.

Think about how a characteristic commented upon in a person (whether accurate or not) may be looked for in that person by others, and how that person may act upon that comment – the comment (or prophecy) comes true.

Experiments indicate that children who can 'pick up' other children's emotions or feelings tend to be more popular. Popular children also tend to perceive situations in a more positive light. Why do you think these factors affect popularity?

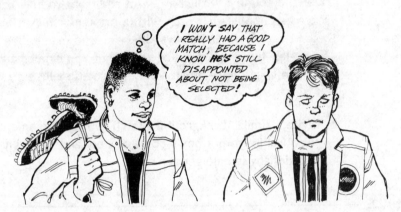

In general terms, girls tend to be more accepting than boys. Boys who are rejected tend to be aggressive and disruptive, while rejected girls tend to be more anxious and withdrawn.

A lot of studies show that self-esteem is rooted in family experience. Praise, affection and treating children as responsible help to boost self-esteem. High self-esteem tends to be linked with:
- high performance
- good relationships with parents
- greater popularity
- the development of an internal locus, or homing mechanism, so that they see themselves as responsible for their own actions and behaviour rather than being ruled by external forces.

Other common factors amongst popular children in school include:
- being friendly
- being outgoing
- being the youngest child rather than the oldest
- success in school
- being physically attractive
- often tall
- often having a specific task activity, for example sport.

Activity 2.3

Give reasons why you think the above factors affect popularity. How are the factors linked?

Androgyny

Another aspect of popularity and positive self-concept concerns **androgyny**. This means a child's ability to perform in both gender roles. Those who don't adopt specific male or female roles entirely tend to be more popular and have higher self-esteem.

Activity 2.4

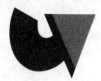

a Read the case study below and explain why Rachel is popular.

> Rachel is 11 years old. She is a county badminton player and enjoys travelling over the country with the rest of the team to play badminton. Once she played an important match with a broken arm – in plaster after she had fallen over playing rounders. She won the match. She likes clothes and hairstyles, but is quite casual about her appearance and far too interested in sport to spend very much time on 'traditionally girly matters'.

b Write a similar background sketch to describe an androgynous relationship from a boy's point of view and his ability to cut across traditionally female gender roles.

Activity 2.5

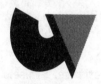

Read the case study about Tony and then answer the questions that follow.

> Tony is also 11 years old, but he is young for his year and small for his age. He has an eyesight problem which makes some sports more difficult. He often feels frustrated because he isn't good at sport and needs to lash out and kick something or someone because he is angry. On non-uniform day in school Tony's mum said he would just have to go in his uniform because he didn't have anything decent to wear. He hated that day. Everyone asked him if he had forgotten non-uniform day. Tony's dad left home when he was little. Tony still sees his dad but sometimes when there is an arrangement to go to his dad's house, his dad rings up at the last minute to say he is busy and can't see him.
>
> Tony's teacher finds him awkward and negative. She says he is sullen, bad tempered and that he doesn't seem bothered about his work. His test scores are quite low. Tony knows his marks are low and that his work is messy. He feels that he is a failure and that's just the way things must be.

a What comments would you make about Tony's self-concept?

b How would you rate his popularity in the class?

c What impact might Tony's father's apparent reluctance to see him, have on him? (Some children are abused by their parent(s) – physically or emotionally or sexually. What effect do you think this might have on self-esteem?)

d What significance would you attach to Tony's appearance and clothing?

e How would you rate Tony's chances of educational success? Would he be one of the ones to put his hand up for a question? Why? Why not?

f How might Tony be making his teacher's life more difficult? How easy is it to rid yourself of the label of 'trouble-maker'?

g What does the final statement of the case study indicate about Tony's feelings of powerlessness to change his situation?

h The passage implies that Tony's family is short of money. What other issues in Tony's life might this affect?

i If the children of the school Tony goes to are not particularly short of money, if they are from a more middle-class or affluent culture, how might Tony's problems be highlighted and what effect will this have on his self-concept?

j What could be done to help Tony improve his self-image?

It is almost as though the different boys have different amounts of money to spend on self-esteem. Tony hasn't much money (literally and as an illustration) he can't risk losing any, whereas James can afford to make a mistake.

Activity 2.6

Read the case study below and answer the questions.

> Joe is 43. He has spent 17 years of his life in custody for various crimes including burglary and grievous bodily harm. His childhood was made difficult by violence and abuse. He grew up with deep feelings of anger, bitterness and injustice. He often found it difficult to control these feelings and this resulted in his offences. Once he 'did someone over' for looking at his girlfriend.
>
> During his time in prison his wife met somebody else. She had had enough of Joe and his tempers.
>
> Since his release from prison seven years ago, Joe has kept straight. He works for the Probation Service touring schools and colleges telling children and young people how it feels to be 'inside'.
>
> His work has given him some financial security, some structure and status but he still feels very lonely.

a What difference has work made to Joe and why?

b Do you think Joe might be tempted to return to his old ways? What might prevent him from doing this?

c What sort of self-image do you think Joe had during his younger days? How did he try to hide his feelings about himself?

d What about Joe's self-image in more recent years?

e What difference do you think age makes to self-concept?

Activity 2.7

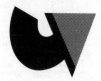

This is a sensitive activity and is probably best carried out with someone you know well. If you are hesitant about this activity omit it and simply answer the questions at the end by imagining what it is like to be someone from a different culture living in Britain.

Choose someone who is of a different culture than your own to interview. Ask them if they mind answering questions which are about them personally. Ask them the following questions:

a How does your culture differ generally from the culture here?

b What specific differences have you noticed or been aware of in terms of family life or habits and customs?

c Did these differences ever really matter – at school or socially?

d How did these differences make you feel?

You might feel it helpful to read the section on the effects of discrimination now, in Chapter 4, page 153.

The impact of changes caused by major events

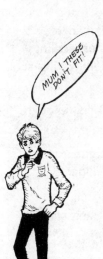

At the beginning of this chapter we noted that life has a habit of pushing us through some changes at particular points. These periods of change or transition are counter-balanced by periods of calm or equilibrium.

Change may be painful but it is *necessary*. Why? If we didn't have change, we would be locked into one stage, we would cease thinking, we would become bored, full of routine thoughts, like automatons.

Change for most people is *inevitable*. Society expects us to change to take on new, different roles. Physically, our bodies change in ways over which we have *no control*.

When we move into a different phase of our lives there may be some awkwardness as we adjust to new roles, new situations and new people. That is why we may feel sad when we leave school even if we are glad to go!

Think about the first time you came to college. How did you feel? Most people are apprehensive because they are learning a new part or role. At first we are conscious of the role, we are eager to play the role as it should be played – like everyone else. We want to wear what everyone else usually wears. We may watch the procedure in the refectory at lunch time before we risk going through ourselves. Once we become familiar with the new roles and routines, we become more confident about performing them as *we* want to.

Anticipatory socialisation

Often the major **life events** we experience have been anticipated through our socialisation experience. The books we read, the films and TV programmes we watch, the discussions we have all help to prepare us for the next event. So that the first time a girl goes out with a boy there is a sort of script that she can follow – an expected way of behaving.

Activity 2.8

Look at the life events listed below and work out specific ways that such events may be prepared for:

a *Starting school* – Think about visits, books, passing the school building, older siblings, going to the toilet independently, dressing independently, parents/carers being around, being patient, comfort toys, favourite foods, inevitable tiredness, reducing other changes, suitable clothes, possessions, equipment.

b *Starting work* – Work experience, possible reduction or increase of social events to give balance or rest, reduction of other changes, new clothes, transport arrangements, knowledge of job, tasks, supervisor.

c *Marriage* – Engagement, marriage preparation classes, books, holidays together, listening, time spent with parents, solid financial and practical base (Research shows that couples who marry with parental approval and have a solid financial basis are less likely to divorce.) Has each individual been independent for long enough? Reached satisfactory points in career? Are they ready to commit themselves solely to each other? Some couples have experienced a lot of difficulties because one or both partners haven't been able to leave their former role of son or daughter to make an emotional bond with the partner.

d *Leaving home* – Breaks away, if young people go on to higher or further education there is a natural break which may reduce the impact of leaving home eventually. In this case, checking out decent accommodation, taking familiar bits and pieces with you, may help – any more ideas?

e *Parenthood* – Parentcraft classes, parenting classes, reading, videos, discussion. Like most life events all practising has to be done on the job – mistakes cannot be rectified!

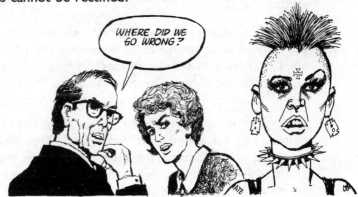

f *Changing jobs* – Often it is difficult to limit other change factors like moving house, changing children's schools; it may even be necessary to change car or learn to drive. Meeting with other people connected with the job may be helpful, if that is possible. Likewise finding out as much as possible about the actual tasks of the job, visiting the area of the job. Working out social contacts, places to go for leisure to provide some balance in the early pressured stages. Keeping as physically fit and healthy as possible by paying attention to diet, exercise and general lifestyle factors, including drinking and smoking.

g *Moving house* – If you have an unsettled base for home this may affect your performance at work. If there is pressure both at work and home then the stress ratings soar. Enlist as much help practically as you can, use as many professional sources of help as you can afford, e.g. full removal service. Make arrangements to see old friends and neighbours. Invite new neighbours to make contacts. Have you ever moved house? How did you manage?

h *Retirement* – Pre-retirement courses, gradual reduction in working hours, increase hobbies and possibly voluntary work. Check financial security, manageability of accommodation, keep in touch with people – more thoughts?

i *Death* – The death of a spouse is a very heavy burden to bear. Women tend to outlive men and may find themselves very bewildered when their husband dies. If they have followed traditional role patterns where the man has dealt with financial matters and household maintenance, the women will have to adjust to this. Conversely some men may find it hard to launder and cater for themselves if their wife dies.

How can people prepare for these life events?

Some life events can never be prepared for because they are *unexpected*. Events such as redundancy, serious illness, disability, divorce or the death of someone close to you happen to other people. Nobody likes to think of these traumas happening to them.

Reactions to life events

Experts have suggested that people go through various stages when experiencing traumas particularly if they are grieving the death of someone close to them.

The early stages involve denial, shock, numbness, disbelief, perhaps a psychological searching for the person, the partner, the job, the health, the ability. There may be questioning: 'Is this really happening to me?'; 'He can't tell me I'm redundant, I've been working here for 25 years'; 'She can't have found someone else – we're married, we've our own children.'

There may be anger, protest, despair: 'She has no right to leave us'; 'I could murder him for making me redundant'. This distances the person from the deceased, the former partner, the old job. The person may feel disorientated as life happens without the partner or the job and they haven't adjusted. They are still attached to the old ways and aspects of the former relationship.

Finally, the person begins to reorganise their sense of self and their life in accordance with the new situation and this is very positive.

Everyone experiences grief differently and it may take some more time than others to recover. If there are complications about the death then the grief process is also more complicated, for example, if the death is very sudden, accidental, if foul play is suspected or murder, if the death is an act of suicide, if there are multiple deaths or if the death is in unusual circumstances. Likewise if a couple had had some tensions in their relationship before the death or there had been a family row then this also makes for a more difficult grief process. The people involved may feel some guilt: 'If only I hadn't said...'; 'I wish I could make it up'; 'I should never have let him go on that camping holiday...'

Similarly with divorce, research shows that the less bitter and acrimonious the break up, the better the readjustment process is for all concerned.

Defence mechanisms
Sometimes people try very hard to get over the shock of redundancy or becoming disabled and repress feelings of anger and frustration. This is referred to as a **defence mechanism**. Research shows that it is best to *allow the grief*, the tears, the sobbing, particularly with children because it is part of the healing process. The 16-year-old girl who loses her sight through a brain tumour has got to grieve the loss of her sight, she has got to mourn all that is no longer available to her before she can begin to work on mobility or learning braille. Repressing the grief may cause many more deep-seated, psychological problems later.

Chapter 3 (page 113) also discusses loss and grief.

It has been said that people who suffer great loss never really completely re-adjust, they just go through the motions of everyday life and that may be true for some people.

In some cultures, it is more accepted to demonstrate grief and bereavement rituals may be more extensive. Families and friends in all cultures support the grieving relative, but in some cultures there is more open, affectionate evidence of this support.

How to manage change
It is presumptuous to advise people who are undergoing major, negative life events, how to conduct their lives, how to cope. People who have shared their reactions to such traumas however might agree that the following points have some benefit:

● Take advantage of friends and family to talk through the problems, but if this doesn't work or relatives are already under pressure, seek professional help. This may also apply to the family members who may worry about the mental health of the bereaved or shocked person. If there is any doubt, seek professional help.
● The professional help may involve a visit to the GP, a referral to a psychiatrist, a therapist or a social worker.
● Professional help may be available through voluntary organisations such as Cruise, Relate, Victim Support, Parent Lifeline, Kidscape or the Samaritans. The list is extensive, phone numbers are generally found in the *Phone Book*. These organisations provide counselling services.

- Practical factors like finance and accommodation problems resulting from the death of a partner or divorce may be dealt with at the Citizen's Advice Bureau. Some local authorities also run Benefits Advice Services.
- Meeting with self-help groups may give support and practical advice.
- Keeping healthy can help you to deal with the impact of major social change – diet, exercise, relaxation.
- Setting milestones for progress in readjustment may help: 'Next week I will go and visit Teresa by myself, I always went with my Joe before.'
- Giving treats may provide some relief and change from the toil of the routine.
- Faith and religious belief can be a great support and renew hope.
- Prayer or meditation can have a calming effect in a pressured life.
- Simply writing comments down in diary form can help to order the inner chaos.
- Often people feel burdened and bewildered by the myriad of tasks that face them while experiencing inner turmoil – so sitting down with a pencil and paper trying to prioritise important tasks and put others into perspective may help.
- Keeping up social contacts helps to keep a sense of balance, whereas withdrawal may increase pressures.
- Reducing unnecessary change and keeping as many familiar routines, possessions and relationships as possible around increases security.
- It is easy to cause more tension in the family because you feel under pressure so that a cycle of arguments and guilt brings you even further down.
- Maintaining some sense of pride in how you look may be a spur for self-preservation when you are feeling low and inclined to neglect yourself.

Activity 2.9

Re-read the case studies on James and Tony in Activities 2.1 and 2.5. Imagine *either* Tony or James is middle-aged. Describe briefly three major life events for either of them. One event must be unexpected and indicate the ways in which the man might manage the social changes in his life.

The section on stress in Chapter 1 is also useful reading in connection with managing the change caused by life events.

Interpersonal relationships and their influence on health and well-being

How early are relationships formed? Early! No one really known how early a baby notices its mother, father or main carer. The significant point is that if a child is denied positive early relationships for a long time, this will affect his or her development. Babies who are neglected or ill-treated, who have had little stimulation, eye contact or physical contact, need a lot of help to become bright and affectionate themselves. Similarly as the child grows, the relationship that develops gives him or her a pattern for future relationships.

The influence of parents

Psychologists hold that a child's early relationship with its parents (particularly the mother) sets the tone of later relationships. Children with secure relationships with their parents are more likely to be accepted by their peers (friends, contemporaries). Sometimes children who have difficult relationships with siblings form closer friendships outside the home.

Activity 2.10

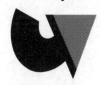

Discuss the following questions and summarise your conclusions for your file.

a Can parents help their children to be accepted? If so, how?

b What makes some children bully?

c Why are some children bullied? Are some children more vulnerable to bullying than others? Why?

d Can parents influence their child's behaviour if he or she is a bully?

e Can teachers prevent bullying?

f Can parents assist their child to develop strategies to cope or deal with bullies?

g What effect might bullying have?

The influence of the family

Although the relationship between parent or main carer and child is a central one, other early relationships soon become significant. The relationship between brothers and sisters may be tempestuous at times, but they do affect development.

Activity 2.11

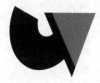

As a class, discuss the following questions.

a Are you an only child? An elder child? From a large family? The youngest child? How do you think this may have affected your development?

b How much contact did you have or do you have with your grandparents? How has this affected your outlook?

Summarise your discussions for your file.

In some cultures the **extended family** (a family which includes grandparents, aunts, cousins) is very much alive. Today, in British society the **nuclear family** is more the norm. This family consists of couples and their children living alone. Relatives, in many cases, may be living long distances from the nuclear family. This is because as people become mobile they tend to move to jobs away from parents and grandparents.

Activity 2.12 ————————————————————————————

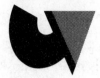

Discuss and write down what you think are the advantages in terms of relationships of:

a the extended family.

b the nuclear family.

Changing relationships

Just as we are continually changing, being socialised for new and different situations, so it is inevitable that the relationships we form need to change. **Transition times**, or times of major change, often test relationships.

Activity 2.13 ————————————————————————————

a Look at the comments below. Can you decide what has provoked them?
   i) 'I thought my Charlie was such a darling until he reached two.'
   ii) 'I can't do a thing right since she's started school even the location of the spaghetti on the plate was wrong.'
   iii) 'I have to walk behind her now she goes to the juniors; she doesn't like the idea of me taking her to school.'
   iv) 'He wants to choose his own clothes now he is in secondary school.'
   v) 'Every time she goes in that bathroom she slams the door and locks it. She is ages in there fiddling about with her hair – at fourteen I ask you!'
   vi) 'She doesn't know what to do with herself. She wants to go to college but she isn't that confident. She sounds off a lot at home of course but that's just me and her dad – we don't matter.'
   vii) 'My mum comes every Saturday night. She used to come to baby sit when they were little. Now we all go out and she watches the television. She says she likes to pop in for the company!'
   viii) 'I used to enjoy going to see my dad but he's become so confused lately . . .'

b The relationships above are all concerned with family life. Why do you think relationships may change in work situations? Work relationships are mainly formal and obviously less deep and personal than those of the family. When might a work relationship become less formal? What are the implications of less formal relationships in a work situation?

————————————————————————————

Relationships change not only because individuals change and develop, but also because of wider issues – a woman may return to work after a period at home, a man may become unemployed, a daughter or a son may go to higher education. The family may have greater affluence, transport, holidays or the reverse.

Why relationships?

People differ greatly in their need for close, informal or even formal relationships. There are those who like to spend long periods by themselves

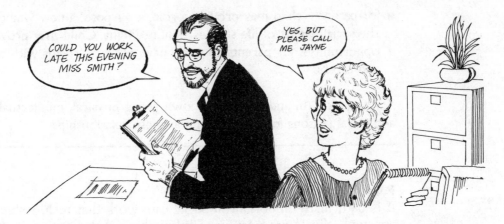

with no one else to be responsible for or share company. Most people, however, need both informal family relationships and more formal ones to thrive and be happy.

Activity 2.14

Think about the relationships that exist in a family situation:

a child–parent

b sibling–sibling

c man–woman.

Write down the physical, intellectual, emotional and social reasons for each relationship, in an ideal world.

Clues to help you with relationship (a):

Physical:
- for child – food, warmth, care, protection, provision of accommodation, care when ill.
- for parent – creation of child satisfies physical need/urge to reproduce. At one time children would eventually provide for the physical needs of their parents as they aged, but this is less common now.

Intellectual:
- for child – parent provides stimulation toys, may assist educationally.
- for parent – may see child-rearing as an intellectual challenge.

Emotional:
- for child – parent provides love, security, affection, guidance, calmness.
- for parent – child provides joy, hope, satisfaction, pride, someone to love and the pleasure of returned love. The parent will feel glad to be needed and loved.

Social:
- for child – parent may provide direction, opportunities, encourage friendships and introduction to wider relationships.

- for parent – child may provide a role, a purpose, a new way of enjoying the social events of life such as Bonfire Night. Child may provide opportunities for parents to make new circle of friends with other parents and carers.

Try to tackle (b) and (c) on your own giving physical, intellectual, emotional and social reasons for participating in these relationships.

Formal or work relationships

It is particularly important in social care work that relationships among staff and with clients are positive. Studies show that poor relationships at work are not good in terms of production or efficiency. Poor relationships or non-existent relationships at work can lead to personal dissatisfaction, depression and ill-health. Many people would say that after the financial incentive to work, the next incentive is the company they have with their colleagues or work mates.

Think about your own experience at school, how significant are/were your relationships with your friends in terms of your motivation to attend school and learn?

Teachers too need to form relationships with the groups and individuals they teach to make learning effective.

Social, informal realtionships

Often we participate in relationships because we enjoy them. We may use our leisure time to play football or badminton. We may go to clubs and discos to meet with friends who are unassociated with work or family. This is because we need to gain a balance in our lives. We need to be free from the responsibilities of home and work for a short time to reinforce a lighter side of ourselves. We go to confirm aspects of ourselves that are sporty, fun loving, creative or even silly.

People who have sincere religious beliefs like to meet together to share thoughts and discussion, worship and praise. This again reaffirms the faith to the individual. One has to be very single-minded to maintain religious belief in isolation.

If people leave their home town or community and live abroad or in another part of the country, they are often glad to meet with someone from their home town or country while they are away. Why do you think this is so?

Family matters: The role of the family in the development of individuals

Parenting is a two-way process. It would be easy for parents if their children simply followed whatever their parents wanted them to do. Children, however, have personalities and wills of their own so it is an interactive, or two-way, process. Two children in the same family can be very different even if their parents have brought them up in roughly the same way.

Activity 2.15

As a class, discuss the following questions and summarise your discussions for your file.

a Does the gender of the child affect the way parents react to him or her?

b Does the position in the family affect the way parents handle children? Think of the eldest and youngest child and how their development may be different because of how their parents have brought them up.

c Are some babies or children more difficult to care for than others? How might this affect parental responses and subsequent development?

d In what ways might babies and children exert power over adults?

Parenting styles

Activity 2.16

a **i)** Write down the possible characteristics of an 'over-protective' parent.
   ii) Why might a parent or carer be over-protective?
   iii) How might over-protection affect a child?

Clues:
- Think about continual monitoring of a child, not allowing play, inhibiting actions, restricting freedom.
- Think of illness in babies, loss of babies, experience of disability.
- Think of timidity, insecurity, inability to cope with small hardships or problems, over-sensitivity.

Parents may move from one style to another depending on mood, situation and child.

b **i)** Now write down the possible characteristics of a 'permissive parent' – one who allows their children to do a wide range of things that some other parents may prohibit.
   ii) How might 'permissive parents' affect child development?

c **i)** Finally write down the possible characteristics of a strict or authoritarian parenting style.
   ii) In what ways may the child be affected by such an approach?

Attitudes to discipline often convey a great deal about parenting styles. Think about your own childhood:
- How were you disciplined?
- Were you ever punished?
- What form did the punishment take?
- Was the punishment effective?
- Does punishment contribute to overall development?

- Is punishment always necessary? Can children be prevented from misdemeanours by careful or thoughtful handling of situations?
- How might children react to punishment?
- Is punishment effective if it is delayed?
- Is verbal punishment effective?
- Are threats to punish effective?
- If parents are inconsistent about what deserves punishment, how might this affect the child?

Activity 2.17

Look at the list of punishments below and comment on the possible pitfalls of such strategies and their possible effects on the child.

a Time out punishment – 'Go to your room...'

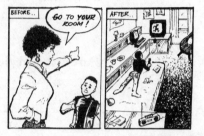

b Natural consequences – 'I told you to eat your meal – you wouldn't, now you are hungry.'

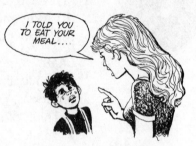

c With adolescents or those old enough to understand – 'I messages'. For example, 'It upsets me when you use such language'; 'I feel weary when I come home from work and you've left the place in a tip.'

d Smacking.

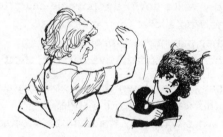

e Denying privileges.

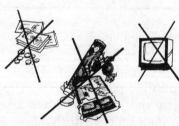

General role or functions of family
- Reproduction – 'it makes it tidier if it's done in families.'
- Socialisation – it is through our socialisation that we learn the norms and values of our culture. Parents are the main agents of socialisation.
- Physical care.
- Emotional support and guidance.
- Education – supporting through school, providing early educational experiences, choosing schools or further education.

Family break-up
Tensions exist in families for many reasons. Studies tend to focus on the divorce of parents, but relationships between parent and child or between siblings (brothers and sisters) are very significant and are often linked with parental separation. You must know from your own experience, it only takes one person in the house to be in a bad mood for everyone to feel put out.

Factors concerning finance, accommodation, work and unemployment are also underplayed in the effect they have on damaging relationships.

Activity 2.18

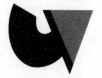

Discuss other possible reasons for family breakdown and make a list of them.

Possible consequences of family separations
- *Practically* – loss of income, different accommodation requirements, change of job or school, arrangements for legalities of separation and access need to be carried out which necessitate time off work and energy which may be reduced because of the trauma.
- *Emotionally* – great feelings of loss, sadness, resentment, anger, anxiety, withdrawal, lack of motivation, drive to work in school or in job situation.
- *Socially* – may be difficult to see old friends because of attachments to 'lost' partner. Former haunts, places of social interest and leisure may be awkward because of associations with former partner.

All studies agree that the more bitter the break up, the more difficult it is for all concerned to readjust. Separations carried out with the minimum of animosity and practical disruption are still painful for everyone, but the effects of the pain aren't as long-lasting and the readjustment process is faster.

Sometimes remarriage makes new demands on families to readjust to step siblings and step parents. It may involve practical upheaval of new schools and accommodation. The new situation may reopen old 'wounds' and this immediately places strain on the new relationship.

Family separations are particularly painful if they occur while a family member is going through a developmental transition, such as adolescence.

Roles
Throughout this chapter the word 'role' has been used to explain the part someone plays, or the function an institution like the family may have – the role of the family.

Activity 2.19

a Draw a role diagram for yourself. Simply draw a stick man or woman with arrows pointing to the different roles you play.

b Interview someone older than yourself, a parent perhaps, and draw their role diagram.

c What do you notice about the role patterns?

d Do you think gender affects role patterns?

How do we know our roles?

We learn our roles through the socialisation process. We absorb by watching, listening and imitating how we should be, what we should say, how we should act. We learn very quickly what is appropriate. Each situation has its own **norms**, or guidelines to behaviour, so that when we first go to school we might rage and kick because we don't want to go. When we reach secondary school we still might not want to go, but we tend not to rage and kick because we know the norms of the situation.

Think of other norms or guidelines to behaviour associated with:
● eating out in a restaurant
● going to church
● dating
● queuing for a bus.

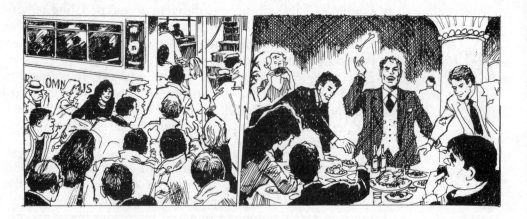

People who don't follow the norms for whatever reason may appear odd, funny and, in extreme cases when they don't follow a legal norm or a law, may be put in court.

Particular groups have their own norms as part of their culture. There are the traditions of dress, ceremonies, festivals and the norms of table manners and courtesy.

People who are interested in house music may have norms that belong to that group. Can you list them?

Norms and roles may change because of factors in society (for example, the availability of contraception changed the role of women) and because of individual development. Sometimes particular behaviours are associated with different social class groupings (see below). This isn't very helpful in that it becomes easy to stereotype people because of the social class groupings they are in.

The influence of social factors on health and well-being

Social class

Social class is a form of social stratification – a system for putting people into strata or layers. In the UK, the Registrar-General, a government official, collects data on all births, deaths and marriages, and census data every ten years. Since the beginning of this century, the Registrar-General has grouped people into five social classes, from a list of 20 000 jobs, as a way of classifying people. The groupings are based on the income, status, skill and educational level of each job.

Classes 1 to 3 are usually what we would call the middle class and Classes 4 to 5 may be referred to as the working class.

The five social classes – the Registrar-General's classification

	Class		Examples
Middle class	1	Professional	Doctors, dentists, solicitors
	2	Managerial	Managers, teachers, nurses
	3	Non-manual Skilled manual	Clerks, typists, travel agents Electricians, hairdressers, cooks
Working class	4	Semi-skilled manual	Postmen or women, farm workers
	5	Unskilled manual	Cleaners, labourers

The Registrar-General's classification has been criticised because:
● It does not take account of unemployed people.
● It does not take account of people (usually women) at home looking after children or dependent relatives.
● It is based on the male's occupation so that even if the wife, or female partner, has a job in a higher class that doesn't count.
● Some occupations don't fit easily into categories and there are lots of grades within individual occupations.
● Individual occupations may be up- or down-graded in society before this is reflected in the scale.
● People are classified by *occupation* – this doesn't necessarily mean that their lifestyle follows a national middle-class pattern because they are teachers in a middle-class bracket.

● The scale doesn't necessarily reflect the power base. The people at the top don't have any more power than those at the bottom. If the refuse workers went on strike, life could become very difficult.

Income

Economic factors like the amount of income we have and how we spend it affects how we live, and is linked to social class.

Activity 2.20

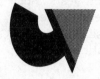

There is a great difference between the income level of a person in Class I and a person in Class 5. What possible differences might there be between two such people in the following areas:

a   diet?

b   health care?

c   housing?

d   leisure?

e   education?

f   holidays?

g   paying for help with house maintenance?

h   paying for help with house cleaning?

i   paying for help with house or gardening?

j   paying for help with child minding?

k   paying for help with catering?

l   stress levels?

m occupational hazards?

Of course, there are individuals in Class 1 who may lead very unhealthy lifestyles and the opposite may be true for Class 5.

Once you have made this comparison you may be able to perceive a scenario with greater extremes. If a person is unemployed, for example, this heightens the difficulties and the need.

In education, research has shown that children lower down the social scale tend to do less well educationally than those higher up. Consider for yourself the differences there may be between the groups in terms of role models (people to base yourself on), encouragement to go on to higher education, private education, extra tuition, a place to study and believing you can do it because you are expected to achieve.

Housing

A home is a very significant factor in an individual's life. The place where we live can affect not only our physical health but also our mental health, and can even affect us socially. The effects are even greater if an individual doesn't have a home!

Activity 2.21

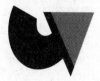

In small groups, consider the possible implications of living in bad housing, cramped, damp conditions or of living in temporary housing for the following people:

a a single parent with young children

b an elderly person living alone

c a teenager living with his or her family.

Tape your discussion or summarise it for your file.

Don't forget to consider the physical, emotional, mental and social aspects of their lives. Think also about what addresses mean – not just where people live but something about *them*. The community that they come from may send messages to other people who may make assumptions about them.

Housing standards have improved a great deal in the UK since the end of the Second World War, but just over 5 per cent of housing is still considered unfit and homelessness is an increasing problem.

In 1991, 70 000 people had their homes repossessed. This means they could not afford to repay their mortgage so the building society had to reclaim the property. Sometimes people's businesses fail and their home is reclaimed by the bank or building society as part payment for the money initially borrowed.

The number of people who have to live in temporary accommodation is rising. This is unsatisfactory for the households concerned because they feel insecure and unsettled. Thousands of people have no home, possibly because they have personal difficulties like alcoholism or mental health problems. Whatever the reason for their homelessness, one thing that is certain is that once they begin to live rough their health declines rapidly. The average age of death for a homeless person is 47 years.

Work

Working conditions can affect health. Think of the risk factors involved in building, refuse collection, working in steel factories or with heavy industrial equipment.

There is no doubt that the higher up the social scale you go the better your life changes are in terms of health, education, career opportunities and personal well-being.

Lifestyle choices

Some people argue that people in the lower socio–economic groups have worse health because of their habits, such as drinking, smoking and poor diet. People in the north, for example, have been accused of eating too many stodgy foods to be good for them. This sort of comment is not helpful because:

- It blames the victim for the situation they are in rather than looking at wider issues such as poverty, which is often the root of many problems to do with lifestyle. The comment could be described as a **deficit model**, one which makes the victim out to be deficient in some way. 'Asian mothers don't know enough about childcare and that is why the mortality rate (death rate) of Asian babies is so high' is another example of a deficit model statement.

- Further questions might be asked concerning what *makes* people lower down the social scale smoke or drink? What pressures are on them to resort to these things? What alternatives have they? Limited income often means limited lifestyle.

People from minority groups may find it more difficult to gain the health care they need when information is not available in community languages, when transport may not be available to attend hospital appointments or the demands of other children make it impossible to sit in long queues for antenatal checks. Similar points could be made concerning white people from lower class groups.

Activity 2.22

Discuss the following questions and statements. Summarise your discussions for your file.

a Why might a child from a lower socio–economic group be five times more likely to be killed on the road than a child from Class 1 or 2?

b Why is the perinatal mortality rate among Asian people very much higher than among white people? (Perinatal mortality rate means babies who die in their first week of life.)

c Why are two-thirds of the students at universities from middle-class backgrounds?

d Children from lower social classes suffer more respiratory infections and diseases, ear infections, squints, and are more likely to be of shorter stature than their more middle-class counterparts.

e Mortality rates for people from Class 5 are sometimes twice as high as for adults in Class 1.

f Black people are more likely to be diagnosed as schizophrenic than white people.

Further information on the effects of negative lifestyle choices can be found in Chapter 1.

Review questions

1 Explain self-concept.

2 Explain role concept.

3 What are the functions of the family?

4 Explain the term 'deficit model'.

5 What is a norm?

6 Explain what is meant by 'time of transition'.

7 Explain the difference between informal and formal relationships.

8 What is socialisation? Give examples.

9 What is the Registrar-General's classification?

10 What criticisms may be made of this classification?

11 What are the possible implications of social class position? Does it matter what class you are in? Why?

12 On what basis is the Registrar-General's classification drawn up? Is this useful or not? Why?

Assignment A2.1
The development of the individual

1 Write a brief report (300 words) on the main characteristics of human development based on the four main stages:
- childhood
- adolescence
- adulthood
- old age.

2 Briefly explain the main factors which influence an individual's self concept.

3 Using the knowledge you have gained from working through the case studies in this chapter, work out three more case studies.

Base one case study on yourself (you needn't give too much away if you're shy), one on someone of a different gender from yourself and one on someone from a different ethnic origin from yourself.

In each case describe an event which is predictable, an event which is unpredicted and how these events were managed.

Assignment A2.2
Interpersonal relationships

1 Using the text and other reading, write a brief report analysing your own relationships. Indicate which relationships are formal or informal and how these relationships have changed. (Some relationships may begin formally but become informal as when you meet a girl/boyfriend). Include family relationships.

2 a Use the case studies of Joe, Tom and James. Imagine they have relationships with women. Explain what they get out of the relationships.
   b Further imagine that James' relationship runs into difficulties. Describe the possible scenario and the consequences of the breakdown of this relationship.

Assignment A2.3
The interaction of individuals within society

1 Discuss the two families described in the case studies below and compare them in terms of their potential health and well-being. Try to put them in social class brackets. Give reasons for your choice and comment on the usefulness of the Registrar-General's classification.

2 Carry out some research in your library in connection with social class and health. *Inequalities in Health*, a government report produced in the 1980s, is a useful book to look at.

3 Write an account of which family you think will have the best health for the longest time. Give reasons for your decision.

Case Study A
The Jones family live in a fairly spacious semi-detached house in a residential area. Mr Jones is a successful solicitor. Mrs Jones is a dentist – she just works part-time. They have two children aged 9 and 11. Mr and Mrs Jones are keen to keep fit, they jog regularly and they are careful about their diet. As a family they enjoy horse-riding and they have recently bought a horse of their own. They are all in good health at the moment, although there is a history of coronary disease. Mr Jones' father died at the age of 50. His mother lives alone in Winchester. Mrs Jones' parents also live in Winchester.

Case Study B

Mrs Smith is a single parent of three children under 7 managing on DSS benefit payments. She lives in a small, terraced house which is in need of some modernisation and is situated on a busy main road. This makes it difficult for the children to play outside. Mrs Smith has little time, money or energy for sporting interests but she is in reasonable health. She is certainly not overweight because of her many chores, but she does feel stressed and exhausted a lot of the time. Her youngest child suffers from asthma. Mrs Smith's mother lives close by. There is no family history of serious illness.

CHAPTER 3

Health and social care services

Element 3.1: Investigate the provision of health and social care services
Element 3.2: Describe how the needs of different client groups are met by health and social care services
Element 3.3: Investigate jobs in health and social care

What is covered in this chapter

- Health care services
- Social care services
- Client groups using health and social care services
- Support for people who use health and social care services
- The role of health and social care workers

These are the resources you will need for your Health and Social Care Services file:

- examples of job descriptions of professionals employed in health and social care services
- a copy of your local authority's annual Community Care Plan
- your written answers to the activities in this chapter
- your written answers to the review questions at the end of this chapter
- your completed Assignments: A3.1, A3.2 and A3.3.

Health care services

We may all work hard at maintaining our health and independence, but there are times when medical or social care is necessary. In the UK, in the 1990s, we have a system of free health care – the National Health Service (NHS). Health care has not always been free, however, and indeed some people today choose to pay into private health care schemes. What is the NHS and how does it work?

Health services before 1948

Before 1948, most doctors worked privately and people had to pay for treatment. Many people took out insurance through friendly societies and trade unions, for example, to help financially in times of illness.

If anyone needed hospital treatment they had to go into one of three types of institution which, by law, the local authority had to provide:

- **pyschiatric hospitals** (or 'asylums' as they were then called), for people with mental health problems

- **isolation hospitals** (also known as sanatoriums or fever hospitals) for people with infectious diseases, such as TB
- **workhouse hospitals** for those who could not afford to pay for health care. Conditions in workhouse hospitals were very poor and many people feared them.

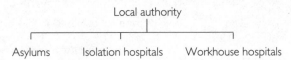

Local authority services before 1948

There were also:

- **voluntary hospitals**   These had much better conditions than workhouse hospitals. Many were very old institutions, founded hundreds of years ago. Doctors worked in these voluntary hospitals for low pay and some ran their own private practices to compensate for such inadequate pay. Patients paid for their treatment according to how much they could afford.
- **cottage hospitals**   These were small, local institutions and were usually based in rural areas. Doctors who treated patients at their local surgeries would also treat them when they were admitted to the cottage hospital. Patients paid for their treatment in cottage hospitals.

Activity 3.1

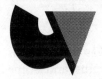

a Use the local history section of your main library and try to find out about the beginnings of hospitals and health services in your locality.

b Arrange to talk to an elderly person about health care before the NHS. Discuss with your class colleagues the accounts you have been given.

The National Health Service 1948–89

In 1948, Aneurin Bevan, Labour Minister for Health, set up a free health service on a national basis in an attempt to provide fair access to health and care for everyone. This new National Health Service brought all the various health and care services under the control of the Ministry of Health. Funding for the service was to come from general taxation, national insurance contributions and charges made to private patients.

The diagram below summarises the administrative structure of the NHS from 1948 until 1974.

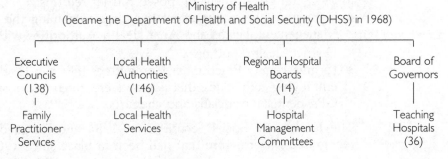

The National Health Service 1948–74

The structure set up at the start of the NHS remained in place for almost 26 years. However, weaknesses began to appear almost immediately. In the late 1960s the government produced proposals for reforming the NHS. The reforms took effect in 1974 under the National Health Service Act (1973). The new structure in England is shown in the diagram below.

Department of Health and Social Security (DHSS)
|
Regional Health Authorities (RHAs)
|
Area Health Authorities (AHAs)
|
District Management Teams (DMTs)
|
Community Health Councils (CHCs)
|
Department of Health Councils (CHCs)

The National Health Service in 1974

The structure in Wales was similar with the Welsh Office combining the functions of a central government department and the Regional Health Authority. In Northern Ireland there were four Health and Social Services Boards linked to the DHSS (Northern Ireland). Each board was split into several districts and was responsible for personal social services as well as health services.

The main aims of the 1974 reorganisation were:
- to unify all the health services under one authority. This was not total as General Practitioners (GPs) retained their self-employed status and some postgraduate teaching hospitals retained separate boards of governors.
- to co-ordinate health authorities (hospitals) and related local government services (social work, health visiting, etc.). For this reason many of the Area Health Authority boundaries were the same as local authority boundaries. Joint consultative committees were set up between the health authorities and local authorities in each area to discuss and plan the delivery of services.
- to improve management. A key feature was the introduction of multi-disciplinary teams (doctors, nurses, accountants, managers) and 'consensus management' (management with the agreement of all the team). It is no coincidence that the management structures borrowed ideas from the private sector as they were devised with the help of the management consultants from outside the local authority or NHS.

In 1979 the government proposed further reforms:
- to remove one management tier, thus combining the functions of District Management Teams and Area Health Authorities within a new body, the District Health Authority
- to give Family Practitioner Committees (FPCs) a level of independence as employing authorities, that is they were given responsibility for employing GPs, dentists, opticians and chemists.

The Health and Social Security Act 1984 encompassed these changes and recognised the structure that had been in place since 1982.

By 1989 the structure of the NHS was as shown in the diagram opposite.

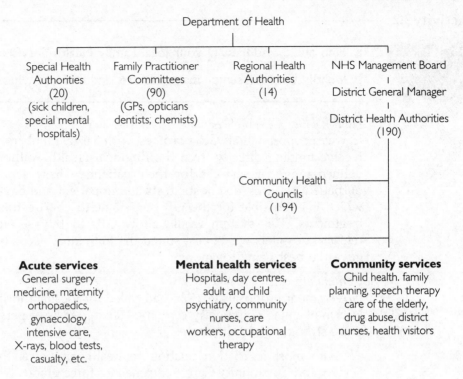

Department of Health

Special Health Authorities (20) (sick children, special mental hospitals)

Family Practitioner Committees (90) (GPs, opticians dentists, chemists)

Regional Health Authorities (14)

NHS Management Board

District General Manager

District Health Authorities (190)

Community Health Councils (194)

Acute services
General surgery medicine, maternity orthopaedics, gynaecology intensive care, X-rays, blood tests, casualty, etc.

Mental health services
Hospitals, day centres, adult and child psychiatry, community nurses, care workers, occupational therapy

Community services
Child health. family planning, speech therapy care of the elderly, drug abuse, district nurses, health visitors

The National Health Service in 1989, England and Wales

The National Health Service 1990–

The National Health and Community Care Act 1990
This Act was the result of a number of proposals put forward in 1989 in a government White Paper 'Working for Change'.

Purchasers and providers
The White Paper proposed that there should be competition between hospitals and other service providers such as Social Service Departments and GPs. It proposed that District Health Authorities (DHAs) should have the responsibility for purchasing services for patients, using funds given to them by the government, based on the population (taking into account factors such as age, sex, etc.). Hospitals would then have to contract with GPs to provide services. The aim was to make the providers of the services (hospitals) more responsive and more efficient as they would have to compete for patients. As a result money would follow patients, as the GPs would pay for services used by their patients. DHAs could in turn could purchase services (such as specialist services or beds in nursing homes) from public, private and voluntary providers.

Health care trusts
It was proposed that hospitals and other units, such as ambulance services, could opt out of health authority control and become self-governing trusts with responsibility for their own budgets.

Family Health Service Authorities
There were also proposals that the Family Practitioner Committees should become Family Health Service Authorities (FHSAs), accountable to the Regional Health Authorities rather than directly to the Ministry of Health.

Activity 3.2

a Find out the address of your local Family Health Service Authority.

b Identify who the senior managers are, and find out what their roles are.

Fund-holding GP practices

It was proposed that GP practices with large numbers of patients should receive funding directly from the Regional Health Authorities to purchase a defined range of services for their patients. These services would include outpatient services, diagnostic tests and in-patient and day-care treatments for which it is possible for the GP or patient to choose the time and place of treatments. This system would allow GPs to buy services from local and regional hospitals which best suited the individual needs of their patients and gave the best value for money.

Community care

Government proposals in 1988 had called for local authorities to be given the lead in planning community care, thus linking areas of personal social services more strongly to health issues.

As with most legislation relating to health and care, the National Health Service and Community Care Act came into force gradually. One of the earliest effects was the formation of 56 hospital trusts in April 1991, with a further 95 hospital and service trusts in 1992. In April 1991 306 fund-holding GP practices were also established. The structure of the NHS in 1991 is shown in the diagram below.

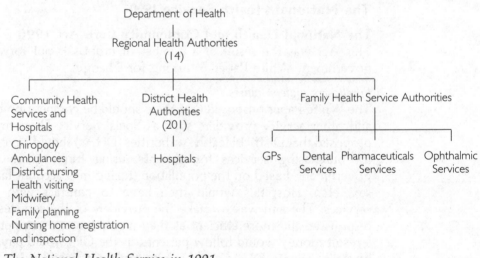

The National Health Service in 1991

Activity 3.3

a Find out who delivers health care in your locality.

b How many hospitals provide services and what type of services?

c Identify where they fit within the structure of the NHS. Are the hospitals trusts? Are the GPs fund-holders?

Hospital and specialist services

Hospitals are traditionally seen as institutions where people who are too ill to be cared for at home go for treatment on an in-patient or out-patient basis. In hospitals the medical personnel are organised into teams of doctors whose role is to diagnose, prescribe and monitor the success or otherwise of treatment. A person is normally referred to a hospital specialist by his or her GP. Many are initially seen by the specialist as an out-patient following this referral, or they may attend hospital for in-patient treatment.

The hospital medical teams are supported by personnel from other disciplines, such as radiologists, occupational therapists and physiotherapists who have specialist knowledge and skills which allow them to provide services to assist the doctor in diagnosis and treatment. This is known as a multi-disciplinary team.

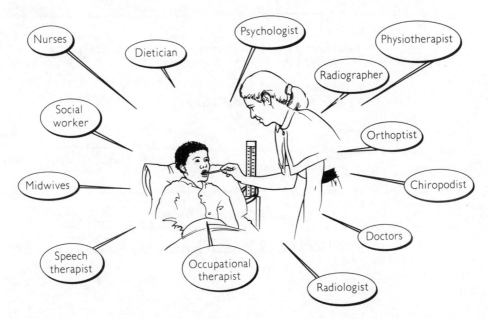

The multi-disciplinary team

Social care services

Social Services Departments (SSDs) are run by local authorities to provide community-based services available to all with a strong orientation towards the family. The main objective of a social services department is to support people in their own homes and enable them to care for themselves and their families and dependants.

The department also provides accommodation, particularly for the elderly, those suffering from disabilities and children who cannot remain in their own homes.

The Social Services Committee, established by the Local Authority and Social Services Act of 1970, has responsibilities in four areas:
- childcare under the various children's Acts and adoption Acts, including the 1989 Children Act

- provision and regulation of residential accommodation for older people and people with disabilities under the 1948 National Assistance Act and the 1984 Registered Homes Act
- welfare services for older people, people with disabilities, those who are chronically ill and statutory powers under the various mental health Acts
- power to delegate some responsibilities to other organisations (usually voluntary organisations) and to provide necessary assistance.

A typical structure of a local authority Social Services Department in England is shown in the diagram below.

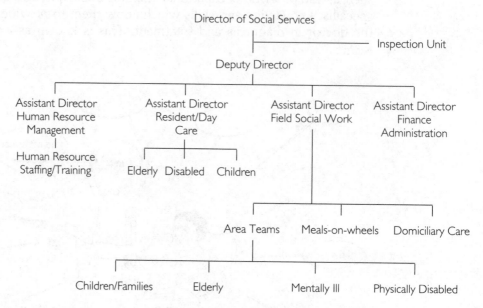

A typical structure of a Social Services Department in England

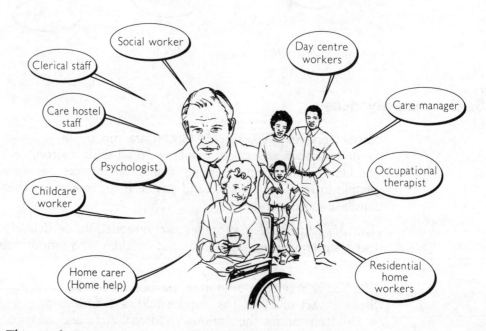

The social services team

Activity 3.4

a Obtain a copy of your local Community Care Plan. You can get this from your local SSD or library.

b Find out what the role of the SSD Inspection Unit is. Obtain from that unit a copy of their annual report and discuss its contents with your class colleagues.

Access to health and social care services

There are basically three ways that a person can be referred to the health or social care services. These are:
- self-referral
- referral through professionals
- compulsory referral.

Self-referral

This is often the first route for most people receiving health and social care. In the health service this may be by simply turning up at the GP's or dentist's surgery. The first point of contact might also be through a health visitor, for example.

Within social care, self-referral may be to a duty social worker in an local office or direct to a care facility, such as a day-care centre or a nursery.

In all cases the initiative is with the person requiring care or a friend or relative making the initial contact. An example of the latter may be a spouse of a person who is depressed seeking professional help for their partner.

Referral through a professional

Unless admitted to hospital as an accident or emergency case, the only way that a person may voluntarily receive hospital treatment is by referral from another professional, normally a GP. Where a GP diagnoses, or suspects, ill-health that requires specialist treatment, the patient is referred to an outpatient clinic or, in more urgent cases, direct admission to a ward may be arranged.

In social care, an example of referral by professionals might be when a teacher in a school suspects child abuse and refers the case to the social services duty social worker. Under the 1989 Children Act all schools should have a named person who makes this referral.

Another example might be through the police who have given a 'warning' to a child who has committed an offence and who they feel should be referred to social services.

Compulsory referral

Some people may have no choice about whether or not they are referred for support or treatment. Severely mentally ill people can be referred compulsorily under the Mental Health Act, as can children who are at risk under the various childcare legislation.

Client groups using health and social care services

How are the needs of client groups met by the health and social care services? We will look at each group in turn:
- families
- people with disabilities
- children
- elderly people.

Families and their needs

Most people understand that 'family' refers to a group of people who may be related to one another by blood and or by marriage. Everyone knows what a family is – mum, dad, brothers, sisters, grandparents. There is no doubt that families are now smaller than they used to be. The average number of children per family has dropped from 2.3 in 1970 to 1.8 in 1991.

People living alone are not considered to be a family. Between 1961 and 1992 the number of people living alone increased by nearly 300 per cent.

There was a four-fold increase in the number of one-parent families from 2.5 per cent to over 10 per cent by 1992.

One-parent families 1971–91, by sex of parent

	No. of families		
	1971	1979	1991
Female	520 000	760 000	1 200 000
Male	100 000	100 000	100 000
Total one-parent families	620 000	860 000	1 300 000

Note: The 1.3 million one-parent families in 1991 contained approximately 2.2 million dependant children.

There is a difference in the spread of one-parent families in the UK. One in 10 families in the North, West Midlands, North West and Wales consists of a lone parent with dependent children, compared to 1 in 14 in East Anglia and Northern Ireland.

All of these figures point to a decline in the number of 'traditional' families (married couple with dependant children).

Activity 3.5

List what you think are the reasons that might contribute to the difference in the number of one-parent families in the regions of the UK.

These changes are making it more difficult for the family to provide the full range of personal care required by dependent groups. The steady increase in the number of one-parent families may be due to the fact that a woman with dependant children may no longer need to stay with her husband. However, as a single parent she is likely to suffer insecurity and loss of income. The increase in one-parent families, and the disruption it brings to married life, not only adds to demands on the social care services, but it also makes it more difficult for families to provide informal care for older people and those with disabilities.

The family and the care of dependent members

An estimated 6 million adults are caring for less-capable friends and relatives at home (informal carers). Around one quarter of those 6 million spend more than 20 hours per week caring for a dependent relative, while approximately 60 per cent spend 60 hours a week doing so.

Women are more likely to be carers than men, but the difference is not very marked. Informal carers are ordinary, untrained people doing an exacting job and like ordinary people they have needs and feelings. They may need support from the social services and health services because of feelings of loneliness, isolation and inability to do heavy jobs, such as lifting or bathing.

Activity 3.6

Write down what you think the feelings of a carer with a dependent relative might be.

Did your list include any of the following:
- embarrassment at the condition or habits of the dependent person?
- embarrassment at having to carry out very personal tasks for close relatives?
- anger at lack of support from the health or social services?
- a sense of loss that the person they are caring for may seem to be a stranger to them because of the nature of their illness?
- feelings of guilt at the possibility that they themselves might need help or counselling?

Informal carers often have a sense of individual, rather then shared and collective, responsibility for their dependent relatives. Many of them suffer physical and emotional stress and ill-health themselves, because of lack of support from the statutory services. When they become ill, the person they are caring for is often left without support. One of the key objectives of the National Health Service and Community Care Act 1990 is the support of informal carers, although it remains to be seen if this occurs to any great extent.

Activity 3.7

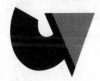

a Find out what types of support your local SSD offers to informal carers.

b List the different kinds of self-help group available in your local community to help carers in their own homes.

The family and abuse

Children are vulnerable members of society. They, like the dependent elderly, are incapable of protecting themselves from adults who may wish to abuse

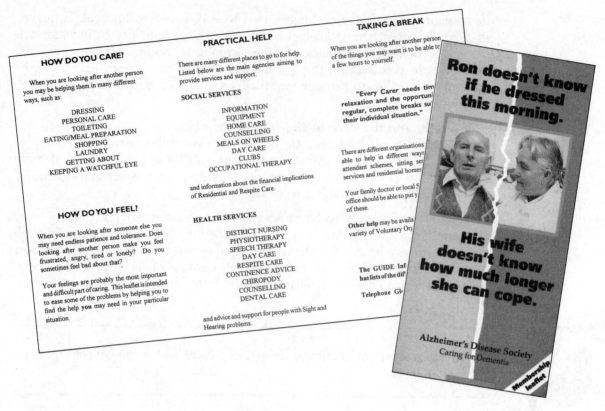

Text from the leaflet image:

HOW DO YOU CARE?

When you are looking after another person you may be helping them in many different ways, such as:

DRESSING
PERSONAL CARE
TOILETING
EATING/MEAL PREPARATION
SHOPPING
LAUNDRY
GETTING ABOUT
KEEPING A WATCHFUL EYE

HOW DO YOU FEEL?

When you are looking after someone else you may need endless patience and tolerance. Does looking after another person make you feel frustrated, angry, tired or lonely? Do you sometimes feel bad about that?

Your feelings are probably the most important and difficult part of caring. This leaflet is intended to ease some of the problems by helping you to find the help you may need in your particular situation.

PRACTICAL HELP

There are many different places to go to for help. Listed below are the main agencies aiming to provide services and support.

SOCIAL SERVICES

INFORMATION
EQUIPMENT
HOME CARE
COUNSELLING
MEALS ON WHEELS
DAY CARE
CLUBS
OCCUPATIONAL THERAPY

and information about the financial implications of Residential and Respite Care.

HEALTH SERVICES

DISTRICT NURSING
PHYSIOTHERAPY
SPEECH THERAPY
DAY CARE
RESPITE CARE
CONTINENCE ADVICE
CHIROPODY
COUNSELLING
DENTAL CARE

and advice and support for people with Sight and Hearing problems.

TAKING A BREAK

When you are looking after another person one of the things you may want is to be able to [...] a few hours to yourself.

"Every Carer needs tim[...] relaxation and the opportuni[...] regular, complete breaks su[...] their individual situation."

There are different organisations [...] able to help in different ways [...] attendant schemes, sitting ser[...] services and residential homes[...]

Your family doctor or local S[...] office should be able to put y[...] of these.

Other help may be availa[...] variety of Voluntary Org[...]

The GUIDE Inf[...] has lists of the dif[...]

Telephone Glo[...]

Ron doesn't know if he dressed this morning.

His wife doesn't know how much longer she can cope.

Alzheimer's Disease Society
Caring for Dementia

Membership leaflet

Carers need support too

them. Children and elderly people may suffer from different types of abuse:

- physical abuse when a person is physically injured
- psychological abuse when a person may be treated and spoken to in a hurtful manner, or neglected or deprived of the emotional factors necessary for a stable life
- sexual abuse of an older person or child when their body is used to gratify another's sexual desire.

All professionals working within or related to the field of child or elderly abuse, such as social workers, teachers, doctors, residential staff, have to face the great responsibility that suspected abuse brings. This creates extra stress for such staff and carers. However, social services staff have the main responsibility for the protection of children and elderly people.

Activity 3.8

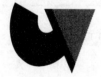

Investigate what services are available in your locality for elderly people in their own homes who have suffered physical or emotional abuse.

The needs of people with disabilities

The main legislation which enables local authorities to support people with disabilities in the community is the Chronically Sick and Disabled Persons Act 1970. For the purposes of the Act, chronically sick or disabled persons are those who are 'substantially and permanently handicapped' by illness, injury

congenital deformity or old age. The Act enables the local authority to provide:
- practical assistance in the home
- assistance in obtaining radio, telephone, TV or library services
- works or adaptations in the home
- assistance with holidays
- provision of meals at home.

What is disability?
There are so many types of disability that the term cannot be defined easily. Disabilities may be the result of:
- genetic or inherited disorders, such as muscular dystrophy, Down's syndrome
- damage at birth, such as cerebral palsy
- accidents (causing brain damage or paralysis, for example), illnesses (such as bronchitis) or disorders (such as Alzheimer's disease) that have occurred during a person's lifetime.

Disability may be either:
- physical, such as arthritis, chronic heart disease, muscular dystrophy, multiple sclerosis, blindness, deafness; or
- mental, now more usually referred to as learning difficulty in children, such as Down's syndrome or cerebral palsy, or in elderly people Alzheimer's disease.

Chronic disability
A condition which develops slowly over a long period or which lasts a long time

Acute disability
A condition which occurs suddenly, which may be severe and which may last for a relatively short time

Congenital disability
A non-hereditary condition which exists at birth

There are degrees of disability. Some people with disabilities, for example, may be able to cope and live at home, while others with the same disability may need much support and may even need residential care.

When discussing support services for people with disabilities we need to keep in mind that each person will react differently to the same disability. For this reason we must always regard each client as an individual with their own strengths and weaknesses. We must focus on their individual needs, both physical and emotional, rather than on their disability.

Value judgements
In the past and, to some extent, in the present services for people with disabilities have been developed on the basis of negative value judgements made by non-disabled people about the meaning of disability and confusion over the role of people with a disability in society. Such judgements are based on prejudice and hearsay. They focus on a person's inabilities, rather than on their abilities. People with disabilities are often seen as objects of derision,

dread, pity and as a burden on society. People with mental disabilities are often denied reasonable access to services. For example, people object to the building of hostels for such people in their community.

Chronic disabilities

Haemophilia

This is an abnormality in which there is a failure of the blood to clot following an injury because the 'clotting factor' is deficient. It is an hereditary condition usually affecting the male. Treatment is by giving the missing 'factor' by injection, either at Haemophilia Centres or in the patient's own home. Serious injury can be caused by bleeding into the joints, which may lead to the patient having to spend time in bed or in a wheelchair while their limbs recover.

Bronchitis

This can exist as an acute illness or a chronic condition. Bronchitis means inflammation of the mucous membrane of the bronchial tubes in the lungs.

Acute bronchitis often develops following exposure to cold, damp conditions or after inhaling irritating dust or vapours in the atmosphere. People experience a painful dry cough accompanied by rapid and wheezing breathing.

Chronic bronchitis is very life threatening in young children and elderly people. It is one of the most common causes of death among elderly people in the UK and occurs as a result of excessive cigarette smoking, bad housing, obesity and recurring chest infections.

Asthma

Asthma is a disorder of breathing. People who experience this illness suffer from severe paroxysms of difficult breathing followed by periods of complete relief. Attacks are in the main sudden and occur usually during the night or in the early hours of the morning. Breathing is performed with great difficulty and is accompanied by wheezing noises. The person's face becomes pale and wet with perspiration, while their arms and legs are cold.

Asthma is usually an allergic reaction to such things as pollens, animals such as cats or dogs, house dust and even certain types of foods. It is more common in males and usually starts in childhood. About one in twenty school children are estimated to suffer from asthma.

How do people react to disability?

Physical disabilities are very real to those who are suffering from them, and there is a wide range of attitudes towards them. Many view the disability as an intrusion into their lives, while others may see the disability as a challenge. This can be seen in people who take up sport for the first time after an illness. Others react in different ways. They may become defensive or want to be more independent than is possible in the circumstances of their disability. Some people with disabilities or severe illness may feel that it is a form of punishment, brought upon them by some misdeed in the past.

Defence mechanisms

People may suffer anxiety – an emotional state which involves feelings of uneasiness, fear or apprehension. We develop a number of strategies to counteract this anxiety which are called defence mechanisms. These are defences against anxiety and are always unconscious, which means that the person is not aware of them. Defence mechanisms are sometimes seen as a protection against the pain of traumatic life experiences such as a severe disability or serious illness.

The most common forms of defence mechanisms which may be used by people with a disability or illness are:

- **Repression and denial**   People may repress from their consciousness any thought of their illness or disability. Because of this they may refuse to come to terms with the change in their lives. For example they may behave as if they were not disabled or ill.
- **Regression**   This involves a return to earlier modes of functioning. The most extreme form may manifest itself by regression to childhood behaviour. For example, a previously toilet-trained child who breaks a leg may revert to incontinence.
- **Projection**   A person uses this defence mechanism when they attribute their own feelings to another person. This is the most common form of defence mechanism. It may be as 'normal' as blaming someone else for some everyday incident, such as seeing all the problems experiences by the disabled person as the shortcomings of others.
- **Sublimation**   This is also a common defence mechanism. A disabled person may may throw themselves into their work or take up some sport in order to keep their mind off a situation.

Loss

A most devastating form of stress experienced by individuals who suffer a severe disability or illness is bereavement. Bereavement is a state characterised by loss, such as the loss of limb, speech or loss of the ability to carry out some actions through illness. Grief is the individual's response to bereavement. It is a complex response which may include such 'symptoms' as fatigue, anxiety, loss of appetite, withdrawal and sleep disturbance.

The most commonly observed characteristics are of grief are shock, denial, anxiety, depression and guilt. Other symptoms include searching behaviour, suicidal thoughts, panic or heightened vulnerability to physical illness.

Stages of grief

- **Denial**   Sometimes the person with the disability will behave as if nothing has happened. They may not believe that they have the illness or disability.
- **Shock**   The second stage begins when the person begins to feel the pain of loss. Some people may cry, but others may feel anger.
- **Acceptance**   The acceptance of the situation usually happens after a short period. Once the person has accepted the reality of the situation they can begin to live their life again with the disability or illness. Most people will not return to their former level of functioning, taking into account their disability. They may move on to a new level where the pain and loss of grieving are incorporated and begin to learn new skills, cooking, looking after themselves or living on their own.

The length of time that a person may spend in each stage of grief will depend upon the circumstances of the loss, the relationship that they had with the thing or person they have lost, and the cultural and religious background of the grieving person.

Most people agree that is desirable for the bereaved to give way to grief. Grief has to be worked through. If it is not, the disabled person will continue to have troubles of some sort. The problems must be brought out into the open and confronted. The bereaved person should be helped and supported at their own pace until they begin to accept their loss.

Children and their needs

The proportion of the population under 15 years of age decreased between 1971 and the mid-1980s – in 1981 it was 1 in 5. In contrast, however, as we shall see later, the population over 65 years of age has risen considerably. This means that the total dependent population (children and elderly people) is approximately 30 per cent of the total population. As the elderly population increases, there will be more and more pressure on social care and health services and less demand for education services.

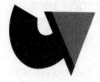

Activity 3.8

Find out how many schools have closed or amalgamated in your area as a result of the downward trend in the school population.

Children with learning difficulties

Until recently, children with learning difficulties used to be termed mentally handicapped. Many factors can cause mental disability. For example, chromosomal defects may cause Down's syndrome, while other factors, such as infections or injury, may cause brain damage.

Cerebral palsy

Severely brain-damaged children may also suffer from cerebral palsy, or spastic paralysis. This is a non-progressive disorder of the brain which impairs motor function. The regions of the brain which control movement and muscle tension are affected. It produces spasticity (or stiffness), floppiness, weakness, involuntary movements or unsteadiness. Children who suffer from cerebral palsy find it difficult to demonstrate their intellectual powers and many such children may in the past have been misdiagnosed as mentally handicapped.

It is important for families to be encouraged to help such children develop their intellectual skills by providing them with a stimulating environment and opportunities to learn, though their ability to move is limited. Children with cerebral palsy may have problems with communicating. Electronic communication systems using voice synthesisers and computers have opened up a whole range of opportunities for people with speech difficulties to communicate.

Deafness

Deafness occurs more commonly among handicapped children than in children without such a problem. Deafness may exaggerate the degree of learning disability, hence the importance of a full assessment of the child's needs and capabilities. The most frequent cause of deafness is nerve deafness caused by brain damage that also caused the mental handicap. In many cases, the child will have missed out on a great deal of speech experience because of their inadequate hearing.

Blindness

This is another disorder which is common among children with mental disabilities. The diagnosis of visual handicap is frequently suspected by the parents at an early stage in the child's life.

Epilepsy

Epilepsy is probably the most common associated disorder that occurs in children with mental disabilities. It can be a major setback in the child's progress. A major fit is very frightening thing for a parent to see. In fact children rarely come to harm during a fit, and attacks look much worse than they really are.

Hydrocephalus and spina bifida

Hydrocephalus (fluid on the brain) and spina bifida (split spine) are not on their own causes of mental disability.

Spina bifida is a congenital abnormality caused by the arches of one of the vertebrae not fusing together so that the spine is split in two. The spinal cord may protrude through this gap. The symptoms of spina bifida may include paralysis of the legs, incontinence and mental disability as a result of hydrocephalus with is commonly associated with spina bifida. Children with spina bifida are very prone to urinary infections which may cause unexpected apathy, vomiting and fever.

Hydrocephalus may occur on its own or in association with spina bifida. It may be present at birth or develop later. In early life the main symptom is an enlarged head. When it occurs in older children and adults, it causes headaches, vomiting, fits or progressive paralysis. Hydrocephalus may be treated.

Many people with hydrocephalus and/or spina bifida have a shortened life span. A few live on into adulthood where the additional problems of increasing weight heighten the risk of bed sores.

The needs of elderly people

Social and medical advances have meant that many more people are living longer. A man born in 1901 could expect to live for an average of 45 years and a woman for nearly 50 years. It is estimated that by the year 2001, a woman born in that year can expect to live for 80 years and a man for 75 years. Life expectancy is currently increasing by about two years every decade. The average child born in 1994 will live about 25 years longer than a child born in 1901.

Population over retirement age, 1900–81

	Percentage of total population
1900	4.7
1911	6.8
1931	9.6
1951	13.6
1971	16.0
1981	17.9

As more people are living longer they become dependent on others for help for longer periods than in the past. The total number of older people over 65 years of age has risen from 2 879 000 in 1911 to 9 711 00 by 1981, with approximately twice as many women in this group as men. The number of the elderly will continue to increase over the next few decades – an increase which will add considerably to the pressures on the health and social care services.

The profile of the elderly population is also changing. The most significant change is the increase in the number of the 'old' old — those aged 75 and over, many of whom are over 85 years of age. In 1975 the number of people over 85 years of age was 515 000. By 2001 this number is expected to rise to 752 000, a 46 per cent increase. Women outnumber men by 3 to 1 in this age group. Of all the women aged between 75 and 84 in 1976, 53 per cent lived alone and of those over 85, nearly 50 per cent lived alone.

The question that managers of health and social care services have to answer is how to meet the needs of people living so long, and the increasing numbers needing increasing levels of support. Current levels of health and social services care to elderly people in their own homes are not sufficient to be a reliable alternative to residential care. What emerges from all the research on provision of support services to elderly people is the importance of the family in the provision of care.

Elderly people and disability

The dramatic increase in life expectancy, and the reduction in mortality rates, would seem to reflect improved medical, social and environmental standards. However, there has also been a growth in physical and mental illness of the elderly, particularly those in the older age groups.

Seventy-five years can be regarded as the point at which many of the problems of dependency associated with ageing become apparent. Many people in the 65–74 age group are not much more dependent than the those in their fifties and early sixties. They have the same hobbies, interests and contacts. However, by the time most elderly people reach 85 years they show a decline in mobility, health and ability to perform personal and domestic tasks. Many elderly people are unable to bath or get into or out of bed unaided.

In 1971 over half of all those over 65 years of age were found to be significantly disabled, with many living alone. The living status of the elderly varies according to the severity of their disability. About 25 per cent need some one to help them with daily living activities, such as feeding, assistance using the toilet, getting into or out of bed, or severe mobility problems. Many old people live alone or with their partner only, many see no relatives or friends for long periods. Those in the 'old' old category are more likely to need domiciliary care from home helps and other services such as meals-on-wheels and chiropody. They also need regular support form the health visitor and social workers. Many are also likely to need hospitalisation for periods of time.

Activity 3.9 ───────────────────────────────────────

Identify as many problems as you can that you think an elderly person might face.

───────────────────────────────────────

Did your list include any of the following?
- rehabilitation/getting better after an illness — even the simplest illness may assume a great importance for an elderly person

- mental deterioration
- loneliness
- accidents and falls
- rheumatism/arthritis
- foot defects – 50 per cent of elderly people have some foot problems, such as ingrown toenails, corns, bunions
- hypothermia
- cardiovascular disease
- hearing loss
- visual defects
- nutrition problems
- bronchitis
- prostate problems.

Loss, disability or illness can occur at any age. However we are only now beginning to appreciate the effect of loss in old age. Many people remain remarkably fit into extreme old age and stay strong and mentally agile. However, there are many losses that affect the elderly including:

- loss of status and defined role
- loss of income
- loss of bodily function
- loss of health
- loss of sexual function
- loss of company, for example the death of a spouse, friends or pets
- loss of independence and home by admission to residential care or hospital.

People of all ages become ill, but when an elderly person falls ill they may suffer from a number of different illnesses at the same time. Older people take longer to recover from illness and are more likely to have an accident in the home. Approximately 70 per cent of home accidents happen to pensioners. When a mother or her children are ill, the family is usually there to help, but this is not always so for an elderly person. The number of visits to people aged 65 and over by home nurses and health visitors has increased significantly since 1971. The number supported by home helps has risen the most sharply.

Elderly people and poverty
The prevalence of poverty among elderly people would indicate that many of them rely on the state health and care services for assistance with daily living.

The association between old age and poverty is well established. The over 65s are the largest group claiming supplementary benefits. About one tenth of the retired population live below the poverty line. Around 1500 people retire every day and their pension should pay for comfortable housing, adequate food, fuel and lighting and a good supply of warm clothes. More and more elderly people have only the state pension and other benefits to live on. Nearly half of all benefits paid in 1992–3 was accounted for by payments to this group.

Activity 3.10

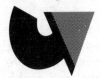

a Visit some elderly people who are living in their own homes. Discuss with them what they spend their income on.

b Make a list and compare the items on the list with what you think a family with children might spend their income on.

Common illnesses of old age

Rheumatism
This is a general term applied to a number of diseases which cause inflammation of joints and muscles. Usually the inflammation is in the joints such as hips, fingers, wrists, knee or ankle joints.

Rheumatoid arthritis is one of the most crippling of all the rheumatic diseases. It usually begins after the age of 40. The onset of the disease is gradual, with pain, swelling and redness of the affected joints. It tends to be chronic and as it is not a fatal disease it is one that many older people suffer from.

Osteoporosis

Osteoporosis is loss of bone substance due to a lack of calcium in the bones, leading to porousness of the main bones. It occurs naturally as part of the ageing process, but there are two severe forms. One form is seen in women at the time of the menopause. The other is senile osteoporosis which affects elderly people of both sexes. It may lead to fractures, particularly of the hips, and possible disability. It is also likely to be caused by prolonged periods in bed or a wheelchair. This is one of the reasons why older people should be encouraged to be as active as possible and also take an adequate amount of calcium, in milk for example.

Support for people who use health and care services

Every person has access to health and social care services but many may not know of their rights because they cannot read or speak English.

Most health and social care organisations have published pamphlets and leaflets describing their services and how people can use them. These sources of information are often published in languages other than English, such as Chinese and Gujerati. Many hospitals have appointed workers to act for patients and take up any complaints they may have. They also provide translators to help clients whose first language is not English.

Many organisations are dedicated to supporting clients in receiving adequate services. For example, MENCAP provides help, support and advice for those with learning difficulties, while the MS Society does the same for those suffering from multiple sclerosis. Sources of help and support can also be obtained from a Citizen's Advice Bureau, local council advice officers and the local Community Health Council.

The Patient's Charter

The Patient's Charter was introduced in 1992 setting out standards that a patient should expect of the NHS. The charter refers to the 'rights' of patients, but these 'rights' or standards are not guaranteed by law. In fact, the charter points out that they are 'not legal rights but major and specific standards which government looks to the NHS to achieve, as circumstances and resources allow'.

One of the new rights is for a patient's complaints to be investigated. The Department of Health says that complaints have risen by at least 35 per cent. However, many Community Health Councils have stated that complaints more than doubled in 1993. Much of the information given by hospital and health authorities has not been found to be user-friendly and is often only provided on request. Many agree that the charter has made people feel good about complaining.

Existing standards specify the following:
● respect for privacy, dignity and religious and cultural beliefs
● availability of services to all including people with special needs

- provision of information to relatives and friends of patients
- waiting time for ambulances (14 minutes in urban areas, 19 minutes in rural areas)
- waiting time for assessment in Accident and Emergency departments
- waiting time in out-patient departments
- what happens when an operation is cancelled
- a named member of nursing staff to be responsible for each patient.

The roles of health and social care workers

Social workers

Social care can be divided into:
- community care
- residential care.

Working in both areas are qualified social workers who have obtained a qualification covering all areas of social work, although they may specialise in one area later. The qualification most of them have is the Certificate of Qualification in Social Work (CQSW). However, recent changes to training have involved the development of a new Diploma in Social Work (DipSW) replacing both the CQSW and the Certificate in Social Service (CSS). This latter was a professional qualification which was undertaken mainly by residential and day care staff.

Field social workers provide support to all types of clients, individuals and families, both in the community or in hospitals (hospital social workers). The social worker provides social rehabilitation and community services, specialising in childcare work, helping elderly people or working with people suffering from mental illness.

The role of the social worker to assess a client's and carer's needs and to organise, with other professionals, services to meet those individual needs. Social workers have access to a wide range of services which they can offer clients.

Key worker	Key client groups
Social worker	All client groups

Activity 3.11

Mr Jones is 85 years old and lives alone. He has just had a bad fall and has broken his right arm.

a List the SSD practitioners that might offer support to Mr Jones.

b Discuss what services that these practitioners could offer him to allow him to stay in his own home.

You may need to do some further research on your own to complete this activity.

Home care assistants

A number of home care staff provide emotional, social and practical support to clients living in their own homes in the community. Local authorities have a duty (this means they must provide this service) to provide home helps (now called home care assistants or home carers).

Working mostly with older people they carry out such tasks as simple cleaning, lighting fires, shopping, cooking and basic personal tasks. They also write letters and provide social support. Most of their work is concerned with supporting elderly people but they do also work with people with physical disabilities and families with young children.

Key worker	Key client groups
Home care assistant	Older people and people with disabilities

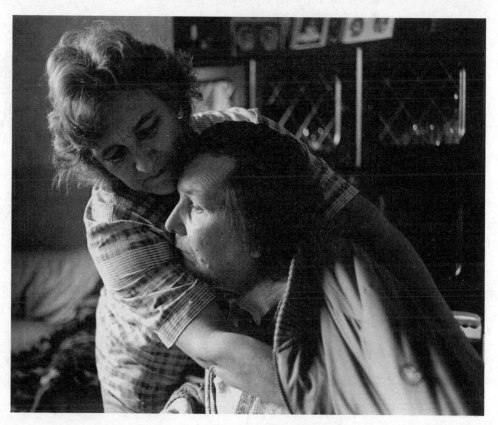

A home care assistant

Meals-on-wheels staff

This service is becoming increasingly important as more and more elderly dependent people choose to live in their own homes. About 33 million meals are provided every year to people in their own homes in England. This service is provided by the local authority in many areas, but it is still also offered by voluntary agencies such as the Women's Royal Voluntary Service or the Women's Institute in rural areas.

Meals-on-wheels is one of the most important forms of community support for elderly people in their own homes. It makes a contribution to their nutritional needs and is often the only social contact that an elderly person has during the week. The service can also improve the moral of elderly people. As the elderly are most susceptible to hypothermia, the daily visit of meals-on-wheels staff can provide a check that all is well.

Key worker	Key client groups
Meals-on-wheels staff	Older people

Activity 3.12

a Find out who runs the meals-on-wheels service in your locality.

b Arrange to interview the organiser. Find out the kinds of client that the service supports and the types of meal delivered.

Hospital doctors

In hospitals patients are looked after by teams of doctors, who specialise in particular areas, such as paediatrics (children), obstetrics (childbirth), geriatrics (elderly people). The role of the doctors is to:
- diagnose – find out what is wrong with the patient
- prescribe – decide on the treatment to help the patient
- monitor – review the condition of the patient and change the treatment if necessary.

Patients are usually referred to hospital doctors by their GPs.

Hospital doctors are supported by other professionals, such as nurses, physiotherapists, social workers – the multi-disciplinary team (see page 105). The senior doctors in the team may be referred to as specialists or consultants.

Key worker	Key client groups
Hospital doctor	All client groups

Hospital nurses

Most nurses are to be found working in hospitals alongside doctors. There are two levels of personnel in the nursing team currently employed in the NHS, Registered General Nurses (RGNs) and Health Care Assistants (HCAs) who support the RGNs. There are still many State Enrolled Nurses, but initial training has ended and so in future all nurses will be at RGN level.

Key worker	Key client groups
Hospital nurse	All client groups

General practitioner

Most people select their own general practitioner (GP) when they are over 16 years old, from the list of GPs kept by the Family Health Service Authority. It has now become very common for several GPs to work together in group practices. Within the group practice are GPs, receptionists, administrative staff, and probably a practice nurse and a social worker employed by the practice. Health visitors may also be based in GP practices.

A number of GP practices (those with over 7000 patients) are now fund-holders and over one third of all patients are registered with such schemes. Fund-holders can spend their money on:
- types of patient care (mainly no-emergency surgery and all out-patient care)
- drugs
- practice staff
- community services, such as district nurses.

Key worker	Key client groups
GP	All client groups

Practice nurses

The practice nurse is usually employed directly by a GP practice, where most of their work is carried out. The practice nurse carries out such routine tasks as dressings, urine tests, and injections. The practice nurse may run 'well woman' and 'well man' clinics and may also offer a counselling service to patients and relatives. At present there are approximately 4000 practice nurses employed.

Key worker	Key client groups
Practice nurse	All client groups

District nurses

District Health Authorities have a responsibility to provide nurses to assist with treatment in a patient's home. There are approximately 20 000 district nurses currently employed, providing support and nursing care for acute and chronic patients of all ages, but predominately for elderly people in their own homes. They also provide the link between hospitals and the primary health care team by referring patients to other carers and services.

Key worker	Key client groups
District nurse	Older people

Health visitors

There are about 13 000 practising health visitors in England, Wales and Scotland. The health visitor is a Registered General Nurse with post-graduate training and the Health Visitor's Certificate. The role of the health visitor is in the area of health education, prevention of illness and promotion of health in antenatal classes, health clinics, monitoring the development of children and with patients in their own homes. The health visitor also has a large part to play in the community care of the elderly.

Key worker	Key client groups
Health visitor	Children and older people

Midwives

Midwives are independent, professional nurses in their own right. They are responsible for supervising antenatal and postnatal care of all women whether they have their baby in hospital or in their own homes. They look after the mother and baby for ten days after birth. They may be based in the community or in a hospital. There are approximately 5000 midwives working in the community.

Key worker	Key client groups
Midwife	Expectant mothers, and mother and baby for 10 days after birth

School nurse

The school nurse promotes positive attitudes to health within the education system. She gives advice on health matters to school staff and looks after the children, carrying out screening checks and giving advice about such matters as immunisation.

Key worker	Key client groups
School nurse	School children

Community psychiatric nurses

Community psychiatric nurses (CPNs) and the community-based mental handicap nurses (RNMHs) provide continuing care and support for people who may have been receiving long-term hospital care and who are now returned to living in the community. The practical interface between health and social care is through social workers and community-based nurses.

Key worker	Key client groups
Community psychiatric nurse	People who suffer from psychiatric or learning disabilities

While the main, face-to-face delivery of care is from nurses and doctors there is a large range of professions allied to medicine.

Radiographers

Diagnostic radiographers use X-rays and ultrasound to visualise internal organs to check for abnormalities. *Therapeutic radiographers* use ionising radiation (such as X-rays and gamma rays) to destroy tissues and help the patient. In particular such treatments are used on a wide range of cancers.

In both cases the radiographer works as a technician, instructed by a *radiologist*. The radiologist is a specialist doctor who, for example, interprets X-ray pictures and produces reports for the doctor requesting the X-ray.

Key worker	Key client groups
Radiologist	All client groups
Radiographer	

Physiotherapists

Physiotherapists have an important role in mobility of patients using supportive and manipulative exercises to develop muscles for movement. Physiotherapists improve the health and function of clients through simple corrective exercises. They often use equipment such as infra-red and ultrasound machines. They work in co-operation with doctors in planning the physiotherapy programmes. There are now approximately 9500 physiotherapists working in the NHS. A number work in private practice.

Key worker	Key client groups
Physiotherapist	Clients needing rehabilitation for physical injuries

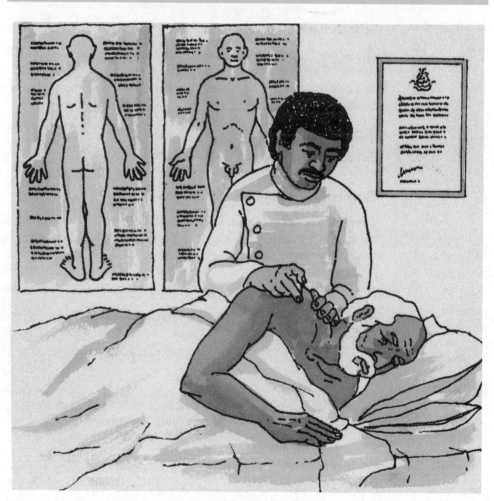

A physiotherapist at work

Occupational therapists

Over 4500 occupational therapists (OTs) work in the NHS to treat illness, both mental and physical, with activity. A large part of their work is with clients or patients suffering from a physical or learning difficulty. They work on a one-to-one basis, with groups and with recreational activities, the aim been to rehabilitate the client and teach them basic living skills. Many OTs work in the community and in Social Service Departments offering advice on aids and adaptations to daily living.

Key worker	Key client groups
Occupational therapist	People with physical or learning disabilities

Speech therapists

Speech therapists help people with speech disorders. These range from children with delayed speech development to older people recovering from strokes. Most of their work is with children.

Key worker	Key client groups
Speech therapist	Older people and children

Chiropodists

Chiropodists work with all client groups dealing with such complaints as corns, ingrown toe nails and hammer toes. Most of the work of the NHS chiropodist is with elderly people.

Key worker	Key client groups
Chiropodist	Older people

Specialist support workers with children

The Children Act 1989 imposed duties on local authorities to provide day-care for children in need under 5 years of age. Day nurseries for children between 6 months and 5 years old are staffed by workers with qualifications in childcare. The special skills required for this type of care are recognised. Nursery nurses have either National Nursery Examinations Board (NNEB) qualifications or BTEC National Diploma or Certificate in Caring Services (Nursery Nursing). There may also have the newly developed NVQ qualifications in Child Care and Education.

National Vocational Qualifications (NVQs) in Health and Social Care

In recent years the UK government has encouraged a new form of training, National Vocational Qualifications (NVQs). At the moment, these new qualifications in health and social care mainly affect those working in the hospital, residential, day or home care fields. NVQs rely on the candidates demonstrating that they are competent to do the job for which they are being assessed. Thus in many areas of social care which were traditionally staffed with untrained, unqualified staff there are now qualifications and recognition of the skills of the work force.

Review questions

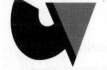

1 What is meant by the term 'GP fund-holder'?

2 How many different ways are there for a client to be referred for support?

3 What were the three main aims of the 1974 health services reorganisation?

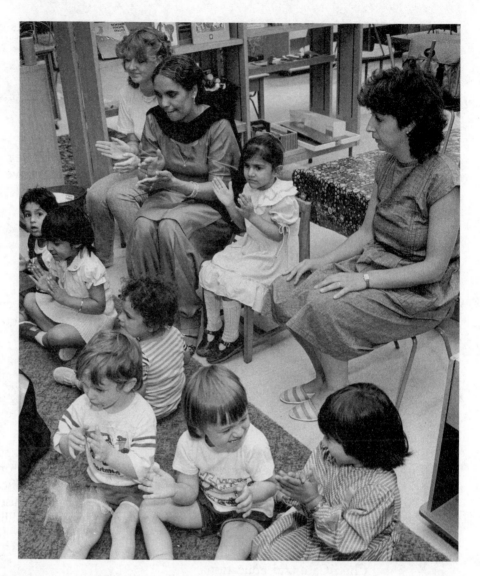

Day nurseries for children between 6 months and 5 years are staffed by workers with qualifications in childcare

4 What was the new name given to Family Practitioner Committees under the National Health and Community Care Act 1990?

5 How do the roles of a hospital nurse and a practice nurse differ?

6 How does an individual choose a GP?

7 What are the four main responsibilities of the Social Services Committee?

8 What are the main responsibilities of a local authority social worker?

9 What is a health care trust?

10 What kind of people are likely to ask for the services of a health visitor?

Assignment A3.1
The provision of health and social care services

You have been asked to write a report for a group of students from overseas on the health and social care services available in the UK. Your report should cover the following specific areas that the students wish to know about:

- an explanation of the organisation of the statutory health and social care services – illustrate your report with organisation charts which will help understanding of the roles of the various organisations
- a description of two services provided by the voluntary sector and two services provided by the private sector
- a description of the different forms of health and social care support provided by informal carers for children with disabilities and elderly dependent people living in their own homes – give a number of examples of support for each of these client groups
- a broad explanation of how the non-statutory and independent health and social care services are funded.

Assignment A3.2
How the needs of different client groups are met

You have been asked to carry out a survey of the needs of three different client groups and show how the services provided meet these needs.

1 Arrange to interview:
   - one elderly person who has used a social care service
   - one person who has used a service provided by the NHS such as a GP, hospital or community nursing service
   - one other person who has used any health or social care service.
   During the interviews you should find out:
   - what difficulties each person had which necessitated their need for the service
   - how they were referred to the service they are now receiving. Was it a self-referral, referral by a professional or by others, or a referral by an emergency service?
   - how the service is meeting, or did meet, their needs
   - how much information they were given about the service
   - how much they knew about how to access the service
   - whether each of them knows about their rights within the service
   - whether they had access to translators, if English is not their first language.

2 Summarise the results of your survey as a short report. Identify the needs of the clients and how they have been met by the services provided for them.

Assignment A3.3
Jobs in health and social care

You have been asked to write a report on the main jobs available in the health and social care services. This should include a profile of three people, one from each of the following three areas:

- support services
- a health and medical care team
- social care.

1 List the main jobs in health and social care under the heading, 'Provision of care'.

2 List the main jobs in the support services of health and social care. (Support services include clinical and technical support, laboratory services, catering services and portering services, for example.)

3 Write a profile of each of the following three workers:
   a a home help
   b a hospital nurse
   c a hospital manager.
   These profiles should include:
   - a description of the day-to-day work
   - a description of the career route for each worker up to the time when you interviewed them
   - a comparison of what they actually do for clients with stereotypes of their roles.

CHAPTER 4

Communication and interpersonal relationships in health and social care

Element 4.1: Develop communication skills

Element 4.2: Explore how interpersonal relationships may be affected by discriminatory behaviour

Element 4.3: Investigate aspects of working with clients in health and social care

What is covered in this chapter

- The importance of communication
- The development of communication skills
- Communication skills in group situations
- The effect of discriminatory behaviour on relationships
- Working with clients in health and social care

These are the resources you will need for your Communication and Interpersonal Relationships in Health and Social Care file:

- notes about opportunities you have taken on work placement to talk to people
- your written answers to the activities in this chapter
- your written answers to the review questions at the end of this chapter
- your completed Assignment A4.1.

Introduction

One of the most probable reasons why you chose to do the GNVQ in Health and Social Care is that you are interested in people. You may be the sort of person friends contact to talk over problems. You may have appreciated someone else listening to you to help you out. Your interest in people and in helping is a great advantage in social care situations when you may be expected to give clients support.

You will probably be part of a team helping to provide this support, but your part is as important as that of anyone else. You may be able to think of examples when you have been in hospital or in a strange situation yourself and you have been glad of someone's warmth and friendliness towards you. That person may not have been the most highly paid or the most powerful in the establishment but they were of enormous significance *to you*.

What are the best ways of supporting people? How can good communication affect you and your relationships? Such questions are answered in this chapter.

Just as people have physical needs, such as the need for food, sleep and warmth and it is necessary to satisfy these needs, they also have emotional needs — the need to be liked, to be loved, to be wanted and respected or to be thought special.

Often physical needs are direct, easy to see and in many cases easy to satisfy. The emotional needs, however, are more tricky to see and satisfy. And perhaps because they are less obvious and more difficult, carers can become preoccupied with physical tasks and fail to pick up on emotional needs. So try not to fall into the trap of providing physical care only. People have feeling, and feelings matter.

It can be considered a privilege if someone relates to you sufficiently well to 'open-up' and talk to you. Their trust in you should not be taken lightly. You may need to refer to someone more senior than yourself for help, but you should never use the person as a conversation point within the establishment or outside.

Be worthy of the trust you have gained from your client. Be discreet but seek help when necessary — either for the client or for yourself, if you feel burdened by what has been said.

The importance of communication

The fact that it is extremely difficult *not* to communicate shows how important communication is. At a fun level, see how long you can manage without communication! On a more serious note, think how hard it is for those in solitary confinement. Our instinct is to communicate with others because relationships hinge on communication, and without relationships living would be mere existence. The word 'communicate' means share and it is a natural, fundamental part of our lives to be social.

We tend to think of communication as speaking, but there are many ways to impart meaning or messages to others. It isn't just what we say that creates impressions, but also how we express the words, what we wear, how we stand, look, behave, listen and respond. Sometimes we may give messages we don't intend.

Individuals and communication

We all know how satisfying relationships can be and also how damaging. Some people can become lonely, unhappy and even mentally ill because they are unable, sometimes through no fault of their own, to establish and maintain social relationships. So one reason why it is important to communicate is that communication is part of a basic drive for us to form relationships.

As we form relationships we are actually affirming and presenting some aspect of ourselves. It is through relationships, and therefore through communication, that we expresss who we are, what we think, feel, know and want. Part of the process of expressing these things actually helps us to identify them. Sometimes it is difficult to know what we think, feel or want; when we can express it, then we know. Try the following activity — you may need some time to prepare for it.

Activity 4.1

Within your group let each person try to express their responses using the following prompts:

- Politically I . . .
- In terms of close relationships I . . .
- I believe . . .
- I am . . .

Communication is necessary to develop self and confirm what we are. On a practical level it helps us to cope with the demands of every day. Danger signs, warnings, notices of information for work and pleasure all form part of the significance of communication. Most of our learning, knowledge and, therefore, control is communicated to us. Education is based on communication.

On an emotional level expressions of affection, pleasure, anger, disappointment define, and often relieve, the intensity of the emotion. To talk about feelings helps us and those we support to come to terms with them. Children and adults who can't express emotion for whatever reason may experience great frustration and look for other ways to vent their feelings.

Communication is important at an individual level because it helps us to:
- live our lives practically
- develop psychologically and intellectually
- express ourselves emotionally
- form relationships socially.

Activity 4.2

a Make a note of people who may have communication difficulties (think about sensory disabilities, mental health and social or relationship problems).

b Brainstorm how the communication barrier may affect the individual:
- practically, during their everyday lives
- educationally – at school
- emotionally – in terms of their feelings
- socially – in terms of relationships with others.

Families and communication

What was your first word? No doubt it was related in some way to those close to you. We form our first set of relationships with our families and these form our first communication patterns. If family members don't communicate with a baby, or communicate in negative ways, this will have an adverse effect on the child and influence how he or she forms relationships with other people.

Communication is a fundamental part of early development and care. Parents or people who are important to us help us to become members of society. They give us a pattern to live to. This is a very gradual, subtle process called **socialisation** (see page 75) and communication is central to the socialisation process.

As we grow our patterns of communication or interaction in families change. Children become less reliant on family members. They have communication with other 'agencies' such as school, friendship groups, media and eventually work.

Sometimes it is difficult for family members to steer a communication path through to each other because of conflicting demands.

Sometimes family members don't realise that individuals have passed through particular stages of development.

Sometimes families just don't communicate.

In most cases, communication breakdowns are resolved by an argument or, in more civil households, by a talk and a family outing or meal. For some families, however, poor communication may lead to tensions which are too set or entrenched to resolve in an obvious way. Individuals may need to change and find it difficult or impossible to alter. Sometimes there are individuals outside the immediate family who create conflict. Sometimes family members may find refuge or happiness in friendships outside the family as in the case of husband and wife. This may in time push the actual family towards a split. Counsellors and family therapists may be involved to try to help individuals communicate with each other.

So communication is important in families because:
- it is an essential part of the care, development and socialisation process
- it affects an individual's capacity to communicate with others
- it may help to resolve family tensions
- it helps us as individuals in our own school or work lives if we have a sound base at home where we can communicate.

Activity 4.3

Just think this activity through – it is a personal exercise and therefore may be difficult to commit to paper.

Think about your own family . . .
- How open or closed are the channels of communication?
- Are there individuals who close the channels of communication more than others – who withdraw or argue or storm off?
- Do the individuals in your family mainly 'do their own thing', or are there times when you all get together to do 'family things' and talk?
- Do you notice any difference in the family atmosphere and relations at particular times, such as holidays, Christmas, Friday evening, Monday morning?
- Are there changes you would like to make in your family patterns or habits?
- Are there changes you would like to make personally in respect of your family?
- How would you like other family members to change?

Communication in groups

Many of the reasons why communication is important for individuals and families apply equally to groups. Think about the groups you belong to socially, in school or college, and work or work experience. It is important to communicate in these groups because you need to express your point of view or how you feel. Other group members formulate judgements about you based on your communication in the group. Sometimes it is necessary to communicate supportive comments in groups if the group members are insecure. Initially groups may need to 'warm up' and get to know one another – communication is important for this. If the group has a specific task to achieve, good communication is vital to the attainment of the goal.

The development of communication skills

There are a number of skills that will help you to communicate effectively with other people:

- taking opportunities to start conversations
- observing
- listening actively and reflectively
- showing empathy
- knowing when to keep quiet
- knowing how to 'read' and use non-verbal communication, such as facial expressions, use of eye contact and posture
- knowing how to ask questions.
- respecting people as individuals.

Take opportunities

Your confidence will grow as you gain more experience. Sometimes it is difficult when you first arrive at a placement to introduce yourself, to take the initiative to talk to someone, to sit down in a staff room, to ask where something is or check out something you don't understand.

A first step to relating to individuals is to remember their names. Listening to what they say and using this to help your conversation the next time you meet makes for positive interaction.

You may develop ways of remembering names. On placement you may see names on rooms or in school registers that you can memorise.

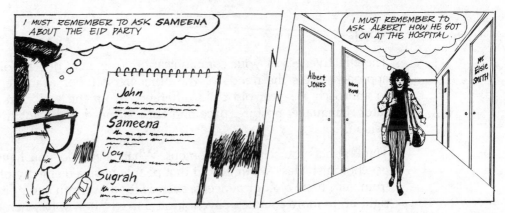

You may develop ways of remembering names

Activity 4.4

Role-play the following situations. Organise a small group to be your 'supporting cast'.

a Your first visit to a home for elderly people where you are going to work for a placement exercise.

b Lunch time in an infant school. You are sitting next to the headteacher.

c You are working on a craft activity with a small group of 6-year-olds.

d You are accompanying a teacher and a small group of disabled children around the age of 7 on a visit to a farm.

e You are working in a playgroup and one group of children is baking some biscuits.

After each role play, stop and discuss the exercise within your group. Were the conversation topics realistic? Did the conversation falter or dry up? Do you need to think more about your language?

Write a brief record of the activity as evidence for your file. Note down where you need to improve.

Activity 4.5

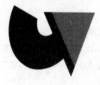

Make sure you note down in your placement record or somewhere in your portfolio the opportunities you have taken to begin conversations and keep them going. Note any improvements that you could make.

Record these improvements as you make them. Record also what you felt about the conversations or interactions you had. Keep this as evidence for your portfolio of relating to a person who is of a different status to you.

Ask your placement supervisor to comment on any interaction you have had with a client as further evidence.

Needs

The effectiveness of your communication skills may depend on how far your approach meets the **needs** of the other person. For example, you will have to approach a 3-year-old child differently from the way you approach your tutor. Language, posture, pace and tone all need to be adapted to the other person.

Think about yourself for a moment. What needs do you have? In 1954 the psychologist Maslow suggested that people have a hierarchy of needs starting from very basic biological needs, such as food, warmth and going to the toilet, right up to more complex psychological needs. It is only when the basic needs have been met that it is possible to work on fulfilling other needs.

Activity 4.6

Look at the diagram below and try to think of an example for each stage of need.

In what ways might people's age and background affect their needs?

Find out more about needs in Chapter 6.

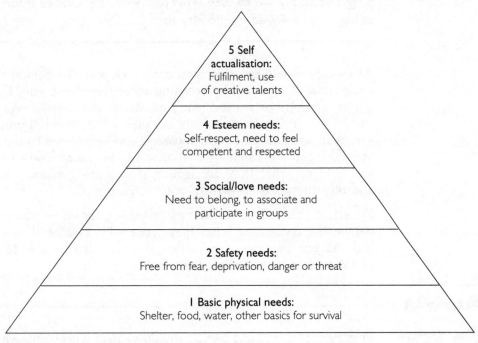

Maslow's hierarchy of needs

Observation

While in placement situations it is useful to take the opportunity to observe how other workers interact with people and learn from them. Really there is hardly a minute which cannot be used to gain some knowledge.

Use your observation skills also to help you to respond effectively to people:
- Is the person happy, sad, dejected?
- What is the person's attitude to other people and to his or her surroundings?
- Is the person anxious or tense?
- Can the person see?
- Can the person hear?
- Can the person talk or is signing used?

Listening

Listen actively. Get ready to listen. Make the shift from speaker to listener a complete one.

You must really focus in and try to remember what the person has said. A good listener hears the *content* of what the speaker says and the *intent* – what the person means.

Activity 4.7

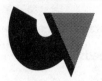

In pairs, allow one person to talk about a topic of his or her own choice for 3 minutes. The partner must listen actively and then report back to the main group what the other has said. Use a different topic to do the exercise the other way round.

Suggestions: My life to date, This past year, My kind of music, I enjoy doing . . . , I enjoyed my holiday in . . .

At an appropriate moment, you can check with the person whether you have understood everything by recalling what they have said. Don't interrupt the person abruptly or ask too many questions otherwise it will be frustrating for the person trying to talk. This is called **reflective listening**. This reassures you that you have the right message and underlines to the other person the fact that you are listening. He or she is far more likely to open up to you and tell you what they are feeling if you are genuinely interested in them and this interest is shown by your reactions.

Reflective listening is sometimes called 'mirroring' − you mirror back to the person the content of what they have said. You need to concentrate to do this. As you become more skilled you will also be able to match the mood of the person by reflecting their feelings.

Activity 4.8

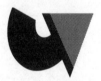

In groups of three, one person should explain a problem, while one person listens and reflects by facial expression what the first person is feeling. The third person observes to see how accurately the listener is reflecting the feeling and writes a brief report for evidence.

Take it in turns to be the speaker, the listener and the observer.

A key to understanding emotions is to describe them! It can be helpful to suggest a particular word to the person which may describe their feelings. This means building up your language skills. Sometimes you need to put what has been said into your own words.

Activity 4.9

List as many words you can think of which describe the following emotions:

happiness   depression
anger   inferiority
shyness   irritation
grief   fear
anxiety

Be on the look out, in your reading and viewing, for new adjectives to describe emotions. Keep the list as evidence for your portfolio.

Activity 4.10

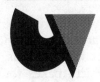

In small groups, think of some responses which might be made to the following people:

a a friend who has had her purse, containing £30, stolen

b a teenager who had just failed her driving test

c a young man who has just been rejected for nurse training

d a mother whose child has been seriously injured in a road accident.

Record the activity for your portfolio. Include a note of points you need to improve on. Ask others in the group to comment on your responses.

Empathy

As you listen actively and try to reflect back to the person their feelings and what they say, you will gradually move towards **empathy**. That is, you will be able to put yourself in the other person's position. You need to empathise in order to be able to help the person effectively.

Activity 4.11

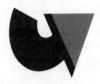

Try to raise the level of your own self-awareness and empathy by thinking back to times when you have been unhappy, hurt, ill, confused or had difficulty in learning a new skill. Describe what you felt. Did anything or anyone make you feel better?

Write a paragraph about your feelings.

Silence is golden . . .

We have so far emphasised the importance of listening, but sometimes people may just need a little space to be quiet. They need moments to pause, to regain themselves, to think of the words they need. It is not always easy to express feelings because it may be painful or embarrassing and there may be silence. Try to use the silence; try not to be tense about it. Even skilled counsellors can find the silences difficult to handle. You may eventually be able to question gently.

Non-verbal communication

A large part of communication is actually carried out without speaking, 'non-verbally' – we call this **non-verbal communication** or body language.

Activity 4.12

Without being rude! List some of the signs or gestures you know which do not involve speech.

Smiling

One of the most significant signs is a smile. Obviously there are times when it would be inappropriate to smile or grin, if people are upset or very anxious, but in introductions smiling shows warmth and openness which makes for positive interaction.

You do need to be aware of your own usual facial expression which can affect the interaction. If you know your group well it may be useful to go round and say how people usually appear. Some people look permanently worried or unhappy – they may not be, but that is the way they come across.

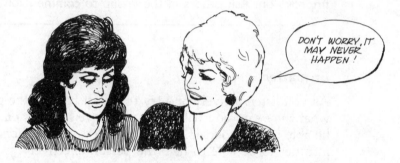

Eye contact

This is one of the most direct ways of communicating. Many of you will have received or made romantic intentions clear without speaking a word!

Certainly there are many phrases in the English language which illustrate the power of eye contact in communication, such as 'she has shifty eyes', 'he had a gleam in his eye', 'he looked daggers at her'. It may be disconcerting at first to try to communicate deeply with someone who is wearing dark glasses!

Where you focus your eyes makes a difference to the interaction, or two-way talk, you achieve. The length of your gaze also makes a difference. It is *not* a good idea to stare the client out but it is necessary to look at the client so that he or she knows they have your attention.

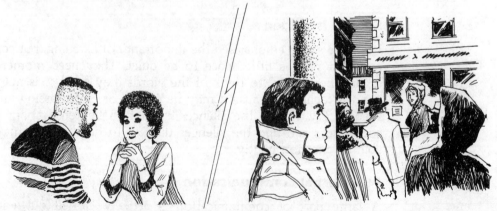

The length of your gaze also makes a difference

People may not be able to return your eye contact for a whole host of reasons. They may be shy, timid, nervous, for example, or unfamiliar with eye contact because they have not been encouraged to look directly at people in their way of life. Some cultures teach that it is impolite to look directly at people particularly if they are above you socially. If someone has a sight problem then you may think about concentrating on the other senses because they miss out on the eye contact. The tone of your voice becomes more important and you may touch an elbow to gain attention or to reassure them that you are listening. In all these cases you may have to take care that you are not 'put off' by the lack of eye contact. There are other ways of developing the rapport, or mutual understanding. If you are talking to an individual child, it is sometimes worth saying gently 'Look at me when I talk to you.'

Posture

Think whether your body language conveys messages like 'Yes, I am listening. I want to hear what you say' or 'No, I'm eager to leave. I'm not interested'. Sitting beside the person you are talking to without distractions or 'blocks' like desks separating you makes the difference between good and poor communication patterns. Stretching back in your chair away from the person sends messages of distance and carelessness, while leaning forward nodding, saying 'yes' or making quiet utterances reinforces your interest to the client.

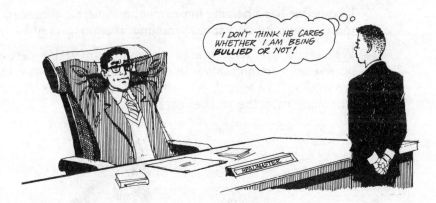

Think whether your body language conveys messages

Gestures

Hands

How do we use our hands in communication? Drumming fingers implies impatience as might jangling keys in pockets or twidding thumbs. Sometimes people use their hands to cover their faces and this may imply they have something to hide – they are being defensive. It is also difficult sometimes to hear what people say if they cover their face!

If you rub your nose or eyes, this may be interpreted as another barrier or form of avoidance. Scratching your head or neck is often a sign of uncertainty. So if someone says 'I know what you mean' while scratching their head, they may not actually understand at all.

If someone clenches their hands while talking, what might it imply? Wringing the hands conveys anxiety and one wrist gripping the other may indicate frustration or that the person is trying to gain self control.

Arms and legs

Folding arms implies that a person has something to hide. This is a negative gesture, it puts a barrier between you and the other person. A partial armfold may indicate being unsure or lacking in self-confidence. This may be reinforced if the head is down. If a person holds their head up, on the other hand, they are more sure of themselves. Notice in group situations if someone disagrees, their head may go down or go from side to side in a 'No, No' gesture.

Like arms, legs can also be positioned in a defensive way, as a barrier. Crossed legs and leaning back from the client may signal avoidance and feelings of superiority. Of course, people may sit with crossed legs because they feel more comfortable that way and not because of any defence mechanism. Crossed legs with a swinging foot, however, may signal flippancy and a tapping foot clearly suggests impatience.

Activity 4.13

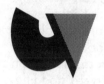

Be aware of other people's body language. Observe how people respond in tense or awkward situations, if they are wearing new clothes, or if they want to impress or attract someone.

Keep notes of your observations for your portfolio.

If someone has a hearing impairment non-verbal communication becomes even more significant and special training in signing may be necessary.

When you are with young children it may be necessary to exaggerate non-verbal communication in order to gain or maintain their attention. If you are working in a school, you will find it useful to observe how much non-verbal communication the teacher uses.

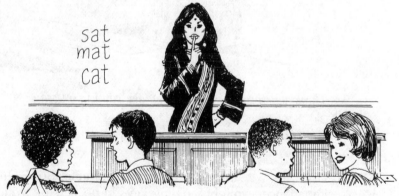

It may be necessary to exaggerate non-verbal communication to maintain their attention

People with learning difficulties may use 'makaton', a form of sign language, which gives them some way to communicate.

Activity 4.14

In pairs discuss the reasons why it is necessary for everyone to be able to find some way of communicating. Make a note of the reasons and share them with the rest of the group. Make a general list for your portfolio.

Touch

Keep your hands off me!
This is a very tricky aspect of non-verbal communication and needs some confidence. Occasionally a hand on someone's shoulder or arm can be very reassuring, and with children giving a hug after a bad fall can be a spontaneous response to a distressed child. You can only act according to the client, the situation, and your own response.

The issue of physical contact can easily be misunderstood or misrepresented if it is retold in the wrong way. This is particularly true if different genders are involved, for example in the case of a male nursery nurse working with children. In this sense your actions must always be above any criticism. Other staff must be involved.

Space

Have you ever noticed how people stand a safe distance apart when they don't know each other? Have you ever felt uncomfortable when somebody you don't know has edged on to your side of the seat on a train or on a bus? Some people actually stand very close to you when they talk and it makes you feel uneasy.

Activity 4.15

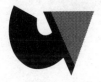

In pairs try to have conversations at different distances apart. Work out which one suits you best. Choose easy subjects of conversation such as hobbies, music, pets or television programmes. What is the preferred distance?

Everyone has their own 'personal space'. That is the space that they need for themselves where only those they know well can enter. When people are compelled to be near each other for some reason, in a railway carriage, for example, they often adopt little mechanisms to avoid catching the eye of the other person, such as staring out of the window, concentrating on the newspaper or a book.

When you are relating to an individual, be careful not to stand or sit too close to them. They may feel their personal space has been suddenly invaded and 'draw back' from being able to talk. On the other hand, you do need to be able to hear each other!

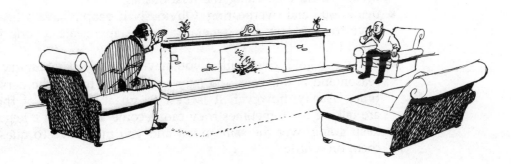

Asking questions

There are more questions than answers . . .
Good questioning techniques can really improve your communication skills.

Some questions can be described as **closed questions**. That is, they don't give the person much opportunity to talk. **Open questions**, on the other hand, give the person more scope for talk. For example, you may ask a friend 'Did you have a good time last night?' She could reply 'Yes' or 'No' or 'OK', but if you ask 'How did it go last night?' she may be awkward and say OK, but she is more likely to give you a fuller answer.

Although it is important to ask questions to clarify the situation or the problem, avoid asking too many questions. Otherwise the person will feel burdened and unable to talk freely.

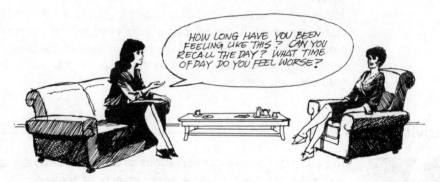

Avoid over-burdening the client with questions

Also avoid:
- telling the person 'Don't worry – you'll soon forget it.' This puts the problem down – it reduces it. To the person the problem is big. He or she doesn't want to have it dismissed but talked through.
- telling the person what to do directly. There may be a course of action which is appropriate, but the person should try and arrive at the decision themselves. You cannot direct the perfect path through a tricky maze. The person has to arrive themselves, possibly with your help. For example a friend of yours may have been seeing someone who you are sure has little real consideration for her. The friend may ask your advice about ending the relationship. You could be tempted to say immediately – 'Ditch him. He's only using you', but it would be more effective to ask the friend questions about examples of his consideration or inconsideration of her. This way she may gradually build up a picture and realise for herself that it isn't worth continuing the relationship.
- being loud and overbearing. Obviously if people have a hearing loss you have to speak up, but generally people appreciate a tone that's easy to listen to.
- rushing to get it over with – you may be in a desperate hurry for a genuine reason and in this case you may have to ask to see the person at another time. Usually, however, it is best to go at the pace of the person you are talking to. Sometimes they can become 'locked' in a negative phase or keep going over the same point and you may have to question to move them on a little.

- shifting the emphasis from the person to yourself and starting to recount your own experiences. Your client doesn't want to know your problems.
- diagnosing 'what your problem is . . .'. By telling someone what their problem or need is you are putting your interpretation on it. It is only the problem as you see it, and not necessarily the whole problem or the problem as it affects their life. You are putting a value or a judgement on the person and the situation they are in. Again you may have it all wrong.

If you can, prepare questions in advance but don't be thrown if it doesn't work out the way you anticipate.

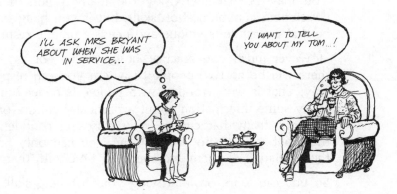

It may be that someone is reluctant to talk to you for a number of reasons or having started to talk, dries up and cannot continue. You may help by asking open questions in relation to the subject and then some more specific closed questions to help you probe a little further. A lot depends on *you* – your understanding of the situation. If you feel a question might be too direct then make a suggestion (a prompt), but be careful, substituting words or giving ideas can be difficult. You can easily distance the person with the wrong suggestion.

Activity 4.16 ───────────────────────────────────────

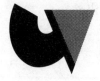

In small groups work out how you might respond to the following situations – what you might say or ask. Tape record your conversations for portfolio evidence.

a You are working in an infant school and a child becomes upset because he cannot do his maths work.

b You are working in an infant school and a child refuses to do the art activity you have been asked to supervise. He says he is hopeless at art and he hates it.

c A member of your college group is finding her placement difficult and tells you that she isn't going to go the next day.

d You are working with a group of 16-year-old special needs students. They are having an aerobics session. Two of the students are finding it difficult to keep up with the others.

e You are in a junior school on the day that the school football team is selected. Some boys are inevitably disappointed.

f You are working in a nursery where there are some children whose first language is not English. You hear one child saying 'I'm not playing with Naseem because she doesn't talk proper.'

Respect for individuals

You may be bewildered by the many points raised in connection with developing communication skills, but if you hang on to one thing it should be that everyone is unique and needs a unique response.

However much you practise, however far you go in the caring profession there will be no two people to whom you can respond in exactly the same way. That is why working with people is never boring. It may be that you study some information about a particular culture or religion and then meet someone from that culture. You may feel confident that you know about them but you do not know *them*. You can only know them by talking to them, relating to them and spending time with them.

So you can work on improving your listening skills, your questioning skills and be conscious of your body language. Other physical or practical factors may inhibit or prevent good interaction with the other person – factors like noise, interruptions from other people or from you, or barriers such as desks or chairs. Sometimes the room temperature may be so cold or so hot that it is difficult to concentrate on the matter in hand. Someone may be very tired or hungry. Children and many others find it hard to take in what is being said if they are tired, thirsty or hungry.

As well as physical barriers affecting your rapport with the other person, there may be language problems or a speech difficulty which slows down the interaction.

There will be many occasions when the other person finds it difficult to talk because of emotional factors such as anger, shame or great sadness. Can you think of other emotional factors which may prevent interaction?

Communication skills in group situations

There are lots of times in our lives when we are members of groups.

Activity 4.17

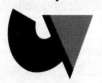

a List five groups that you now belong to and the reasons why you chose them.

b Explain to others in your class why the groups you chose to highlight are important to you.

You may have included some of these groups in your list:

- church
- family
- sports club
- political party
- ethnic group
- voluntary organisation
- football team
- student group.

Why do people form groups?

For security
People form groups for security as they are naturally sociable and want to be with others, sharing common ideas, values and pleasures. As a member of a group, people enjoy the companionship of others with the same interests, ideas and attitudes. They feel safe and confident as one of a group sharing similar aims and objectives.

To share or help
People may join a group to help others out of some commitment. This could be a voluntary group or charity. Alternatively, they may want to share an experience with others in a group, such as the desire to play football well in a team. These needs are different from joining a club simply to enjoy the company of others.

To get things done
Personal objectives may be more easily attained in a group. Individuals can often achieve aims as part of a group that they would not otherwise manage alone. One person may not be able to stop a development in a nature reserve, but as a member of a pressure group this aim may be achieved.

Activity 4.18

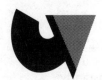

Choose one group to which you belong. Write down what you believe to be:

a the aims of the group

b how the group works

c what your contribution is to the group

d what the group demands of you

e what kind of group it is.

Primary groups

Primary groups are usually small enough to allow the members to form close personal relationships. As a result the whole group develops a strong sense of solidarity and individuals rely on each other. The family is one important primary group, but others include sports teams, street gangs and small groups of people, such as a few black families in a street containing a majority of white families, or disabled students in a class with a majority of able-bodied students.

Secondary groups

Secondary groups are large bodies in which the members have looser ties than in primary groups. Many secondary groups are joined on a voluntary basis, such as football supporters' clubs and trade unions, but many others have involuntary membership, such as racial groups, schools or social class. Both primary and secondary groups have unity and share many of the same rules and pressures.

Activity 4.19

a What regulations and rules apply to the groups that you belong to?

b How did you get to know of the group?

c Do you have to wear a uniform, badge or special clothes, or speak a special language?

d Do you have to carry out certain rituals or admission procedures?

How do groups work?

People who belong to a group usually have a strong bond which makes them feel very differently about people not in their group, the 'out group'. Members of a group may discriminate against those who are not in their group. Think of your class group. Are there any members who are always picked on or blamed for anything that goes wrong?

Activity 4.20

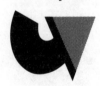

Discuss as a class how you would deal with a colleague who constantly interrupts the class

Summarise your discussion for your file.

Group pressure

Pressure on group members to conform to the group rules is very strong, resulting in people doing things that they would not normally do. If the group drinks, individuals who do not normally do so may drink. Normally placid individuals may become very violent and aggressive in a group. Some members fear the consequences if they do not follow the will of the group. Think how you would feel if all your classmates decided not to involve you in their activities. Belonging to a group can lift from you the responsibility for making decisions. It is much easier, in many cases, to follow group thinking or activities than to take your own stance on an issue.

Activity 4.21

Form a group of five or six in the class. Imagine that you have belonged to this group for a long time. Your friends in the group want you to smoke a cigarette – something you have never done before.

How would you go about resisting this pressure? Make a note of your thoughts for your file.

Why belong to a group?

Membership of a group can result in the following benefits:
- pleasure and satisfaction from sharing a common interest
- security which can engender confidence
- learning opportunities – individuals can learn skills in the group which can be practised in personal life
- opportunities to develop leadership skills
- experience of democratic processes.

Activity 4.22

The aim of this activity is to enable half your class colleagues to observe the other half in achieving some group tasks. The whole activity may take about two hours.

Read through the whole activity before you begin.

The tasks are:

a As a group, decide how to assess an assignment that you have just been given.

You may wish to consider some of the following assessment strategies:
- percentage marks
- pass or fail (no marks given)
- fail, pass, merit, distinction (no marks given).

b As a group, decide who should assess the assignment and why. The assessor may be:
- college staff
- college staff and students
- students as a group
- other students on the course
- another option.

Recording interaction within the group
Procedure
One group performs the tasks and the other observes them. The performing group sits in a circle. The other group members place themselves where they can see the interaction between the members of the first group.

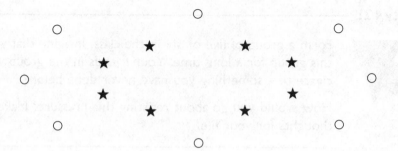

★: Members who perform tasks
○: Members who observe.

What to observe
● Who speaks to whom?
● How often do they speak?

Recording interactions
Use a diagram like the one illustrated below to record the interaction between group members.

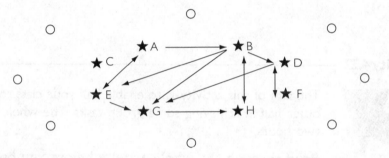

★: Member of group performing tasks
→: Direction of communication

Member **B** is leader of this group; member **C** seems to be left out.

Another method you can use is to draw up a table to record:
● who communicates non-verbally
● who started the discussion
● who speaks a lot
● who said very little
● who needs to look up more
● who covers their face with their hand so that it masks their voice and inhibits interaction
● who speaks too quickly
● who drones on
● who asks too many questions.

Said little	Started discussion	Speaks a lot
A F	D	B

How can you record non-verbal communication in a group? You could draw up a table to record who did what. For example:

Folded arms	Sat back in chair	Waved hands for emphasis
B	A	D

Procedure to measure contributions

The simplest measure of behaviour in a group is how much each member says. One way to record this is to record a mark for each time a member makes a statement. The results will indicate who speaks a great deal or is silent most of the time. This procedure will *not* tell you how valuable any contribution may have been.

Contributions are usually recorded in a *tally* such as the one shown below:

A	B	C	D	G
⁜⁜ ⁜⁜ ⁜⁜ ⁜⁜	⁜⁜ ⁜⁜ ⁜⁜ ⁜⁜ ||	⁜⁜ ⁜⁜	⁜⁜ ⁜⁜ |	⁜⁜ |||

In many social care situations staff work as teams, or groups, such as the staff in a residential home for elderly people. Groups may be used to help and support people with similar situations like parents of children with special needs or 'Weight Watchers'.

Groups can be used for therapy when they are managed by skilled people. Questions are prepared and structured to enable people to work through their difficulties in the group situation. The members benefit by releasing their emotional energy and hopefully make some progress in coming to terms with their problem.

One of the best ways to learn how groups work is to carry out a task in a group situation and then reflect on how the group has operated. Some of your assignment work may be carried out in this way.

First ask yourself which statement, if any, best describes how you feel in groups?
- 'I find it difficult to speak out in groups.'
- 'I find it difficult to express myself well in groups.'
- 'I don't like working in groups. I prefer working on my own.'
- 'I like groups. I feel more secure.'
- 'I'm afraid in groups. I think I might show myself up.'

Another question, which may be best asked indirectly in order to save embarrassment, is whether you have observed other people in group situations who could be described as:
- the know-all type?
- the quarrelsome type?
- the shy type?
- the talkative type?
- the highbrow type?

One of the reasons why people might be quarrelsome, overbearing or shy is that they don't feel secure within the group. The shy person doesn't feel that he or she can contribute because they lack confidence. The quarrelsome one has to pick arguments to assert his or her point of view because they haven't the confidence to back down. Everyone brings something to a group situation and they can work best when they feel least threatened. They need to have a sense of their own worth. They need to know that they can contribute.

Sometimes the work rate of groups can be reduced because group members stereotype others. They may make an assumption that a particular group member will not contribute.

Questions to establish the group
1 Does everyone know each other's name?
2 Does the group need more information?
3 Does the group need a leader?
4 Does the group need a contract or agreement?

Then later:
5 Does the group feel safe?
6 Are people sticking to the contract?
7 Does everyone speak?
8 Does everyone feel valued?
9 Is anyone opting out?
10 Are members being honest?
11 Are members being positive?

Practical tips to help you organise the group
1 Clarify the situation at the end of each meeting and make a note of what was agreed.
2 Pin down tasks – make sure that the individuals know their responsibilities.
3 Check everyone is clear.
4 Decide the time, date and place of the next meeting.

Assess yourself on your group skills and your personal skills in Activity 4.24.

One of the ways in which you can provide more effective emotional support is by being aware of your own strengths and weaknesses. Work through the following exercises to help you do this.

Activity 4.23 ───────────────────────────────────

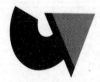

You may talk the questions over in pairs and note the answers briefly on a piece of paper.

a Consider times when you have needed help yourself.
   i) What sort of help was given?
   ii) How valuable was the help?

b Consider the way you usually respond to people when they express strong emotions like anger, fear or distress.
   i) Are you:
      ● embarrassed?
      ● cross?

- distant?
- calm?

ii) Do you look for practical solutions?

iii) Do you try to:
- get away?
- ask questions?
- listen?
- offer a cup of tea?

Activity 4.24

Read through the list of communication skills below and indicate with a tick which skills you feel weak, confident or really confident about.

When you have done this go back and look at the ticks. Make a note of your confidence points. Then look for specific evidence of these skills over the next three weeks. Record your evidence.

Communication skills	Weak	Confident	Really confident
Talking in the group			
Thinking before I talk			
Keeping my comments to the point			
Bringing quieter members of the group in			
Starting conversations			

Observation skills

Sensing the feelings of individuals
Being aware of reactions to my comments
Being aware of group tension
Noting who is being left out in the group

General

Telling others what I feel
Showing interest in others
Helping people reach an agreement

Defending the rights of an individual against group pressure

Counselling skills
Introducing myself
Listening
Responding to anger
Coping with silence
Asking open-ended questions
Expressing support
Ending sessions in a positive way

Interpersonal style

Interpersonal style is something we all have. The effective counsellor must explore his or her style and be familiar with it. In this way he or she will have greater awareness of the impact they make on others, have knowledge of, and be prepared to confront negative aspects of the style and have clarified their value system.

Activity 4.25

a Complete the following sentences – don't spend a lot of time on them. Do it relatively quickly. Let the sentence act as a stimulus and put down whatever arises naturally.

1 One thing I really like about myself is . . .
2 I dislike people who . . .
3 When people ignore me I . . .
4 When someone praises me I . . .
5 When I relate to people I . . .
6 Those who really know me . . .
7 My moods . . .
8 I am at my best with people when . . .
9 When I am in a group of strangers I . . .
10 I feel lonely when . . .
11 I envy . . .
12 I think I have hurt others by . . .
13 Those who don't know me well . . .
14 What I am really looking for in my relationships is . . .
15 I get hurt when . . .
16 I am at my best with people when . . .
17 I like people who . . .
18 What I feel most guilty about in relationships is . . .
19 Few people know that I . . .
20 When I think about intimacy . . .
21 One thing I really dislike about myself is . . .
22 I get angry with . . .
23 One thing that makes me nervous with people is . . .
24 When I really feel good about myself I . . .
25 When others put me down I . . .
26 When I like someone who doesn't feel the same about me I . . .
27 I feel awkward with others when . . .
28 I feel let down when . . .
29 In relationships what I run away from most is . . .
30 I hate people to see that I am . . .

b Did any of these questions give you a problem? If so, which?

c Which questions did you find hardest to answer? Why?

d Which question(s) were easiest to answer? Why?

e Would you like to add any other question? What?

The effect of discriminatory behaviour on relationships

Stereotyping

Unless you treat each person as an individual you are likely to make assumptions about them – that is make a judgment about them based on something you have seen or read. The judgment may be wrong but it affects your interaction with that person. The assumption grows to a **stereotype** – we make the person fit the image we have of them rather than accepting them for what they are. The stereotypes act as barriers to good communication. Good carers try to be aware of the stereotypes they may make particularly when the person they are trying to help may be from a different social class background, a different ethnic background or the opposite gender. Here are some examples of how we can easily misjudge people and get the wrong message.

Judging on appearance
'The guy looked so punk I thought he was very threatening but he was really gentle when he worked with the toddlers.'

Day nursery assistant

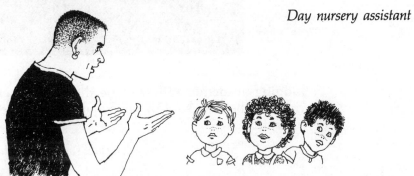

Judging age
'Old people don't care about their appearance so I don't bother if the hem of her underskirt falls below her dress or Pop walks around with his fly undone.'

Care assistant in elderly persons' home

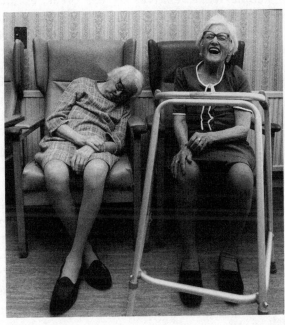

153

Judging disabled people – see the wheelchair and assume total immobility
'I was really surprised when I pushed the wheel chair to the toilet block and she got up and walked to the toilet on her own.'

Tutor in a college when a disabled student joins a course

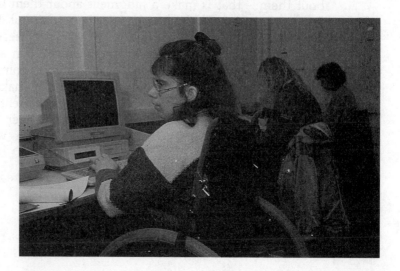

Judging academic ability to be the same as emotional and social
'Some of them are so slow you wouldn't think they'd be interested in anything romantic.'

Student working alongside some other students with learning difficulties

By responding to people as individuals you are respecting who they are and what they want. You are giving them some scope to make a choice and exercise control.

An old people's home, offering respite care or temporary care for elderly people while relatives have a break, admitted a man of Jewish background. The staff could have assumed that he wouldn't mind just eating like everyone else for his fortnight stay. They could have assumed that he was no longer practising his religion. They did, however, check his dietary requirements and took trouble to obtain the right Kosher food. This made a huge difference to his stay.

Activity 4.26

Making judgments – checking values
a As a group discussion, consider the following people and ask yourself how you would feel about helping them. Follow through by asking why you felt that way.
   i) a lonely elderly person with financial problems and bad housing
   ii) a mother of four who is depressed and has assaulted one of her children
   iii) a group member who frequently misses time from college because of some emotional problems

iv) a teenage boy from a private school whose parents are rich but he has financial difficulties

v) a man suffering from depression after a driving accident in which someone was killed (the man had been drinking)

vi) a man who is living rough, who smells and pesters you for money.

Keynote:
assumption → stereotype → prejudice → discrimination → denies individuality

Make a note in your file about your feelings and how they might link with assumptions and stereotyping.

b In your group discuss possible areas of stereotyping.

c Work out how stereotyping might lead to prejudice.

Prejudice

Everyone stereotypes to a certain extent. We make judgments about people in our minds so that we can interact with them. For example, if you met a young male wearing sports clothes you might assume he enjoyed playing sport. If you met a teenage girl wearing trendy clothes you might assume she liked listening to music and socialising. You might be very wrong in both cases, but the misjudgements are probably not damaging.

When is stereotyping damaging and when does stereotyping become discrimination? These are not easy questions to answer because there may be only a subtle difference between stereotyping being helpful or being damaging to the other person. Categorising people is *not* helpful when it leads you to assume people who look or behave like the mental image you have of them fit in this category. When people make assumptions like this we call it **prejudice**. It means someone has prejudged the other person or group, or made up their minds beforehand. They have a **personal bias**, based on something they have heard or seen. It is confirmed and perpeturated in their response to people and their interactions with them.

Look at these comments – you can understand that there is prejudice and unhelpful categorisation in them:
● A woman's place is in the home.
● People with AIDS have got what they deserve.
● Disabled people shouldn't have children – it's not fair to the children.
● Lesbians and gays shouldn't teach in schools.

Activity 4.27

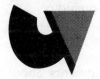

a Working in pairs try to detect prejudice in yourself or your partner by completing these sentences.
   i) All police are . . .
   ii) All lesbians are . . .
   iii) All football supporters are . . .

    iv) All black people are . . .

    v) All teachers are . . .

    vi) All students are . . .

b Look out for general statements in newspapers, magazines or on television which could lead to prejudice. Cut the statements or articles out or make a note of the television quotes and programme.

c In a small group discuss a particular area of prejudice – any prejudice will do even if someone supports a different football team from you.

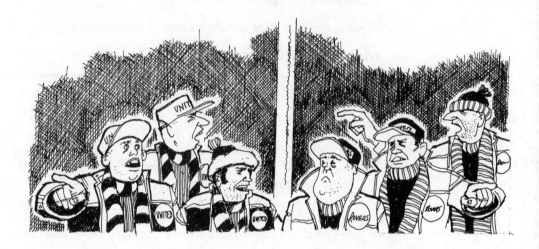

Put yourself in the place of the person who 'suffers' from the prejudice. Ask yourself how it might feel to be disliked, ignored or bullied because you didn't have the same colour skin or football scarf.

Examine your own prejuduces – being aware of them is halfway to overcoming them.

Sometimes articles or programmes can take a particular slant which categorises people in a certain way, 'The Disabled', 'The Elderly'. The article may be patronising (making the people seem as children) or give a lot of coverage to something a disabled person may achieve, however minor. This approach may have the effect of cutting disabled people off from mainstream society.

Discrimination

While prejudice is what a person *thinks*, **discrimination** is what a person *does* – how they treat another person or group unfairly, based on their prejudice.

Forms of discrimination

Visual clues often guide our first impressions. We make judgments about people based on what we see. Look at the list below and select the factors

which you might decide from sight:
- nationality
- age
- religion
- skin colour
- politics
- race
- married or single
- overweight, obese
- accent
- disability/ability
- problems with alcohol
- problems with drugs
- sexual orientation
- social class or status
- criminal record
- occupation
- employed/unemployed
- gender.

Why do you think that:
- fat people may be more likely to receive negative treatment than slim people?
- black people find it more difficult to secure accommodation than white?
- women who dress in a very masculine way may find it more difficult to succeed in a job application if interviewed by men?
- teachers may devote less time to female pupils than male pupils in mixed classes?

Activity 4.28

Make your own list of possible areas of discrimination, using the clues in this section and others you can glean from class discussion. Check your own feelings about the areas you have listed. Why do you think people in the above list may be treated unfairly?

Mind your language
On a cultural level our language is peppered with both sexist and racist terms which are indirectly discriminative. Often the words 'man', 'he', 'him' are used to refer to both genders.

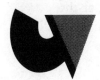

Activity 4.29

Work out alternatives for:

businessman	manning	man hours
man power	man-made	fireman
to a man	headmaster	foreman
chairman	cameraman	ice cream man
salesman	newsman	
dustman		

Language and race
In the first part of the twentieth century the terms 'negro', 'coloured', etc. were commonly used. The development of black movements in the 1960s led to the use of the word 'black' as a good term so it has been kept and used.

Negative uses of the word 'black' which have come from a racist situation, such as 'working like a black', should be avoided. Several phrases are negatively associated with 'black', such as 'black magic', 'black sheep' or the use of the word 'black' to mean dirty. Such uses need to be avoided.

Levels of discrimination

Prejudice or discrimination can arise at:

- **an individual level** where people may have personal attitudes and beliefs which they use to prejudge other groups negatively.
- **an institutional level** where the systems and practices of an organisation exclude certain groups from access to resources. For example, if publicity about antenatal classes was not produced in community languages in a multi-racial area, this could be seen as institutional racism.
- **a cultural level** when people have so absorbed values, beliefs and ideas that they don't challenge negative stereotypes in media images. These people accept racist or sexist remarks.

Behaviours indicating discrimination

These are obviously direct behaviours which are blatantly prejudiced like using offensive language, denying people rights or being rude. A young black girl was sitting on the inside seat of a bus. Her white friend sitting beside her stood up to let an older woman sit down. The woman refused the seat saying she would rather stand that sit next to 'one of them'. The young black girl was the victim of **direct discrimination**.

Indirect discrimination is more subtle and less easy to report, but equally damaging. The director who may have decided he doesn't want to appoint a female assistant director may find ways of undermining her confidence so that she doesn't even feel she can apply for the post. She becomes the victim of indirect discrimination.

Devaluing someone by not taking them seriously or not respecting what they say is a form of indirect discrimination.

Activity 4.30 ————————————————————————————————

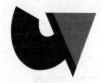

Racism is the belief that some 'races' are superior to others. Sometimes actions are clearly racist, other times it is less easy to tell. Look at the situations below and decide whether:

- the intention is racist
- the method is racist
- the effect is racist.

a A housing department has a policy of spreading black tenants throughout its estates. The reasons given for this policy are to ensure that there is no discrimination against black applicants, leading to their being allocated to worse estates, and to encourage racial mixing.

b A company finds it has more applicants for unskilled jobs than it has vacancies. In the past some of these jobs have been given to Asian workers who do not speak English fluently. They have been able to do the work satisfactorily and there haven't been any problems. Now that there are more applicants, the company have decided to ask all applicants to pass a test in basic written and spoken English before they can be offered a job.

c A company has a vacancy for a supervisor's post in a department where 60 per cent of the workers are Asian. The supervisor's job includes explaining to the other workers what to do, filling in forms, report writing, etc. The company says all applicants for the job must pass a test to show that they have a good level of spoken and written English.

The answers are on page 177.

So it is necessary to check out not only what we intend but also our methods and the effects of our actions. Policies should also be checked out in this way.

The ways in which groups may be stereotyped

Gender

We are socialised into our gender roles from the minute we are born, by the colour of the blanket that is wrapped around us and the sort of cards which are sent to greet us.

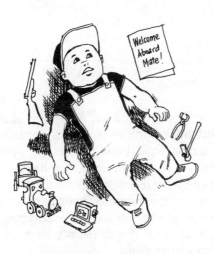
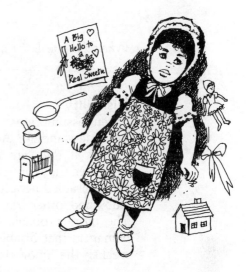

Activity 4.31

Write down the gender that you think is best suited to the following occupations/careers:

a	nanny	**h**	footballer
b	nurse	**i**	car mechanic
c	engineer	**j**	financial adviser
d	domestic worker	**k**	electrician
e	builder	**l**	plumber
f	joiner	**m**	caterer
g	counsellor	**n**	councillor

Age

When did you last run a marathon? Negative stereotyping about age highlights sickness, dependency and not being able to be sociable. Older people may be seen by others as retarded, slow or inefficient. If they show interest in sexual matters this may be regarded as odd, funny or dirty.

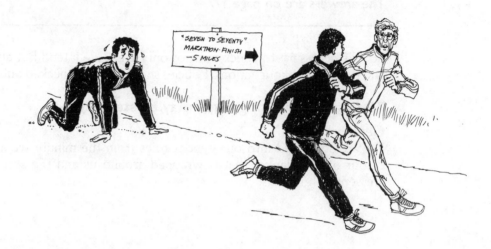

When did you last run a marathon?

Disability

Often assumptions are made about disabled people's abilities based on misunderstanding. Access and opportunities are very significant to disabled people. If they are denied access to a building or the opportunity to do a job then they cannot demonstrate the capabilities they have. Similarly, socially some disabled people have experienced difficulties concerning access to night clubs and other 'rave' venues on the tenuous reason of increased fire risk. The more probable explanation is the negative stereotyping of night club managers that disabled people are not 'good' people to have around – they weaken the 'good time' image of the place.

Activity 4.32

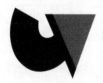

Use your list of possible areas of discrimination from Activity 4.28 and try to think of ways in which particular groups may be stereotyped. Discuss examples in your class and share stereotypes you have heard and seen.

The effects of discrimination

The possible effects of discrimination are so pervasive and wide-ranging that it is impossible to explain or describe them in depth or with accuracy. Reading novels, poems, watching films or television programmes and listening to personal experiences can inform us about the possible effects of discrimination.

Activity 4.33

Consider the physical, intellectual, emotional and social implications of discrimination for the following groups of people. Make a list of the groups and give examples of how discrimination may affect them. Some clues are provided.

a Women

Clues:
- *Physically* May never achieve full physical potential because of traditional notions of weakness. May be barred from participating in particular sports. May be unlikely to gain employment in certain occupations. May be denied career or promotion opportunities because of their biological capacity to bear children.
- *Intellectually* May be considered as intellectually less capable in some areas and therefore not given opportunities educationally, 'My father encouraged my brother but he didn't think it was worth educating a girl.'
- *Emotionally* 'I wanted to apply for the promotion but I didn't *feel* it was right, management posts are nearly all men. I should concentrate on things at home; my mother said it was wrong to leave the children and she's probably right.'
  'I would like to learn French at evening classes but there is so much to do at home what with the family and Grandad needs more help now.'
- *Socially* The traditional roles of women are often underpaid and undervalued. 'Anyone can look after children.' 'There is no need to cook or do housework.'

b Black and minority group members

Clues:
- *Physically* May be discriminated against in terms of access to health care. Health service runs mainly on white, middle-class systems and culture.
- *Intellectually* In classrooms, racist tensions among staff and pupils can affect educational progress and intellectual development.
- *Emotionally* Feelings of being different or singled out, like the black boy who wanted to wash his hands white.
- *Socially* Jobs – the unemployment level for black people is significantly higher than for white people. There are still few black people in senior positions in professional occupations. Similarly, black people have encountered racism in terms of housing, lodgings or temporary accommodation. It is only relatively recently that black footballers have played in league teams.

c Disabled people

Clues:
- *Physically* Good access often denied so life becomes more difficult.
- *Intellectually* May be regarded as intellectually weak even if their disability is physical.

- *Emotionally* Dependence may have been encouraged from childhood and this is usually well-intentioned, but creates a situation where the person feels dependent on others and fails to develop independence, even over matters like choice of clothes or hairstyle.
- *Socially* Disabled people may have been subtly dissuaded from holiday centres, clubs, pubs and cinemas.

d Lesbian and gay people

Clues:
- *Physically* Abuse, bullying.
- *Intellectually* May be discriminated against in education by staff or pupils, which could affect intellectual progress.
- *Emotionally* Reactions to comments about being odd or different – general stigma and unkind responses may all combine to produce low self-esteem, isolation and withdrawal. Such negative emotions affect on individual's general outlook and world view.
- *Socially* Jobs, promotion, even accommodation with, for example, shared housing or lodgings.

Research shows that discrimination, both sexual and racial, is still strong and widespread despite legislation (see page 166).

Racial discrimination

Activity 4.34

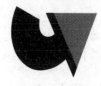

Consider how much such discrimination may affect the people making the comments below. Discuss your thoughts and record your answers.

a At school – intellectually, educationally
  i) 'It's hard being the only black boy in the class. I'm noticed especially if I do anything wrong.' *Black 12-year-old boy*
  ii) 'It's hopeless with these second language speakers, they'll never get through the exam.' *English teacher*
  iii) 'The PE staff keep asking me to play for this and that – they think because I'm black I'm really sporty, but I'm much more interested in history.' *Black 12-year-old boy*
  iv) 'Sometimes I feel angry and resentful when I read about what white people did to blacks in the past and what still happens today. I don't feel like being co-operative at school.' *Black 14-year-old girl*
  v) 'People are just waking up to the fact that there are so few black people in senior positions in education, in commerce and industry . . . . The unemployment rate amongst black youths is so much higher than for whites looking at the situation in proportion to the numbers in this population.' *Careers officer*

b In the community – socially

   i) 'Sometimes I know people view me differently because of the colour of my skin. The other day I was sitting on the bus. The person sitting next to me stood up to give an elderly lady the seat. The lady refused the seat mumbling that she would rather stand than sit next to a Paki. I didn't realise how it had affected me until I arrive at school – I went to the toilets and had a good cry.'   *Young Asian girl*

   ii) 'As jobs are scarce they've got to blame someone and we are the easiest target. Most of my family actually run their own businesses.'   *Young Asian boy*

   iii) 'I saw a black family looking round the empty house up the road. That's all this neighbourhood needs.'   *Mrs Snodgrass*

c Physically – in terms of health care

   i) 'We must have these leaflets about immunisation and surgery hours printed in community languages.'   *GP Smith*
'Oh what's the point? They'll do their own thing anyhow – we've enough to do as it is.'   *GP Jones*

   ii) 'I find it so difficult to communicate sometimes with the Asian families. The babies usually thrive but I wish there were more Asian workers to relate to them more easily. I'm sure they'd open up more.'   *Health visitor*

   iii) 'I can't understand why the Asian women will never look you directly in the eye when you're trying to make a point to them.'   *Community psychiatric nurse*

   iv) 'Hospitals are such busy bewildering places it's easy to be put off unless you really need medical attention.'   *White male out-patient*

How did you get on? Perhaps your discussion showed that it is easy for back people or minority groups to be nudged out of health care services and therefore discriminated against almost by chance without people noticing. Similarly in schools, attitudes are set and may create tensions before any learning takes place. In the community people are worried about employment and house sales and these fears are often directed against minority groups. Securing housing and employment therefore becomes more problematic for black people and, coupled with potential educational difficulties, such groups become disadvantaged through discrimination.

Sexual discrimination

Ask the people in your group 'Which would you rather be – male or female?' Ask someone to keep a record. Then ask 'Which would you, or your partner, rather have – a boy or a girl?' Again keep a note.

Some research shows that more people actually want boys rather than girls. Why do you think this may be true?

People evidently have images of boy or girl children in their minds and what those male or female roles mean in life.

Think about the moment a child is born — Is it all right? Is it a boy or girl? The pink or the blue blanket covers the little body. The cards arrive conveying good wishes for the bouncing boy or the darling daughter. Soon, room decoration, clothes, toys, language, attitudes and responses all work to reinforce male or female roles. Later books, films, television programmes and expectations of relatives, parents and teachers may further confirm these roles. There doesn't seem anything wrong with this, but consider the following questions.

Activity 4.35

Tape your answers to the questions, or write them down.

a Why are there so few male nurses, secretaries, child minders, nursery teachers? What difficulties would a man have if he tried to do any of these jobs?

b What happens if a girl wants to follow a traditionally male-dominated career?

c Why are there so few women MPs?

d Why are there so few women in senior positions?

e Why do we know so many more famous male authors and artists than female?

f In co-educational schools who receives the greatest share of teacher attention?

g Who takes on the greatest amount of childcare and domestic responsibility?

h What are the problems for women who want to work and have a family?

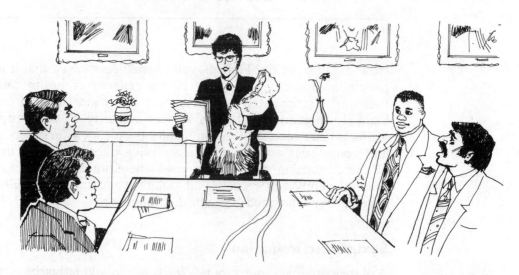

When you answer these questions it becomes clear that by pre-judging people on the basis of gender, we are actually discriminating against them. We are not allowing them to develop in the way they wish to go. We stifle their choice and their ability to control. We stereotype them, we put them into a box in our minds which may say 'She is a woman who should take care of her family before she thinks about her career.' This limits development and in some cases stops people aspiring, or going on to, jobs or promotion.

Discrimination and disability

A similar process occurs in relation to disability. It is easy to see a wheelchair or a white stick and categorise that person as being unable to cope. We may not even know what that person is capable of until further explanation.

Many disabled people feel that one of the worst aspects of being disabled is how other people perceive them. Very often it is assumed that disabled people cannot do things. For example, if someone is in a wheelchair there is a tendency for a speaker to address the person pushing the wheelchair rather than the person in the wheelchair. Of course, it is naive to suggest that a disabled person can do everything despite their disability, but if appropriate access, services and support are provided new avenues can be opened up. There is also a lot of evidence of disabled people achieving physical and academic feats that some able-bodied people would never dream of.

Since 1970 all public buildings must by law provide wheelchair access. Similarly, pathways, walkways and staircases should not restrict wheelchair users. In reality, there are still enormous difficulties in terms of access. This limits disabled people socially and in connection with employment. Similarly with housing, if a disabled person has an adapted home which they can manage this increases their independence. If funds are low and they have to rely on other people then they are limited.

Sometimes a person's disability is not evident. They may have a mental health problem, but the same discriminatory practices may still occur. People may be refused jobs or promotion, be disadvantaged socially or educationally because of attitudes formed by focusing on negative stereotypes.

What about you? Have there been times in your life when you have been unfairly treated because of your age, colour, social class, appearance or gender? How did you feel? Could you do anything about it?

Preventing discrimination

Personal prejudice

Most people have preferences. It is helpful if you are aware of your own preferences so that you can work on them to prevent prejudices. When you make decisions or choices you must try to avoid your own personal bias or preference affecting your judgements. This is particularly important when you are out on work placement. It is easy to like the attractive, well-dressed infant at the local school in preference to some of the others, and to assume they are more intelligent and treat them accordingly. Some of the less obvious pupils may be equally or more capable, however, and deserve recognition. Read the section on self-concept in Chapter 2 and consider where attention may be best placed in such a school situation.

For most people first judgements are made on visual impressions. You may be able to recall times when you have judged somebody on sight and then later, when you have got to know them, realised how wrong your first impressions were. We categorise on sight. Research shows that:
- fat people are more likely to get negative treatment
- in mixed classes teachers devote more time to male pupils than to female
- women who dress in a very masculine way are less likely to succeed in a job application if interviewed by men

- supervisors sum up young workers' behaviour in the first couple of weeks and don't change their opinions.

The first step must be to check your own prejudices and try to be aware of them in reacting in social care situations.

Working with children

If you are working with young children you can try to counteract stereotypical practices and language by:

- encouraging role reversal – the boys play in the wendy house and the girls with Lego
- selecting books and posters reflecting positive images of black children and non-sexist attitudes
- presenting toys and equipment in a non-sexist way
- avoiding sexist, racist language yourself but also monitoring children's conversations
- never saying things like 'Big boys don't cry' – it's probably better for the child to have a good bawl, male or female!
- being firm about racist actions or language from children – act quickly to report it to a member of staff if you don't feel that it is appropriate for you to deal with it
- not separating children on the basis of gender – grouping often sets up tensions and there is enough tension without creating more. Use birthdays or names with particular letters
- pointing out role models if you can find any, such as a female garage hand, a female doctor or a male nurse.

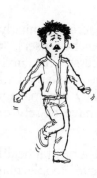

At work

Most establishments have equal opportunities policies and codes of practice for dealing with racist remarks, attitudes or actions. Make sure you know who to report to if you see or hear anything you regard as racist. If matters are dealt with promptly it is less likely that feelings will run high and escalate into violence.

If situations of violence do break out because of racism then obviously this is a matter for the police and the courts.

Legislation relating to discrimination

The Race Relations Act, 1976

This Act made racial discrimination illegal in public life. It says people can take action in circumstances like employment, housing, education, provision of goods and services.

The Act outlines:

- direct discrimination – treating a person less favourably on the grounds of race
- indirect discrimination – applying certain criteria which work to the disadvantage of one person over another.

It also makes victimisation illegal – it is illegal to treat somebody unfairly for being involved in making a complaint about discrimination.

The Commission for Racial Equality can help in the preparation of Race Relations Act cases. The Citizen's Advice Bureau can also assist with these matters.

The Chronically Sick and Disabled Persons Act, 1970
This Act attempted to reduce discrimination against disabled people. It instructed local authorities to provide services for disabled people and legislated (made it law) that any new public buildings must provide access for disabled people.

The services that the Act recommended should be available to disabled people include:
● home care workers (home helps)
● meals-on-wheels
● adaptions to homes
● telephones
● aids to daily living
● occupation at home and at centres
● outings
● provision of transport.

The Act stated that local authorities had to know how many disabled people there were in their area.

The National Health Service Act, 1977
This Act went on to make it a duty of the local authority to provide some home help services and recommended the provision of laundry services for people who need them.

The Disabled Persons Act, 1986 (Services, Consultation and Representation)
This Act reinforced the need for assessment for disabled people and services. A disabled person or their representative may request an assessment.

The Sex Discrimination Act, 1975
The Act applies to men and women. It states that it is unlawful to discriminate in the areas of recruitment, selection, promotion and training. It is also unlawful to treat a person less favourably because they are married. Like the Race Relations Act, it separates direct and indirect discrimination as well as victimisation.

The Equal Opportunities Commission and the Citizen's Advice Bureau can assist with complaints.

Equal Pay Act, 1970
This Act should be considered alongside the Sex Discrimination Act. The Act was amended in 1983 to comply with the (then) EC law. The main point of the Act is that equal work must be rewarded with equal pay.

Employment Protection Act, 1975
This Act meant that employers had to recognise unions by law, but the Employment Act of 1980 repealed this.

Disabled Persons Act, 1944 and 1988
Both Acts obliged companies employing more than 20 staff to employ 3 per cent disabled people.

Employment Protection Act, 1978
This consisted of rights to guarantee pay, medical suspension, time off work, maternity rights, sick pay and access to computerised data. Unions could be

recognised at the discretion of the employer. Recognised unions can insist on equal opportunities policies, analysis of data to indicate how many black and white, male and female, disabled and non-disabled workers.

Although legislation or laws exist, discrimination continues because it takes a long time to change people's attitudes and ways of thinking. We can only challenge bad practice when we see it and try to promote as much good practice as possible.

Working with clients in health and social care

Much of our interpersonal interaction is guided by our personal values and attitudes. What we think is right and true affects the views we hold. Many of the ideas and assumptions we have are based on what we were told as children and later through what we have seen and heard on television or read about. We hinted at this earlier when discussing stereotypes and discrimination. Sometimes our own prejudices or personal fears and values are more subtle but are still significant in affecting how we relate to people.

Activity 4.36

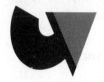

This can be quite an invasive task so everyone should carry it out on their own and time should be allowed for students to 'debrief' and reconnect with the class.

Have a piece of paper ready but if you feel the questions are too deep to write answers to then just think through each question.

Think about your childhood . . .

a What are the times you enjoyed most?

b What were the times you hated most?

c Where was your favourite place?

d What was your favourite toy or possession?

e What sort of things frightened you?

f Who were your favourite people?

g What were your playmates like?

h What sort of things made you feel guilty?

i What was your favourite book?

j What was your favourite television programme?

k Was there a particular phase or saying that was said to you repeatedly which you have carried through with you?

When you have answered the questions, you may find that you have a clearer picture of the sort of childhood you had and how these experiences may have affected your life now.

Activity 4.37

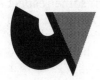

As a class, discuss a book, a film, a television programme or documentary which you know has influenced the way you think. Tape your discussion or make a brief note for your file.

Gradually you can appreciate how complicated individuals are and how much we need to be aware of our own values and attitudes. Activities 4.36 and 4.37 highlight how different experiences can create different attitudes. The next activity is demanding because it asks you to try and crystallise some of your values.

Activity 4.38

Write down your own ten personal statements or values. If you stop at less than ten, try to think why.

Once you have established what you think about key issues try the next activity.

Activity 4.39

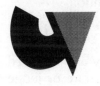

In groups of four, look at the list below and try to decide whether you would be willing to help these people with their problems. Give reasons for your decision. Make a note of your decisions and reasons.

a An adolescent who is in trouble for hooliganism at football matches.

b A man suffering from depression after killing a child in a road accident. The man had been drinking.

c A mother of three who is very low.

d A mother of three who is very low and has assaulted one of her children.

e A teenage girl who continually makes suicide attempts.

f A mother who has left home because she felt she couldn't cope and now desperately misses her children.

g A man who has a drink problem and continually hounds you for money.

h A man who has convictions for molesting young boys.

i An unemployed father of two who wants a job but seems reluctant to go and find one.

j A boy with a public school background and a drugs problem.

A factor which influences many people's willingness to help others with their problems is the extent to which they believe individuals are themselves responsible for the predicaments they are in. Sometimes it is difficult to find any respect for individuals who are so at odds with the values you hold. The irony is that these are usually the people who need to be shown some respect because their own self-respect has been so damaged. Think about small ways in which respect can be shown in any counselling situation – introducing yourself, in some situations a handshake may be appropriate, listening, eye contact, body language . . .

Usually, the relationship between client and counsellor or person and helper is unbalanced in terms of power. The helper or counsellor often has an advantage over the client. He or she knows the situation, they may have background notes about the client, and the meeting may take place in familiar surroundings to the counsellor. The counsellor may not feel under any pressure because they are not in the wrong or the one with the problem.

The counsellor may also be advantaged in terms of material position, status, clothing and confidence level. Effective communication skills can help to redress the balance of power in such a situation.

Look at the clues below and think about how they can be incorporated into the interpersonal interaction setting so that the interaction becomes more effective:

- discretion, keeping confidences or informing the client when confidence has to be broken
- introduction – names
- eye contact
- talking down
- physical space – position of furniture

- reassurance
- tone of voice
- language
- being patronising
- giving attention
- showing respect
- using observation skills.

In some situations, for example in court, distance and formality are increased to emphasise the wrong-doing of the client so that the magistrate or judge never introduces himself or herself. There is always physical distance between the accuser and the accused. The language is formal and may be difficult to understand. All business is carried on openly in court, although there are safeguards in juvenile courts concerning information being reported by the press.

When working with clients in residential settings, respect can be demonstrated by relating to them as **individuals**. Individuals usually show their individuality by the decisions and **choices** they make. Think about yourself . . . how many decisions have you made since you woke up this morning? Decisions about what to eat, what to wear, whether in fact to get up, where you were going, what time to leave – we are continually making choices in the routine of our everyday existence. We exercise a lot of control over what we do.

Activity 4.40

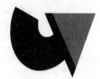

Divide into three groups. Each group should choose one of the following:
- a child around school age
- an elderly person in a residential situation
- a person with a physical disability.

a As a group, compare your situation with that of the individual you have chosen. Discuss, and keep a note of your discussion.

b Imagine you are working with one of these individuals. Trace a potential day in the life of him or her, paying attention to possible ways that choice could be maximised. Make brief notes for your file.

Once you have completed this activity you should be able to see how there are lots of small ways in which choice can be built in to each day. When choice has been established, the client feels more independent, more in control of his or her own life. To deny choice has the opposite effect. Then the client has little control, has to abide by the rules, sees little point in thinking because someone else has made the decisions.

Giving people choices to encourage independence is not always straightforward, It may involve some element of risk.

Activity 4.41

a An elderly woman lives alone. She has a condition which means she often falls over. She desperately wants to live in her own home. She has an open fire and has in fact received treatment for burns from a fall on to the fire.

You are the social worker in charge of the case. What do you do?

b Your are the parent of a 17-year-old girl who has very little vision. She wants to travel from Sheffield to Oxford to stay with a friend for the weekend. The girl has been almost blind since she was 5. She has good mobility and has travelled on buses before, and trains from Sheffield to Derby.

Do you say she can go?

c You are a teacher on a school holiday with a group of 12-year-old boys. Most of the boys are busy with supervised organised activities. Four boys are unoccupied and want to have a look around the village where you are staying. They are sensible boys. There are some dangerous cliffs near to the village. Your fellow teachers urge you to take a break and have a coffee with them.

What do you do?

d Sally is 11 years old. Most of her friends go to town on a Saturday morning or after school. If you were Sally's parents would you let her go? If you were her childminder or nanny would you let her go?

e Who is taking risks in the situations above?

f Who has responsibility?

g What difference does professional position make?

Activity 4.42

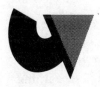

Make a note of the words below and explain how they link:

Respect; relinquishing control; giving choice; independence; improved self-esteem; risk

---

Responses to care

Good carers are sensitive to the needs and wishes of individuals. It is arrogant to assume need or to think that you are necessarily doing someone a favour by providing care. It is a good feeling to know that you have helped someone, but don't be fooled into thinking you can always give the right help or that the person wants to accept the help.

Activity 4.43

a Read the case study below. Write a brief report about how Mrs Atkin may be feeling and what her initial responses to care may be.

> Mabel Atkin suffers badly with arthritis and has a heart condition. She has lived most of her life in a council house where she brought up her three children who are now married and have moved away. She found the house too difficult to keep clean and tidy in spite of being extremely houseproud. She had a serious heart attack and much against her will decided she needed care in a residential situation. She watched her house being packed up; there wasn't time for a preliminary visit to the home arranged by her son. Her belongings and furniture were mostly put in a skip as they were too old and tatty for her family. Sadly she had to say goodbye to Jasper, her pet dog. She hates the restriction of the room in the home after being in the big house. She smokes and is very much overweight so the staff are trying to do something about this. She is upset that someone has marked her clothes and underwear with 'Room 13'. She doesn't know one care assistant from another – they keep changing and some of them are only slips of girls telling her what to do. She thinks she should be doing her own washing and cooking. She always thought of homes as workhouses.

b Look again at Mrs Atkin and work out what support she needed. How might her admission to the home have been made less traumatic? How might her feelings be demonstrated?

Think of her seeing the principal of the residential home in her own home. How could the situation have been made easier? How could the staff of the home have been briefed? How far are the staff right to try to do something about Mabel's smoking and eating?

Activity 4.44

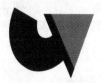

Read this case study.

> An 8-year-old boy is continually badly behaved in school. He often bullies younger children and even older ones. He cannot concentrate, he hates quietness and creates havoc if there is any sort of working atmosphere or structure. Even in PE he runs wild shouting, screaming

and laughing. He seeks attention constantly. He found his father dead in the car – he had committed suicide through carbon monoxide poisoning.

Work out what sort of support the boy needs.

Activity 4.45

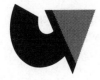

What sort of support would be appropriate in the case study below?

A mother of three children under 5 is struggling to manage on her husband's low income. She feels harassed and depressed with the workload of the children and her low income. The family live on a council estate which has a reputation for vandalism and the house itself is in a bad state.

Ethical issues in health and socal care

At the beginning of this chapter we mentioned confidentiality in the sense of betraying trust. If someone trusts you sufficiently to talk to you deeply about themselves or their problems, then this trust should never be broken. It is demeaning to the other person if you chat about them openly. It would also be very distressing to anyone who knew the other person. If you need help yourself because of what the client has told you, then you must go to the supervisor in private. There are two levels of confidentiality. The first is that there are many things you need never speak about to anyone. If it is your task on placement to help an elderly man who has wet himself to change his trousers, you do the task and say nothing. It is unprofessional to moan on the bus about what a fuss it was. How would you feel if it was your father, or indeed have you ever been in an embarrassing situation yourself?

The second level is when someone is discussing an issue with you and you need to warn them that if what they say cuts across legal boundaries or the rules of the residential/establishment you are in, then you will have to pass the information on. For example, if someone was about to tell you in a hostel that they sniffed glue, then you would have to say that you would need to speak to someone more senior. If they had already told you, then the same rule would apply.

There are times when client confidentiality has to be limited.

Activity 4.46

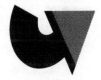

a You are attempting to help a very disturbed and disruptive girl of 15. After many failures you eventually win her confidence, or appear to. During a casual conversation she implies, but does not say outright, that she has been having sex with a 17-year-old boy who has left school.

What do you do?

b Your 14-year-old girl friend is very sharp with you one day. When you tackle her about it she gets very upset, apologises and says she needs to talk to you. She swears you to secrecy because she knows the rows and damage that will follow if her story is revealed. She tells you that her father has made sexual advances to her. She thinks she can cope and distance him – she says he is really kind to her and never forces her. She feels very mixed up. She isn't even sure if she has misinterpreted his attitude towards her. The last thing she wants is for the story to be known.

She loves her mother and doesn't want her to be upset by this, particularly as her mother has been very ill. Her two younger brothers would also be badly affected by allegations.

What do you do?

c You are approaching A-level examinations. Your friend's dad is very ill but your friend doesn't know that his dad has only a few months left to live. Your friend's mother doesn't want her son to know the seriousness of the situation because of the impending exams. Your friend keeps talking about the holiday he wants to go on after the exams with the whole family, when his dad is better.

Could you continue the pretence?

It may be helpful to discuss these situations with the whole group before moving on to the next activity.

Activity 4.47

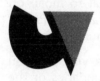

Write down examples of when client confidentiality may be limited by law, client safety, the safety of others and the rights of others.

Review questions

1 Explain the difference between primary and secondary groups.

2 Explain emotional need and give examples.

3 Give reasons why discretion is very important in social care situations.

4 What is reflective listening?

5 What is non-verbal communication?

6 What is a stereotype?

7 Why is observation important in communicating with individuals?

8 Give two ways in which you can convey to an individual that you are interested in them personally.

9 What is personal space?

10 Explain and give examples of:
   a open questions
   b closed questions.

11 What is:
   a direct discrimination?
   b indirect discrimination?

12 Explain institutional discrimination.

13 List three possible effects of racial discrimination.

14 Describe four ways of avoiding gender stereotyping when working with young children.

15 When was the Chronically Sick and Disabled Persons Act passed, and what did it state?

16 When was the Sex Discrimination Act passed?

17 Why is legislation (laws) not the total solution to the problem of discrimination?

18 In what situations might confidentiality be broken?

Assignment A4.1
Developing Communication Skills

One of the benefits of a vocational course is the opportunity to develop skills in work placement situations. It is often necessary to reflect and analyse your own performance in the caring situation in order to improve. **Read this assignment before you go on placement** so that you can plan and prepare.

Produce a placement report. It should include:
- **details about the establishment** – size, location, numbers of clients, staff, routines, systems
- **a record of your interaction in a one-to-one situation** at the beginning of the placement, with notes on how it develops through to an evaluation of the interpersonal interaction at the end. You may choose a client or a member of staff.

Record how you might improve the interaction as you go on – think of points like listening, reflective listening, non-verbal communications, questions and respect for individuals.

Ask your placement supervisor to observe your interaction when they can so that you can include their feedback in the report.

- **a record of your interaction with a group.** You may plan a group activity for children or older people. Again ask for an observer – you could arrange this with your tutor.

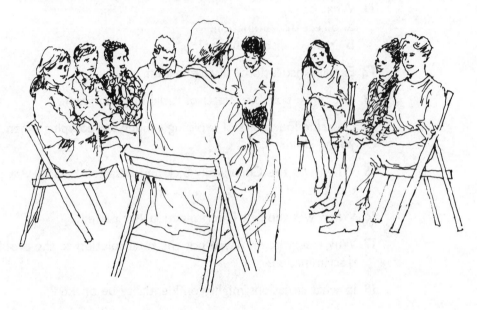

A group at work

- **a consideration of the possible effects of discriminatory behaviour** in your work placement:

  - an explanation of discrimination
  - imaginary examples of four bases of discrimination that *might* be found in the work place
  - a description of how the groups you are working with *might* be stereotyped
  - a brief description of the possible short- and long-term effects of such discrimination on an individual or a group
  - some statements concerning the policies and practices which exist inside and outside the establishment where you work to uphold equal rights

- **a comparison between your role in the care situation and in a purely social situation**. Think about how different you are in the workplace and at home. Think about the way clients respond to care, with examples from your work placement (while young children are at school they are within the care of the staff), the support systems you learnt about, the need to be a good communicator, the ethical issues which may have occurred and the *need for confidentiality*, particularly in the writing of this report. There is no need to use real names.

Answers to Activity 4.29, page 159

	Intention	Method	Effect
a	not racist	racist	racist
b	not racist	not racist	racist
c	not racist	not racist	racist

CHAPTER 5
Application of science in health and social care

Element 5.1: Explain the basic organisation and functions of human body systems

Element 5.2: Investigate observation and measurement of individuals in care settings

Element 5.3: Investigate the ways science is applied in care contexts

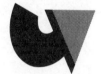

What is covered in this chapter

- Cells, tissues and organs
- The body systems
- Observation and measurement of clients
- Food, work and energy
- The effects of reduction of pressure in care contexts
- Muscle movement and levers in the body

These are the resources you will need for your Application of Science in Health and Social Care file:
- your own notes and observations
- evidence of research carried out and your responses to the activities in this chapter
- your answers to the review questions at the end of this chapter
- your completed Assignments A5.1, A5.2 and A5.3.

Introduction

In this chapter you will find biological and scientific information which will help you to understand some of the health problems and physical difficulties experienced by the people you will be looking after.

Look at any group of people and you will notice that individual humans look very different from each other. However, all contain the same basic features.

The final human form is influenced by:
- the size of the skeleton
- the shape of the muscles
- the amount of fat
- the age and sex of the individual.

There is a tendency for males to be taller than females. They have broader shoulders and more body hair. The fat is differently distributed: females are not as muscular as males and they have a wider pelvis to allow for childbirth.

Cells, tissues and organs

Cells

Most of the human body is made up from a jelly-like substance called **protoplasm**. It consists of about 80 per cent water, with the remainder being proteins, fats, oils and sugars.

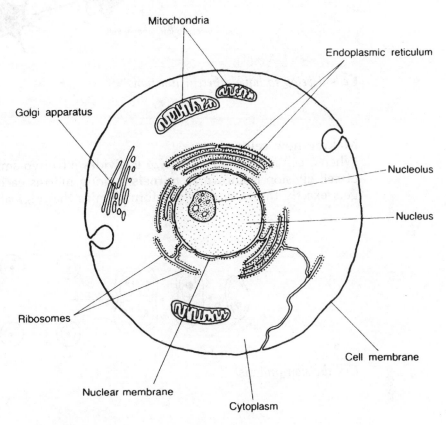

A typical animal cell

The protoplasm forms small units called **cells**. There are millions of cells.

> There are 50 000 000 000 000 cells in the human body. Most are so small it would take 100 000 to cover the head of a pin.

The cells make up the bones, muscles, skin and all the parts of the body. Everything we do involves millions of cells working together.

Each cell has its own function. For example, muscle cells are designed to move, skin cells to protect. Cells live, grow and finally die. And although they are so small, many are quite complex.

As the body grows, more and more cells are produced. Even when we are fully grown adults, new cells continue to be made to replace those which have worn out.

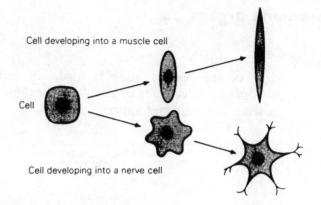

Cells develop to have different functions

Making new cells

When a cell reaches a certain size it divides into two smaller cells. This kind of cell division is known as **mitosis**. During mitosis each new cell produced gets exactly the same genetic information as the original cell.

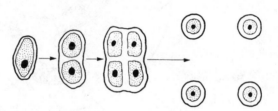

Cell division (mitosis)

Tissues

As we have already seen, not all cells are alike. Most cells are specialised to perform certain functions. For example nerve cells are specialised to conduct nerve impulses and muscle cells are specialised for contraction. Groups of specialised cells are called **tissues**.

There are four types of tissue:
● **epithelial tissues** – layers of cells which cover the external and internal surfaces of the body and line the insides of glands
● **muscle tissues** – made up from fibres which contract. The fibres are bound together with connective tissues which also connect muscles to bones and skin.
● **nervous tissues** – cells which conduct messages called nerve impulses. The cells are called **neurones**.
● **connective tissues** – cells which are embedded in a substance called matrix which they produce. Connective tissues connect tissues and organs together giving support and protection.

Organs

An **organ** consists of several tissues grouped together, for example the heart, which is made up of nervous tissue and cardiac muscle. Most organs are found in the body cavities:

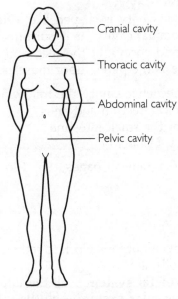

The body cavities

The cranial cavity
The main organ of the cranial cavity is the brain.

The thoracic cavity
The organs in the thoracic cavity are:
- trachea
- two bronchi
- two lungs
- heart
- aorta
- inferior and superior vena cava and numerous other blood vessels
- oesophagus
- lymph vessels and nodes
- nerves.

See the diagrams on pages 190, 192 and 195.

The abdominal cavity
This is the largest cavity in the body. It is oval-shaped, situated in the main part of the trunk between the thoracic cavity and the pelvis.

The organs in the abdominal cavity are:
- stomach
- small intestine (includes the duodenum, jejunum and ileum)
- large intestine (includes the caecum, appendix, colon and rectum)
- liver
- gall bladder

- bile ducts
- pancreas
- spleen
- kidney and ureters

- adrenal and suprarenal glands
- blood vessels
- lymph nodes.

See the diagram on pages 195 and 196.

The pelvic cavity

The pelvic cavity is shaped like a funnel and extends from the lower end of the abdominal cavity. It is surrounded by the pubic bones at the front, the sacrum and coccyx at the rear, and the innominate (hip) bones to each side. The base is the pelvic floor muscles.

Inside the pelvic cavity the following structures are found

- the colon, rectum and anus
- part of the small intestine
- urinary bladder

- lower parts of the ureters
- urethra
- male/female reproductive organs.

See the diagram on pages 195, 196 and 197.

The body systems

Where several organs work together, a **system** is formed. The systems in the human body are:

- **the skeletal system** – all the different bones in the body
- **the muscular system** – all the different muscles in the body
- **the central nervous system** – the brain, the spinal cord, cranial and spinal nerves
- **the respiratory system** – the lungs, the windpipe and the diaphragm
- **the cardio-vascular system** (or the circulatory system) – the heart, blood vessels and blood
- **the digestive system** – the oesophagus, stomach, intestines and associated glands, liver, pancreas, gall bladder
- **the urinary system** – the kidneys, ureters, bladder and urethra
- **the reproductive system** – male/female reproductive organs
- **the endocrine system** – the glands which release hormones into the bloodstream and which control many body functions
- **the skin.**

The skeletal system

The skeleton is the framework of the body. It is made up of 206 bones. The bones are rigid but the skeleton as a whole is flexible allowing the human body the full range of movement.

What does the skeleton do?
- Acts as a framework and support for soft tissues.
- Gives attachment to the muscles.
- Protects delicate organs.
- Makes red blood cells in the bone marrow.

The skeleton can be divided into two parts:
- **the axial skeleton** This is made up of:
  - the skull
  - the vertebral column (the spine)

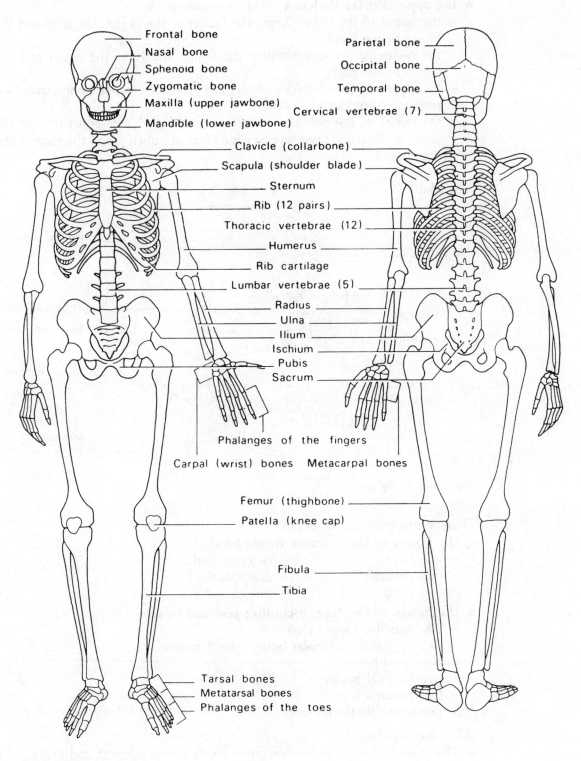

Frontal bone
Nasal bone
Sphenoid bone
Zygomatic bone
Maxilla (upper jawbone)
Mandible (lower jawbone)

Parietal bone
Occipital bone
Temporal bone
Cervical vertebrae (7)

Clavicle (collarbone)
Scapula (shoulder blade)
Sternum
Rib (12 pairs)
Thoracic vertebrae (12)
Humerus
Rib cartilage
Lumbar vertebrae (5)
Radius
Ulna
Ilium
Ischium
Pubis
Sacrum

Phalanges of the fingers
Carpal (wrist) bones   Metacarpal bones

Femur (thighbone)
Patella (knee cap)

Fibula
Tibia

Tarsal bones
Metatarsal bones
Phalanges of the toes

The skeletal system

— the sternum (breast bone)
— the ribs
— the thoracic cage

● **the appendicular skeleton** This is made up of:
  – the bones of the upper limbs: the humerus, the radius, the ulna and the bones of the hand
  – the bones of the lower limbs: the femur, the tibia, the fibula and the bones of the foot
  – the bones of the shoulder girdle: two clavicles (collar bones) and two scapulae (shoulder blades)
  – the bones of the pelvis: two innominate (hip) bones consisting of the ilium, ischium and pubic bones which fuse at puberty, and the sacrum and the coccyx.

The skull

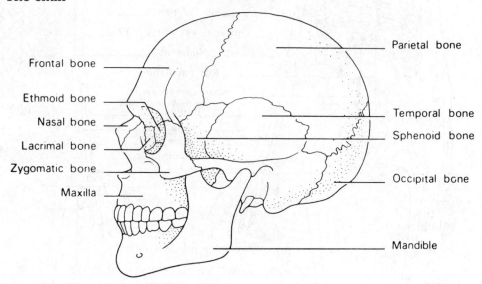

The bones of the skull

There are two groups of bones:
● **the bones of the cranium (brain box):**
  – one frontal   – one ethmoid
  – two parietal   – one sphenoid
  – two temporal   – one occipital
● **the bones of the face, including jaw and nose:**
  – two maxillae (upper jaw)
  – two zygomatic or malar bones (cheek bones)
  – two nasal bones
  – two lacrimal bones
  – two palatine bones
  – one mandible (lower jaw)

What does the skull do?
● The main hollow chamber has three levels which support and protect the brain.
● The bony eye sockets protect the eyes against injury and give attachment to the muscles which move the eyes.
● The temporal bones protect the delicate structures of the ears.
● Resonance is given to the voice by the sinuses in the bones of the face.

- The teeth are embedded in the upper and lower jaw.
- The mandible is the only movable bone in the skull. Food is chewed when it is raised and lowered by muscle action.

The vertebral column

The vertebral column, or spine, consists of 24 individually-shaped, moveable bones (vertebrae) with the sacrum and coccyx at the bottom.

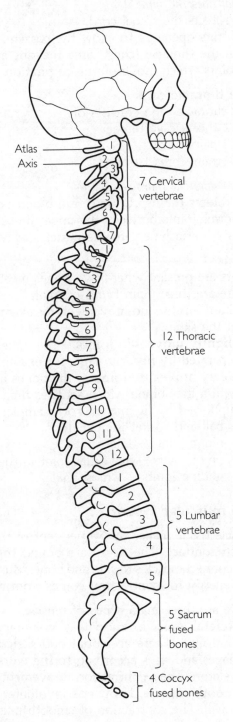

Atlas
Axis

7 Cervical vertebrae

12 Thoracic vertebrae

5 Lumbar vertebrae

5 Sacrum fused bones

4 Coccyx fused bones

The bones of the spine

The bodies of the bones are separated from each other by intervertebral discs made up of a jelly-like substance surrounded by fibrous material.

The vertebral column is divided into five parts. The bones of each part are numbered from the top downwards.

The first cervical vertebra is called the **atlas**, it articulates with the skull and rotates with the second cervical vertebra which is called the **axis**.

What does the spine do?
- Protects the spinal cord.
- Forms openings to allow the passage of the spinal nerves.
- In the thoracic (chest) area the ribs articulate with the vertebrae forming joints which move during respiration.

The thoracic cage
The thoracic cage consists of:
- 12 thoracic vertebrae
- 12 pairs of ribs
- sternum (breast bone).

What does the thoracic cage do?
- Protects the heart, lungs and blood vessels.
- Forms joints between the upper limbs and the axial skeleton.
- Gives attachment to the muscles of respiration.

Joints
Joints are present where two bones meet. They differ in the way they move. There are three main types of joint:
- **fixed joints** – no movement, for example sutures (joins) between the bones of the skull
- **slightly moveable joints** – the bones held together by strong ligaments separated by fibrocartilage, for example the sacroiliac joint
- **freely moveable joints** – the bones are in a fibrous capsule which is lined with a membrane which secretes fluid which acts as a lubricant. Joints are supported by ligaments. For example:
  - ball and socket joints – hips
  - hinge joints – knees
  - pivot joints – axis–atlas joint in the neck
  - gliding joints – wrists, ankles.

The muscular system

Muscle tissue makes up 50 per cent of the body weight. It consists of fibres which contract. The fibres are bound together by connective tissues which also connect muscles to skin and bone. Muscle cells contain contractive proteins. The energy for contraction comes from respiration.

There are three main types of muscle:
- **skeletal muscle**, known as voluntary muscle as it can be consciously controlled. There are about 600 skeletal muscles in the body, of different shapes and sizes according to the work they do. They are attached to the skeleton. Their contraction (movement) is rapid and powerful.
- **smooth muscle**, known as involuntary muscle, and cannot be controlled at will. The contraction of smooth muscle is smooth and slow. It is found in the walls of the intestines, blood vessels, uterus and bladder.

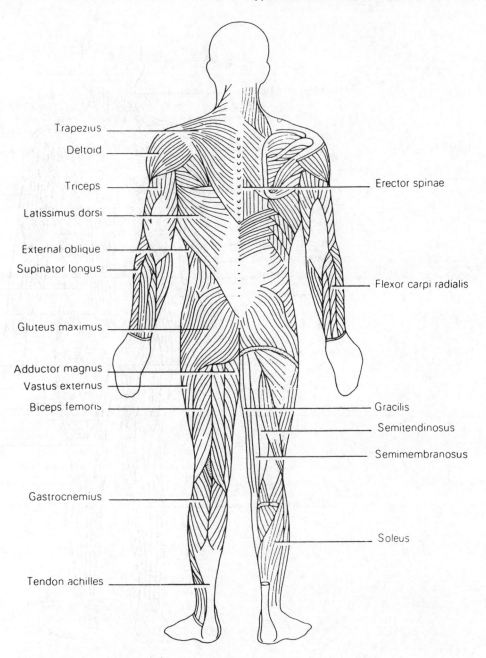

Trapezius

Deltoid

Triceps

Latissimus dorsi

External oblique

Supinator longus

Gluteus maximus

Adductor magnus

Vastus externus

Biceps femoris

Gastrocnemius

Tendon achilles

Erector spinae

Flexor carpi radialis

Gracilis

Semitendinosus

Semimembranosus

Soleus

The skeletal muscular system (viewed from the back)

- **cardiac muscle**, found only in the heart and arteries. The contraction of this muscle is rapid, powerful and continues rhythmically throughout life. It cannot be consciously controlled.

What do the skeletal muscles do?
Tendons attach skeletal muscles to bones. The muscles work in opposing pairs, one muscle contracting while the other relaxes in order to produce body movement.

What do the smooth muscles do?
They are involved in the movement of food through the intestines (peristalsis,

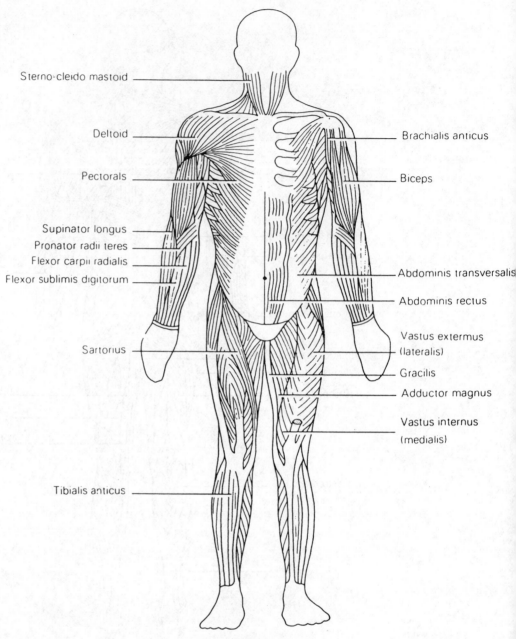

Sterno-cleido mastoid

Deltoid

Pectorals

Supinator longus
Pronator radii teres
Flexor carpii radialis
Flexor sublimis digitorum

Sartorius

Tibialis anticus

Brachialis anticus

Biceps

Abdominis transversalis

Abdominis rectus

Vastus extermus
(lateralis)

Gracilis

Adductor magnus

Vastus internus
(medialis)

The skeletal muscular system (viewed from the front)

see page 194), pumping blood through the blood vessels and contracting the uterus during childbirth.

What does the cardiac muscle do?
Its rhythmic contractions pump blood around the body.

For more about how muscles act as levers and move bones, see page 219.

The central nervous system

The central nervous system is made up of:
- the brain
- the spinal cord
- the spinal nerves
- the cranial nerves.

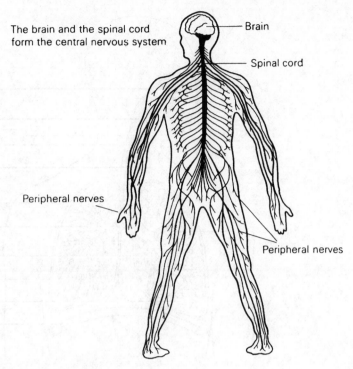

The central nervous system

What does the central nervous system do?
The central nervous system is the electro-chemical communications network of the body. Nerves transmit impulses between the central nervous system and other regions of the body. Each nerve is made up of neurones. Each neurone has three parts:
● cell body
● dendrites, which receive messages from other neurones
● an axon, which sends messages to other neurones or tissues.

Chemical signals are received from other neurones and these are conveyed as electrical impulses.

The brain
The brain weighs about 1.36 kg and contains ten thousand million nerve cells. There are three main regions in the brain:
● the **medulla oblongata** which controls vital body functions, such as breathing and digestion
● the **cerebellum** which maintains posture, balance and co-ordinates body movement
● the **cerebrum** which controls intelligence, the senses, memory, reasoning, etc.

What does the brain do?
It is the control centre for all the body's voluntary and involuntary acts.

The respiratory system

The parts of the system:
● nasal cavities
● pharynx
● larynx
● trachea

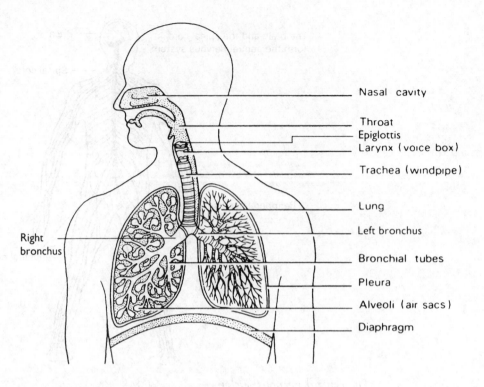

Nasal cavity

Throat
Epiglottis
Larynx (voice box)

Trachea (windpipe)

Lung

Left bronchus

Bronchial tubes

Pleura

Alveoli (air sacs)

Diaphragm

Right bronchus

The respiratory system

- lungs, which are made up of bronchi, bronchioles and alveoli, all surrounded by the pleura (a protective lining)
- intercostal muscles (between the ribs)
- diaphragm

What does the respiratory system do?
It supplies oxygen to the body cells and removes carbon dioxide. When we breathe in, air passes via the windpipe (trachea) through the narrower tubes (bronchi) to the lungs.

> During normal breathing, approximately 0.5 litres of air flows in and out of the lungs. This is known as **tidal air**.

What happens in the lungs?
The rib muscles and the diaphragm below the lungs operate the lungs like bellows, drawing air in and forcing it out alternately.

Each lung is made up of fine branching tubes called bronchioles which end up as tiny alveoli (air sacs). Gases cross the thin walls of the alveoli to and from the network of tiny blood vessels which surround them.

The lungs are grey in colour and spongey in appearance. The right lung has three lobes (sections) and the left lung has two lobes.

The diaphragm
This is a dome-shaped muscle which separates the thoracic and abdominal cavities. It is attached to the bones of the thorax (chest) and, when it contracts, it assists with inspiration.

Rate of breathing

Adults breathe about 15 times per minute. Each breath consists of:

- an inspiration (breathing in)
- an expiration (breathing out)
- a pause.

What controls respiration?

There is a special centre in the medulla oblongata of the brain. Nerve connections pass to the diaphragm and respiratory muscles.

The respiratory centre is very sensitive to the amount of carbon dioxide in the blood. If the amount rises, the centre is stimulated to send out impulses to the respiratory muscles to produce deeper and quicker breathing so that the carbon dioxide can be excreted more quickly.

The difference between air we breathe in and air we breathe out

	Inspired air	Expired air
Oxygen	21.0%	16.0%*
Carbon dioxide	0.04%	4.0%
Nitrogen and rare gases	78.0%	78.0%
Water vapour	Variable	Saturated

*Notice that expired air still contains 16 per cent oxygen, which is why mouth-to-mouth resuscitation is so effective.

The cardio-vascular system

The parts of the system:
- the heart
- the blood vessels:
  - arteries and arterioles
  - veins and venules
  - capillaries
- the blood
- the spleen.

What does the cardio-vascular system do?

The heart and the blood vessels together keep a continuous flow of blood around the body. It is also known as the circulatory system.

The heart

The heart is a muscular, conical organ which is situated in the middle of the thoracic cavity. A muscular wall, the **septum**, divides the right and left sides of the heart. A valve divides each side into two chambers: the **atria** and the **ventricles**

What does the heart do?

It pumps blood round the body to supply the cells with oxygen and nutrients.

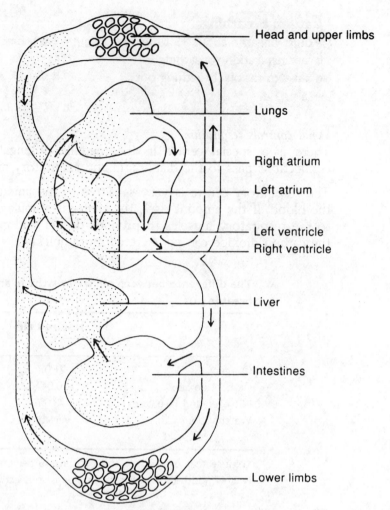

How the heart pumps blood around the body

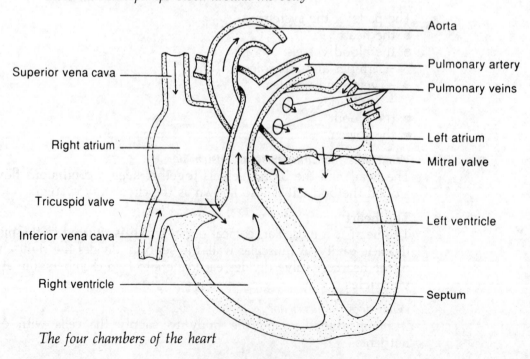

The four chambers of the heart

The heart muscle contracts, blood is squeezed through the atria and then through the ventricles.

Blood rich in oxygen from the lungs flows from the pulmonary veins into the left atria, through the left ventricles and then leaves the heart via the **aorta** to all the different parts of the body.

Blood which has been round the body and is lacking in oxygen flows from the **vena cava** into the right atrium, through the right ventricle and then via the pulmonary artery to the lungs to pick up more oxygen.

The direction of blood flow in the heart is controlled by valves:
- The valve between the right atrium and the right ventricle is called the **tricuspid valve**.
- The valve between the left atrium and the left ventricle is called the **mitral valve**.

These valves are supported by special tendons called chordae tendineae. In addition, semilunar valves are situated in the channels leading from the ventricles to the aorta and pulmonary artery.

> **Average heart beat per minute**
> 60–80 for adults, faster for younger children and babies. Exercise, stress and excitement all increase the heart rate.

The blood vessels
Blood is pumped to all parts of the body through a network of tubes called **arteries** and smaller tubes called **arterioles**.

Blood is returned to the heart by small tubes called **venules** which lead into larger tubes called **veins**.

Arterioles and venules are linked to each other by a network of very small blood vessels called **capillaries**.

Oxygen and carbon dioxide are exchanged between the body cells and the capillaries.

The blood
Blood is made up of straw-coloured transparent fluid called **plasma** in which different types of cells are suspended:
- red cells – carry oxygen and some carbon dioxide
- white cells – produces antibodies
- platelets – contribute to blood clotting.

Plasma makes up 55 per cent and cells 45 per cent of the blood volume.

What does blood do?
- It carries oxygen from the lungs to the tissues and carbon dioxide from the tissues to the lungs.
- It carries nutrients from the digestive tract to the tissues and waste materials to the excretory organs.
- It carries hormones to their targets.
- It carries antibodies to areas of infection.
- It carries the clotting factors to ruptured vessels to stop bleeding.

Blood is about 7 per cent of the adult body weight, with the proportion varying for women and children. A man weighing 70 kg would have 5.6 litres of blood. A new baby would have approximately 300 ml of blood.

The spleen

This dark purple organ which is 12 cm long and 7 cm wide is found in the left side of the abdomen under the diaphragm, between the stomach and the duodenum.

What does the spleen do?
- It breaks down worn out blood cells.
- It forms lymphocytes (white cells).
- It is part of the body's immune system.

The digestive system

Parts of the system:
- **the mouth**, including teeth, tongue and salivary glands
- **the pharynx**, a muscular bag concerned with swallowing and passing food onwards
- **the oesophagus**, a tube which receives food from the pharynx and passes it to the stomach
- **the stomach**, which lies in the upper part of the abdominal cavity. The entrance from the oesophagus is called the cardiac sphincter muscle and the exit to the small intestine is called the pyloric sphincter muscle.
- **the small intestine**, which is 6 m long and has three parts: the duodenum, the jejunum and the ileum. It leads to the large intestine.
- **the large intestine**, which is 1.5 m long. It consists of the caecum, appendix, colon, rectum and anus.

The system, which is 9 m in length, extends from the mouth to the rectum. Smooth muscles (see page 186) in the walls of the system force food along. This process is known as **peristalsis**.

What does the digestive system do?
The food we eat is broken down by the digestive system so that it can be absorbed into the blood stream.

What happens?
1 Food is chewed
2 Chewed food travels by the oesophagus to the stomach where it is churned up and liquidised.
3 Liquidised food passes through the small intestine where digestive juices from the pancreas and gall bladder break down the food particles further.
4 Absorption of nutritional materials takes place from the villi in the walls of the small intestine to the blood vessels.
5 Further absorption takes place in the large intestine.
6 Undigested food in the colon forms faeces that leave the body through the anus.

Organs which help with digestion
- **The liver**   This is the largest organ in the body. It weighs about 1.5 kg. It is found in the upper part of the abdominal cavity just below the diaphragm. It has two lobes, right and left.

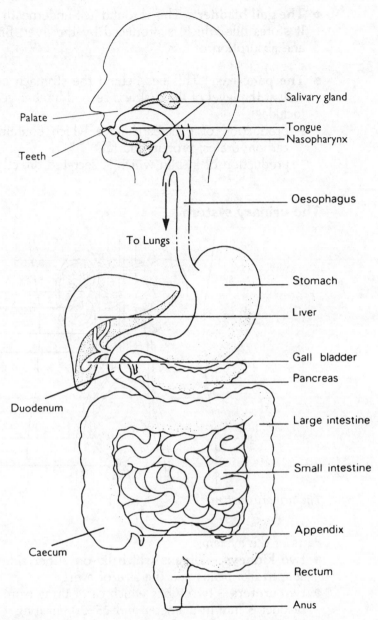

Palate

Teeth

Salivary gland

Tongue
Nasopharynx

Oesophagus

To Lungs

Stomach

Liver

Gall bladder
Pancreas

Duodenum

Large intestine

Small intestine

Appendix

Caecum

Rectum

Anus

The digestive system

The liver is a very active organ. Its main functions include:
- heat production
- secretion of bile
- converting stored fat into a form which it can be used by the tissues to provide energy
- breaking down protein from worn-out cells to form uric acid
- converting glucose to glycogen and vice versa thereby regulating the blood glucose level
- storage of vitamins including vitamin B_{12}, the anti-anaemic factor
- storage of iron and copper
- de-toxification of drugs and noxious substances
- metabolism of ethanol in alcoholic drinks.

- **The gall bladder**   This is found just underneath the right lobe of the liver. It stores bile which is produced by the liver. Bile assists in the digestion and absorption of fats.

- **The pancreas**   This lies behind the stomach across the back abdominal wall at the level of the first and second lumbar vertebrae. Its main functions include:
  - production of pancreatic juice which contains enzymes which digest carbohydrates, protein and fats
  - production of insulin which is secreted directly into the blood stream.

The urinary system

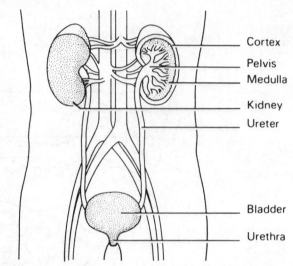

The urinary system

Parts of the system:
- two **kidneys** – organs which lie on either side of the vertebral column, shaped like beans and the size of a fist
- two **ureters** – two tubes which carry urine from the kidney to the urinary bladder 3 mm in diameter and 25–30 cm long
- **bladder** – a reservoir for urine which lies in the pelvic cavity
- **urethra** – a tube which extends from the neck of the bladder to the exterior. In the female the urethra is 4 cm long. In the male the urethra is part of the urinary and reproductive systems.

What does the urinary system do?
It gets rid of body waste in the form of urine.

What happens?
1 The renal arteries carry the blood to the kidneys.
2 The blood is filtered in the kidneys and urine is produced.
3 Urine is passed via the ureters to the bladder where it is stored until it is passed through the urethra.

- **150–180 litres of fluid are processed by the kidneys each day.**
- **The urinary system passes 1.5 litres of urine each day.**

The reproductive system

It is useful to know the correct names for the various parts of the male and female reproductive organs and to understand their functions.

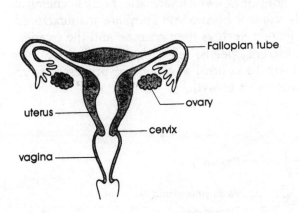

The female reproductive system

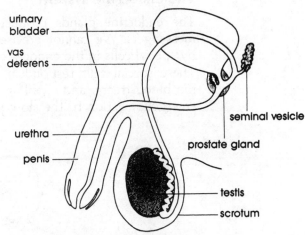

The male reproductive system

The sex organs of males and females are located in the pelvic cavity (see page 181):

● **Sperm** are produced in the testes.
● **Ova** (egg cells) are produced in the ovaries.

Each month one ovum (usually, but sometimes several) becomes ripe and is released from the ovaries into a nearby fallopian tube where tiny hairs help the ovum drift down towards the **uterus** (womb). The ovum remains in a state of ripeness for about two days. If it does not meet a sperm cell during this time, it dies. Like the nucleus of the sperm cell, the ovum contains only one set of chromosomes.

Fertilisation of the ovum

During sexual intercourse, a small amount of fluid containing millions of sperm cells is expelled through the man's penis and deposited in the woman's vagina, just below the uterus. The sperm make their way to the ovum which is present in the fallopian tube. Assisted by movements of the vagina and uterus, some of the sperm manage to swim into the uterus. Only the very strongest sperm pass through the uterus into the fallopian tubes. Finally, a few hundred sperm approach the ovum, although only one sperm cell will be successful in fertilising the ovum.

Stages of fertilisation

1 The sperm cells release digestive enzymes to help penetrate the ovum's jelly coating.
2 A few sperm cells pass straight through the jelly coating and reach the ovum.
3 One sperm cell penetrates the membrane surrounding the ovum. Other sperm are prevented from entering by changes in the membrane and protective jelly-like coating.

4 The nucleus of the sperm cell moves towards the nucleus of the ovum and the two nuclei merge into one.

5 The fertilised ovum moves from the fallopian tube and implants itself in the uterus.

The endocrine system

The endocrine glands produce hormones, which are the body's chemical messengers. We cannot precisely control hormones. They are manufactured by special cells in the endocrine glands, such as the pancreas, and the ovaries. These special cells respond at different speeds, releasing them directly into the bloodstream, and enabling them to control a variety of processes from emergency action to the slow process of growth.

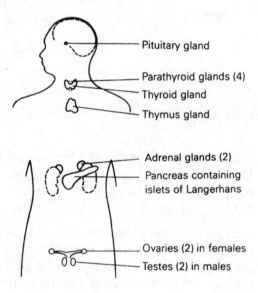

The endocrine system

The hypothalamus (in the brain) and the pituitary glands control the hormone system by regulating the amount of each hormone present in the blood. They do this using a balancing mechanism called **feedback**. Virtually all body processes controlled by hormones involve feedback systems.

Sometimes hormones work together, **synergism**, and sometimes against each other, **antagonism**

Some glands produce several hormones which control different processes. The table opposite summarises the processes controlled by hormones.

Hormones and health
Medical conditions related to hormonal imbalance include:
● diabetes mellitus – too little insulin
● diabetes insipidus – too little ADH
● pituitary dwarfism – too little growth hormone
● cretinism in children – too little thyroxin
● myxoedema in adults – too little thyroxine
● thyrotoxicosis – too much thyroxine.

Processes controlled by hormones

Gland/organ	Hormone	Process
Pituitary gland	Trophic hormones	Stimulate production of hormones from other glands
	Somatotrophic (growth hormone or GH)	Growth of long bones in limbs
	Prolactin	Milk production
	Luteinising hormone (LH)	Controls menstrual cycle, triggers ovulation
		Controls sex hormones from testes
	Follicle stimulatory hormone (FSH)	Control of menstrual cycle
		Starts the ripening of ova
		Assists in control of sperm production
Hypothalamus	Hormone releasing factors	Stimulates pituitary gland to produce hormones
	Anti-diuretic hormones (ADH) (stored in the pituitary gland)	Control of water balance
	Oxytocin (stored in the pituitary gland)	Helps uterine contraction in childbirth and stimulates the let-down reflex for breastfeeding
Thyroid gland	Thyroxine	Controls rate of body processes and heat production and energy production from food, controls the growth and development of the nervous system
Parathyroid glands	Parathormone (or parathyroid hormone)	Controls the amount of calcium in blood and bones
Pancreas	Insulin	Controls blood sugar
Adrenal glands	Adrenaline	Controls emergency action, response to stress
	Cortisol	Stress control
		Conversion of fats, proteins and carbohydrates to glucose
	Aldosterone	Acts on the kidneys to control salt and water balance
	Androgens	Stimulates male sex hormones and characteristics (bear growth, deepening of voice, muscle development)
Testes	Testosterone	Control of sperm
		Growth and development of male features at puberty
		Beard growth
Ovaries	Progesterone	Helps control normal progess of pregnancy
		Interacts with FSH and LH and oestrogen to control the menstrual cycle
	Oestrogen	Controls the development of female features at puberty
		Interacts with LH and FSH and progesterone to control menstrual cycle
	Placental hormones (pregnancy only)	Control normal progress of pregnancy
		Oestrogen and progesterone start milk production
Stomach wall	Gastrin	Starts acid production by stomach
Small intestine	Enterogasterine	Turns off acid production by the stomach
	Secretin	Triggers release of digestive enzymes from pancreas

199

Activity 5.1

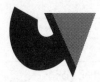

Find out as much as you can about one of the medical conditions related to hormonal imbalance. Write a concise report of the effects of the condition on the sufferer and the treatments which may be given.

The skin

The skin is the largest organ in the body.

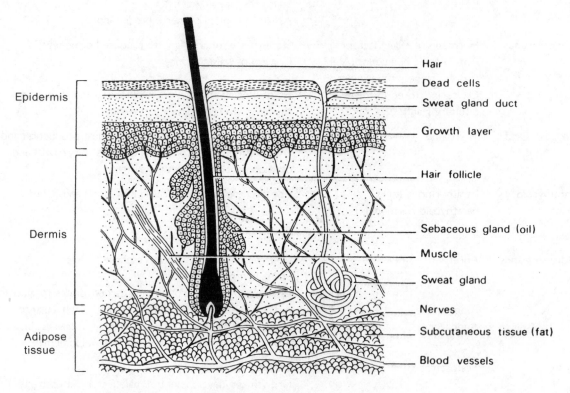

The structure of the skin

The parts of the skin:
- **Epidermis** This is made up of several layers:
  - The top layer is the cornified layer. It consists of flat, dead cells which are constantly flaking off.
  - The lowest layer is the malphigian layer. It is alive and growing. It contains the skin pigment melanin which helps to protect the skin from damage caused by ultra violet light.
- **Dermis** This is a very complex layer of tissue. It contains irregular ridges (dermal papillae) which give each individual a unique set of finger prints. Contained in this layer are:
  - blood vessels
  - lymph vessels

  - sensory nerve endings (touch, pain, pressure, temperature)
  - hair follicles
  - sebaceous glands
  - sweat glands
  - connective tissue for elasticity of skin.
- **Adipose tissue** A layer of subcutaneous fat which acts an as insulator and also as a source of stored food.

What does the skin do?
- It helps to maintain a constant body temperature.
- It also gives protection from:
  - injury
  - sunlight
  - water loss
  - disease.
- It contains sense organs to detect:
  - pain
  - pressure
  - temperature.
- It makes vitamin D.
- It makes hair.

Observation and measurement of individuals

Observation and assessment of individuals in care settings is an intrinsic part of caring because:
- clients must be assessed so that carers can make appropriate responses and work out and modify individual care plans
- measurement of body parts and functions can be noted and compared with norms and averages
- improvement or deterioration in a client's condition can be detected.

How do we know where to start? Firstly carers must have a lot of commonsense. As you become more experienced as a care worker, your observational skills will develop. You will learn to use your initiative.

What is normal? What is not normal? What is the person who is being cared for usually like? Again experience and knowledge of the person will help you. Listen carefully to what clients and relatives have to say.

Remember when carrying out any task or procedure you should:
- make an initial **assessment**
- **plan** what to do
- **implement** your plan (do the task)
- **evaluate** what has taken place.

Your observational skills will help you to modify care plans.

Observation

Intuition or 'gut feeling'?
Sometimes you might think that things are not quite right. It is always worth taking an extra look or investigating further. Ask someone who is more experienced for help or advice.

Use your senses

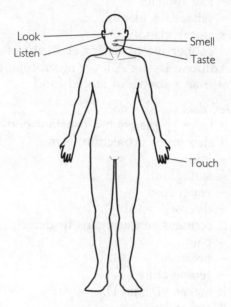

Here are some of the observations carers should make during their day-to-day care of clients:

- Is the client happy, sad, bored, dejected?
- What is the client's attitude to other people and his/her surroundings?
- How mobile is the client?
- Is the client anxious or tense?
- Can the client see?
- Can the client hear?
- Is the client able to smell and taste?
- Is the client able to talk or are methods of non-verbal communication used?
- Is the client clean? Is there any body odour?
- Does the client suffer from halitosis?
- Does the client have a good appetite? Are there any difficulties with eating and drinking?
- Does the client suffer from excessive thirst?
- Does the client have dentures?
- Is the client mentally alert?
- Are there any abnormal behaviour patterns?
- What is the state of the skin? Are there any spots, rashes or pressure sores?
- Is the client incontinent?
- Is the client in any pain?
- Are there any abnormalities in urine, faeces or sputum?

More specific observations of temperature, pulse, respirations, urine and body measurements may be required.

Body measurements

We are all familiar with our own body size and shape. Looking around we can see there is an immense variation in others' sizes and shapes. We are all individuals.

Factors influencing body measurements include:
- inheritance
- age
- sex
- nutrition
- environment
- economic circumstances.

Average or 'normal'?
What do we mean? Always remember, it is possible to be different from the average height, weight, length, etc., but still be within normal limits.

The following measurements are used as a guide to an individual's progress:
- height
- weight
- head circumference
- body fat
- vision
- hearing.

Measurement and assessment of babies and children

Measurement and assessment starts immediately after birth with the Agpar score which assesses a newborn baby's condition.

The Agpar score
The method is based on heart rate, respirations, muscle tone, colour and reflex response to stimulation recorded 1, 5 and 10 minutes after birth. If the score is less than 7 at 1 minute, less than 8 at 5 minutes and less than 10 at 10 minutes, then resuscitation and special care are needed. The Agpar score is used in conjunction with other methods of assessment.

The Agpar scale

Heart rate	Respiratory effort	Muscle tone	Colour	Reflex irritability	Score
Over 100	Strong cry	Good, active movement	Completely pink	Vigorous withdrawal of leg, normal cry	2
Below 100	Slow, irregular breathing	Fair, some limb flexion	Baby pink, limbs blue	Slight withdrawal, whimper	1
Absent	Absent	Limp	Blue/pale	Absent	0

Weight
The average weight for a newborn baby is 3.5 kg. The largest recorded live-born baby weighed in at 9.3 kg (20 lb 8 oz)!

Babies should be weighed regularly, as weight gain and contentment are signs that they are being fed adequately.

Suggested times for weighing:
- months 1 and 2 – weigh once a week
- months 3 to 12 – weigh once a month
- over 12 months – weigh at six-monthly intervals.

A baby can be expected to double his or her birth weight in the first six months, and treble it by the end of the first year.

Too fat?
Children will become fat if they over-eat and do not have enough exercise. Both children and adults can tend to over-eat if they are worried, bored or insecure. It is unwise to give a small child excessive quantities of sweets or fattening foods. Excessive weight gain in the early months makes it more likely that a child will be overweight in later life.

Height

The average length of a new baby is 50 cm. By the second birthday, a child is likely to have reached half his or her eventual adult height.

The table below shows height and weight from birth to 5 years.

Average heights and weights – birth to 5 years

Age	Weight		Height	
	kg	lb	cm	in.
Girls				
Birth	3.4	7.5	53.0	20.9
3 months	5.6	12.3	—	—
6 months	6.9	15.2	—	—
9 months	8.7	19.2	—	—
1 year	9.7	21.4	74.2	29.2
2 years	12.2	26.9	85.6	33.7
3 years	14.3	31.5	93.0	36.6
4 years	16.3	35.9	100.4	39.5
5 years	18.3	40.3	107.2	42.4
Boys				
Birth	3.5	7.7	54.0	21.3
3 months	5.9	13.1	—	—
6 months	7.9	17.4	—	—
9 months	9.2	20.3	—	—
1 year	10.2	22.5	76.3	30.0
2 years	12.7	28.0	86.9	34.2
3 years	14.7	32.4	94.2	37.1
4 years	16.6	36.6	101.6	40.0
5 years	18.5	40.7	108.3	42.6

It can be dangerous for parents or carers to become pre-occupied with a child's size. If a child is happy, contented, growing and energetic there is nothing to worry about.

Activity 5.2

a Within your group, ask everyone to find out what their birth weight was. Work out the average birth weight for the group.

b Ask your parent(s) what length you were when you were born (perhaps you still have a record). Compare your length at birth with your height now.

c What is your present height and weight? Compare them with the graph below. Are you the appropriate weight for your height?

d Within your group, calculate the average heights and weights.

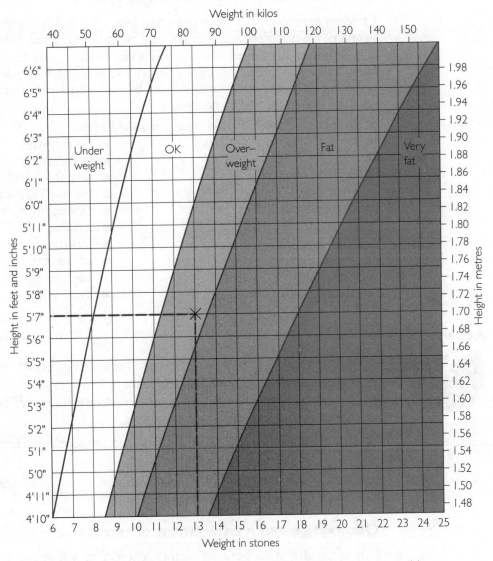

- - - For example, a person who is 5'7" tall and weighs 13 stones is overweight

This is a graph showing the heights and weights of adults. To find out whether you need to lose or gain weight, draw a line up from your weight and across from your height. Put a cross where the two lines meet.

Head circumference

The average head circumference of a new baby is 35 cm. The size and shape of a baby's head can cause anxiety to carers or parents. Larger babies will have larger heads and parents with large, small or unusual-shaped heads may find babies take after them.

There are some important conditions, however, which relate to head size and which require immediate diagnosis:
- hydrocephalus, characterised by an enlarged head, often associated with other conditions, such as spina bifida
- microcephaly – small head, may be associated with brain defects.

Keeping records

Health care workers plot children's height, weight and head circumference on special charts, called **centile charts** (see opposite).

Children are monitored from birth to 5 years by health visitors (see page 122). In many cases parents and carers will be given a Child Health Record. This is a working document about the child's health, growth and development. Health staff and parents or carers participate in filling in the details. The parents or carers keep the book and it may be shown to other child care workers, such as a child minder if necessary.

Contents of a typical child health record include:
- child's name and address
- family details
- health problems
- birth details
- when to call the doctor
- well-baby services and screening tests
- immunisations
- growth charts
- review pages
- hearing test
- heart check
- hospital visits
- teeth and dental visits
- development
- feeding
- services for children
- advice on aspects of care, such as feeding
- local information.

Activity 5.3

a In your local area, find out how child health care records are kept. See if you can obtain a copy of a typical record.

b Do your parents still have your own child health record? Look at it and compare it with a more recent record.

Medical and developmental checks continue throughout childhood through local doctors, clinics and the School Health Service.

Observation and measurement of excreta

It is often useful to observe clients' excreta as variations from normal may indicate certain medical conditions. Highly specialised tests are carried out by laboratory staff.

The table on page 208 shows some of the normal values and variations which carers should note and report.

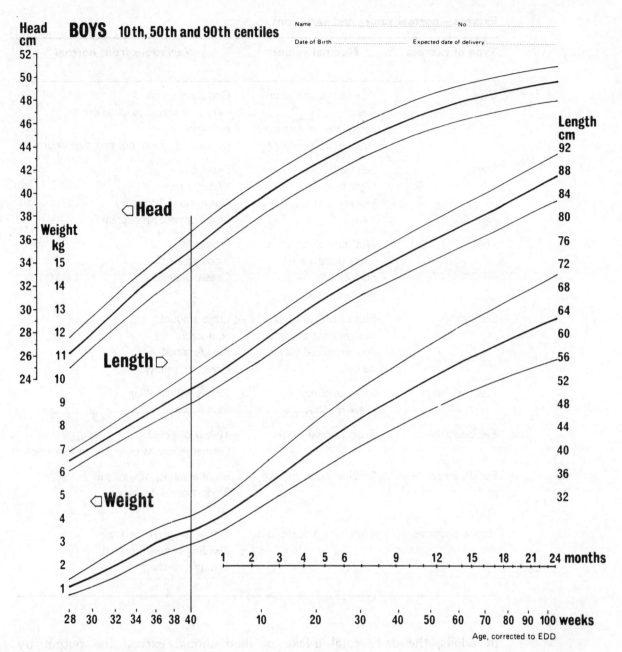

An example of a centile chart for a boy. This one combines all three measurements (weight, length and head circumference) on a single chart

Measuring output

To find out whether a person is drinking and excreting enough fluid, it may be necessary to measure their urinary output over a 24-hour period. In addition, if all drinks consumed are measured and recorded, fluid intake and output can be compared. This is known as a **fluid balance**.

Times when intake and output are carefully monitored include:
- an elderly person who is reluctant to drink
- an elderly person or small child who is suffering from diarrhoea and vomiting.

Excreta – normal values and variations

Type of excreta	Normal values	Variations from normal
Urine	Pale yellow in colour Clear Faint smell of ammonia Amount 1500 ml/day	Dark concentrated Very pale and copious amounts Evil smell Containing blood, pus or other debris
Faeces	Semi-solid Light brown Usually passed once a day	Diarrhoea Watery, green Constipated: hard, dry Blood or mucous present
Vomit	Not normal to vomit Small possets are normal after feeds in small babies	Projectile Blood-stained Green, watery
Sputum	Not usually produced in significant amounts Any produced would be clear	Large amounts Foul smell Blood-stained Green or yellow
Nasal discharge	Small amounts Clear mucous	Green, evil-smelling Blood-stained
Eye discharge	Tears normally clear	Yellow or green Discharge, crusts especially in morning
Ear discharge	Small amounts of wax	Large amounts of wax, pus Blood-stained discharge Foul smell
Vagina discharge	Clear or white mucous	Yellow or green discharge Bleeding between periods Irritating discharge

In adults, the daily total intake of fluid should exceed the output by approximately 90 ml, as fluid is also lost by respiration and sweating.

In hospital, fluid balance charts are used to record all intake, including intravenous fluids and all output, including vomit and watery stools.

Chemical tests
Sometimes special tests are used to detect the presence of specific substances in urine:
- protein
- blood
- sugar
- acetone
- bile
- pus.

The presence of such substances will indicate an abnormality. Small, chemically-impregnated sticks are used for these tests. The stick is dipped in the urine and the colour change is compared with a chart.

Special bags and collecting devices are available for people who are unable to co-operate in producing a specimen and for collecting urine from babies.

Measuring body temperature

The normal body temperature is between 36 and 37°C. Even when the environmental temperature changes markedly a human's body temperature will stay constant. A healthy adult is able to maintain body temperature by balancing heat loss from the skin with type of food eaten and the clothing worn.

Problems arise when the balance of heat loss and heat gain breaks down. This may result in:

- **pyrexia** – a body temperature of 40°C or more is considered to be dangerously high. At 41°C death will occur.
- **hypothermia** – a body temperature below the normal range may accompany exposure or shock. A body temperature of 34°C or below is dangerously low. Death occurs at 28–30°C.

For more about the regulation of body temperature, see pages 211–12.

Four main types of thermometer are available for measuring body temperature:

- **clinical thermometers** – the traditional thermometers made from glass, containing mercury
- **digital thermometers** – very accurate thermometers, operated by batteries, giving a digital readout
- **disposable thermometers** – not as accurate as clinical or digital thermometers but very safe and easy to use. When the thermometer is placed under the tongue the dots representing the temperature change colour. The thermometer is discarded after use
- **forehead thermometers** – heat-sensitive strips or discs which are placed on the forehead for 15 seconds. They are re-usable.

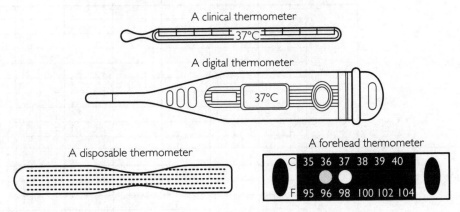

Types of thermometer

The type of thermometer used will depend upon the circumstances and degree of accuracy required.

The thermometer should **never** be placed in the mouth in the following situations:

- if the client is unconscious

- if the client is a baby or small child
- if the client suffers from fits
- if the client is confused
- if the client has injuries to or infection of the mouth.

When taking temperatures, follow the instructions specific to the type of thermometer you are using. Note the temperature carefully, excessively high or low temperatures must be brought to the attention of the carer who is in charge immediately.

Recording body temperature

In hospital, temperatures are recorded on charts at regular time intervals. Often several observations can be shown on the same chart (see below).

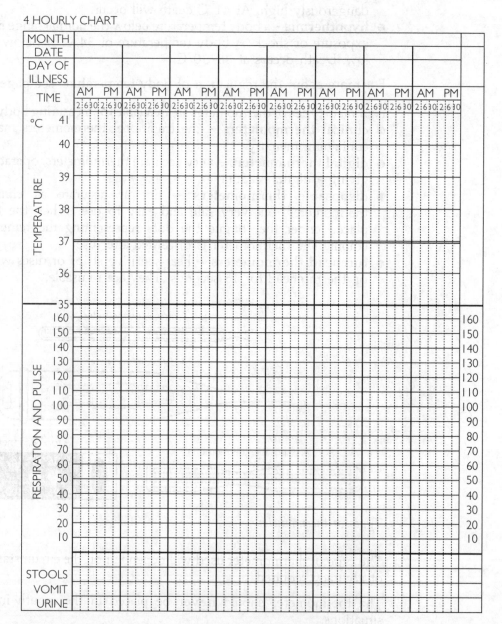

An example of a recording chart used in a hospital

The regulation of body temperature: What happens?

- A system of cells in the hypothalamus of the brain respond to the temperature of the circulating blood and information from temperature receptors in the skin.
- Vascular changes take place in the skin. When blood vessels constrict heat is conserved and when they dilate heat is lost.
- Sweat evaporates from the skin and has a cooling effect.
- Heat is also lost in the air we breathe out and excreta passed.

Problems arise when the balance between heat loss and heat gain are disturbed. The body's response to infection is a rise in temperature above 37°C, known as **pyrexia** (fever). If, on the other hand, the body loses more heat than can be produced and the temperature falls below 35° C **hypothermia** results.

Observation and treatment of hypothermia in an elderly person

The body temperature can fall below normal bringing about a sleepy state which can lead to death. Elderly people who live alone are prone to suffer from hypothermia.

Signs of hypothermia include:
- drowsiness
- slurred speech
- pale, cold skin
- unsteady movements
- slow, shallow breathing
- body temperature 35°C or below (a special low reading thermometer will be needed to check this).

This is a very serious situation and medical help should be summoned. Meanwhile, the elderly person should be wrapped in blankets and given a warm drink and the room should be warmed.

Observation and treatment of hypothermia in a newborn baby

Until the heat regulating mechanism in the brain is fully developed, a baby relies on the temperature of his or her surroundings to maintain body temperature. If the room where the baby is seems cold to you, it is certainly far too cold for the baby. A baby who is suffering from hypothermia may actually have quite rosy cheeks, but the skin will feel very cold to touch. Typically, the baby will be:
- lethargic
- immobile
- unresponsive
- not feeding.

Urgent medical help is required in this situation. Meanwhile, warm the room and warm the baby gradually.

- Large amounts of heat are lost from the head – elderly people may have thin hair or be bald, and the head of a baby is a large proportion of the body. Therefore the head should be kept warm.
- Special room thermometers are available for use in homes of elderly people or in babies' bedrooms.

Treatment of fever (pyrexia)
The aim is to prevent the temperature from rising to a dangerously high level:
- give cool drinks
- remove excessive clothing and bed clothes
- you can cool the client further by sponging with tepid water or use an electric fan.

The effects of excessive heat
In dry conditions, when we sweat evaporation from the surface of the skin takes place quickly. In humid conditions, where there is very little breeze, sweat evaporates and cools the skin very slowly. In these sort of conditions the body temperature may rise out of control and if it exceeds 41°C collapse and death may occur.

If people take a lot of exercise in a hot climate they lose large amounts of water and salt causing the blood to become thick and fail to circulate properly. The loss of salt causes muscle cramps.

Long periods of hard physical work in hot climates can result in a sudden failure of the ability to sweat. This is known as **heat stroke** which, if not reversed by moving the victim to a cool place, can result in an uncontrollable rise in temperature and possible death.

Activity 5.4

a Explain the signs you would see in an old person suffering from hypothermia. How would you deal with the situation?

b What do you consider to be a suitable temperature for a room in an ordinary home?

Measuring the pulse
Each time the heart beats to pump blood (see page 191), a wave passes along the walls of the arteries. This wave is the **pulse** and it can be felt at any point in the body where a large artery crosses a bone just beneath the skin.

The pulse is usually counted at the radial artery in the wrist or the carotid artery in the neck (see page 61).

Taking a pulse
The finger tips (but not the thumb tips) are placed over the site where the pulse is being taken. The beats are counted for a full minute and then recorded. Normally the rhythm is regular and the volume is sufficient to make the pulse easily felt.

The three main observations which are made on the pulse are:
- rate
- rhythm
- strength.

The average adult pulse rate varies between 60 and 80 beats per minute, while a young baby has a heart rate of about 140 beats per minute.

An increased pulse rate may indicate recent exercise, emotion, infection, blood or fluid loss, shock and heart disease.

Activity 5.5

a In your group, practise taking pulse rates.

b Make an accurate recording of each group member's pulse rate.

c Calculate the average pulse rate for your group.

Measuring respiration

Changes in the volume of air breathed in and out of the lungs can be measured. This is useful for detecting any obstruction to the air flow. Various measurements can be taken, including **vital capacity**.

Vital capacity

This is the volume of air which is breathed out after a person has breathed in as fully as possible. Normal vital capacity is approximately 4–5 litres for healthy, young adults. It is higher in males than females. It is reduced in cases of lung disease, such as bronchitis.

Measurement of vital capacity is made using a spirometer.

Exercising regularly will increase the maximum amount of air that can be breathed in per minute. Breathing becomes more efficient so that fewer breaths are taken to move the same amount of air.

Observations on respiration

The most important observation to be made concerning respiration is to establish that it is in fact taking place and that it is effective. You will probably have learned about this in First Aid.

The average adult respiratory rate is 16–18 breaths per minute. A child will breathe more rapidly, 24–40 times per minute. Respiratory rates should be recorded when clients are not aware that a count is taking place.

When respiration is failing:
● the client's skin will look pale or blue
● he may gasp for breath,
● he may produce deep sighing breaths or short shallow breaths
● his limbs may twitch
● unconsciousness may occur
● finally, respirations may cease completely.

Make sure you report any adverse changes in ill clients to your supervisor immediately.

Activity 5.6

a What do you understand by 'being observant'?

b List ten observations which a carer might make about an elderly client.

c List ten observations that a carer might make about a nursery school child?

d What is the normal body temperature?

e   What is a dangerously high body temperature?

f   What is a dangerously low body temperature?

g   State one instance when the body temperature would be raised.

h   Describe two types of thermometer which you have seen.

i   How could you tell if a person's temperature was raised if you did not have a thermometer?

k   When would you **not** place a thermometer in a client's mouth?

l   State three sites other than the mouth where the body temperature could be recorded.

m   On graph paper plot the following information:

Time	Temperature (°C)
1 p.m.	37
2 p.m.	40
3 p.m.	36
4 p.m.	37.8
5 p.m.	39
6 p.m.	35.5
7 p.m.	37.6
8 p.m.	36.8

Convert the times to the 24-hour clock.

n   What is the average adult pulse rate?

o   What is the average pulse rate for a baby of 6 months?

p   Name three observations which are made when checking the pulse.

q   When would you expect a client to have a very rapid pulse rate?

r   What is the average respiratory rate for an adult?

s   What would you observe about a client's breathing?

Food, work and energy

Nutrients and dietary requirements are discussed in Chapter 1. The food which humans and animals eat comes originally from green plants. Plants make their food by a process called **photosynthesis**.

Photosynthesis

In this process, the green parts of plants use energy from sunlight to combine carbon dioxide with water, making sugar. Oxygen is given off as a waste product during the process.

What do plants do with the sugar?
- They use it for energy.
- They make carbohydrates.
- They store it as sugar starch or fat.

How plants and animals differ

Plants	Animals
Contain chlorophyll, making them green	Do not contain chlorophyll
Make their own food (photosynthesis)	Eat ready-made food
Give out oxygen by day and carbon dioxide by night	Produce carbon dioxide but not oxygen
Grow in length	Grow in all parts of the body
Rooted to the spot	Move about
No nervous system	Have a nervous system

Food chains and webs

Green plants are known as **producers**, because they make food. The plants are eaten by an animal (the **primary consumer**). That animal may then be eaten by another animal (the **secondary consumer**). This feeding relationship is known as a **food chain**. Humans are at the end of the food chain.

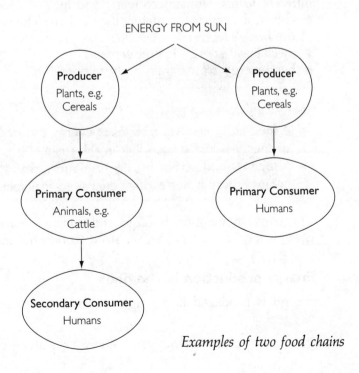

Examples of two food chains

Food chains are quite simple to follow. However, most animals have several sources of food, some eating both plants and other animals. This complex feeding relationship can be shown as a **food web**.

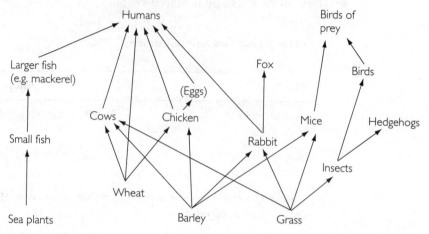

An example of a food web

Decomposers

These are organisms which break down the bodies of dead plants and animals so that they can be absorbed by plants and then pass back into the food chain. Examples of decomposers are bacteria, fungi and scavengers.

Transfer of energy

Energy gives us the power to do work. Our body cells are hard at work all the time and without energy they would die. Food is a means of transferring energy as well as materials. As energy is transferred it is converted into different forms. Humans convert food into:

- chemical energy for metabolism (all the chemical processes that occur in the body)
- mechanical energy for movement
- heat energy to maintain body temperature.

More about food chains

- A food chain involves a series of energy transfers. A considerable amount of energy is lost at each link in the chain.
- A food chain does not usually have more than three or four links, because there is not enough energy to maintain more.

The world population is large and constantly increasing. If there is to be enough food for everyone, we need to become more energy efficient.

Energy production in the body

Energy is produced if the right substances are present: food (glucose) and oxygen:

$$\text{glucose} + \text{oxygen} = \text{energy} + \text{water} + \text{carbon dioxide}$$

What happens to the energy which is produced?

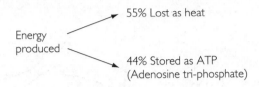

Energy
produced → 55% Lost as heat

→ 44% Stored as ATP
(Adenosine tri-phosphate)

But what is adenosine triphosphate? It is a compound which combines with energy to allow the energy to be easily transported to the parts of the body which need it.

Energy in food

Foods produce different amounts of energy. The total amount of energy required by a person each day varies according to:

- sex
- age
- occupation
- body size.

Measuring energy

Energy is measured in either joules (1000 joules [j] = 1 kilojoule [k]) or kilocalories (kcal). Of the nutrients, fats are the richest source of energy.

Activity 5.7

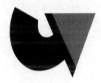

Find a table of energy requirements for people of different ages and occupations. Compare the daily energy requirements for:

a a labourer

b a pensioner.

Write up your findings.

The effects of reduction of pressure in care contexts

Friction is the force that stops materials sliding across each other. There is friction between our hands when they are rubbed together and friction between shoes and the ground when we walk. Friction is necessary to give our shoes a grip on the ground. Friction is partly due to minute bumps in the surfaces and partly due to atoms in the two materials which tend to stick together.

If clients have impaired mobility and are constantly sitting or lying in one position, possibly needing a lot of help to change position, they may be prone to pressure sores. A pressure sore is a break in the skin caused by pressure or friction. Certain types of client are most likely to develop pressure sores, including those who:

- are very ill
- are overweight
- are unconscious
- have broken bones
- are paralysed
- are dying
- are incontinent
- are emaciated.

217

Some parts of the body are more prone to pressure, and pressure sores, than others:

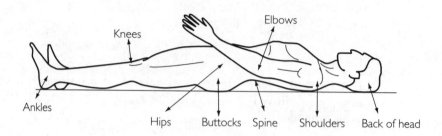

The areas of the body which are subject to pressure

Prevention of pressure sore

- Relieve pressure every two hours by altering the position of the client.
- Keep the skin clean and dry.
- Make sure sheets, cushions, etc. are clean, dry and free from crumbs and other irritants.
- Use rings, fleecy pads and pillows to relieve pressure.
- Barrier cream is useful to protect the skin of incontinent clients.
- Great care should be taken when moving and handling clients.
- Signs of redness or soreness should be reported to the person in charge immediately.

Muscle movement and levers in the body

To help you to understand the principles of safe lifting and moving, it will help to know about the body's mechanism for lifting and moving.

How muscles move bones

The skeletal muscles (see pages 187–8) are attached to the skeleton (see pages 182–6), and their job is to pull on the bones to produce movement and to keep the body in the right position. They work under instruction from the brain, their movement is voluntary and they tire quickly.

Skeletal muscles are attached to bones by pieces of non-stretch tissue called tendons. One end of the muscle (the origin end) is always attached to the bone which does not move. The other end (the insertion end) is attached to a bone near a joint.

When a muscle contracts it pulls on the bones and the one near the joint moves in the direction of the pull. This movement is produced by a lever:
- the joint acts as the fulcrum (the point around which movement takes place)
- the bone acts as the lever
- the muscle provides the effort to overcome the load
- the weight of the arm is the load.

Muscles work in pairs. The muscle which bends the joint is called the **flexor**. The muscle that straightens it is called the **extensor**. Flexor and extensor muscles are known as an antagonistic pair of muscles.

The diagram below shows how the biceps muscle (the flexor) moves the bones in the lower part of the arm. To straighten the arm out again the triceps muscle (the extensor) pulls the bones at the opposite side of the elbow joint.

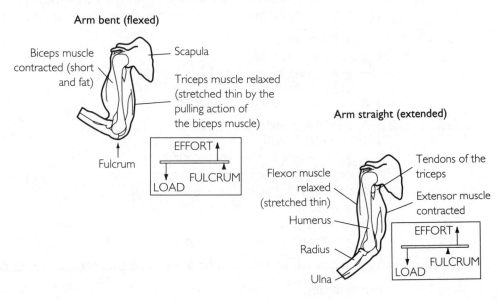

How muscles make the arm move

Skeletal muscles give the body its basic shape. They are responsible for maintaining posture. They are always slightly contracted (muscle tone). Without regular exercise and nutrition, muscle tone will deteriorate, posture will become poor.

Mobility, moving and handling techniques

Movement, or assisting with movement, of clients and loads, frequently becomes the responsibility of the carer. Since back problems can so easily occur when moving and handling clients, it is very important that you learn the techniques involved.

Your back allows you to do everything from sleeping to mountain climbing. People who experience back problems suffer pain and often have to take time off work. This can result in diminished earnings, inconvenience and even permanent disability.

Did you know that...?
- At some time in their lives four out of five people will suffer from back pain.
- 24 million working days are lost each year at a cost of over £1 billion per annum.
- Approximately 5 per cent of people have to change the nature of their work completely because of back problems.

Back pain and back problems can be caused by:
- sprains due to faulty lifting
- disc trouble
- poor posture
- lack of exercise
- being overweight
- injuries
- diseases.

Working safely when moving and handling clients

You can help yourself to avoid back problems by ensuring that you maintain a good posture and that you rest your muscles when you stand, sit and sleep.

Follow these simple rules:
- Stand correctly with:
  - your head high
  - your chin in
  - your chest forward
  - your abdomen flat.
- Sit correctly with:
  - your knees higher that your hips
  - your lower back firm against the backrest.
- Sleep correctly with:
  - a firm mattress
  - a bed board
  - your knees bent and lying on your side.

You may wish to follow a back exercise programme designed for carers.

Before lifting:
- Assess the situation.
- Know when to get help and advice.
- Predict potential difficulties.
- Follow the rules and methods your supervisors have explained.
- Use new and improved methods and equipment, and keep up to date with developments.
- Wherever possible **do not lift** – allow the client to help him or herself, use a hoist, slipmats, transfer boards.

EU regulations state that **two** women must not lift weights in excess of 50.8 kg.

General rules when lifting any object

In situations where lifting is unavoidable follow these rules:
- Think and assess the situation.
- Examine the object.
- Clear the immediate area.
- Know how and where to position the item to be lifted.
- Get help if necessary.
- Follow the steps for safe lifting in the diagram below.
- Avoid sudden, jerky movements.
- Lift with a smooth action.
- Bend your knees **not** your back.

Rules for lifting or moving a client

When lifting or moving a client some specific rules apply:
- Prepare a detailed assessment checklist (see below).
- Always wear flat shoes.

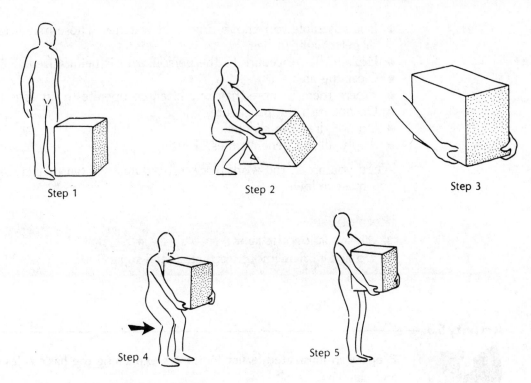

Step 1   Step 2   Step 3

Step 4   Step 5

Safe steps to lifting an object

Lifting action plan and evaluation			
Human/Physical factors	Factors which must be established	Action to be taken	Evaluation
The client	Height, weight, shape Ability to help self Previous experience of being lifted Age, culture, clothing being worn Existing medical or physical conditions Painful areas Appliances, drainage bags, plasters Ability to communicate, understand and co-operate Ability to hear and see		
The surrounding area	Any obstruction Floor surfaces Lifting height Space available Equipment available Degree of privacy which must be afforded		
The care worker	Have they appropriate skills and confidence Appropriate dress, no jewellery Flat shoes Able to explain procedure to client Able to co-ordinate effectively with workers		

An example of a lifting checklist

- It is advisable to remove rings and watches. These may scratch the client or get caught in hair.
- Explain the procedure to the person who is being lifted.
- Clear the area.
- Where there is more than one lifter, co-operate to lift together.
- Do not rush the procedure.
- Do not drag the client.
- Apply all the general rules of lifting

When you are in the work place, procedures will have been drawn up which you must follow.

Remember!
- Always follow the rules.
- Do not work without instruction and supervision.

Activity 5.8

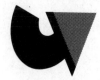

Prepare an illustrated leaflet for carers explaining the basic rules of moving and handling.

Review questions

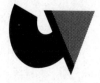

1 List four functions of the skeleton.

2 List four functions of the spine.

3 Name the bones which form the thoracic cage.

4 Name the organs which are contained in the thoracic cage.

5 The diaphragm is a large _____ which separates the _____ from the _____.

6 List the hormones which are produced in the human body.

7 What factors influence human body size and measurement?

8 What is assessed using the Agpar scale?

9 What is:
   a the average weight for a newborn baby?
   b the expected weight of a baby at 1 year?

10 Name two medical conditions which relate to a child's head size.

11 What is a centile chart?

12 What do you understand by the term pyrexia?

13 What do you understand by the term hypothermia?

14 Which body functions does the skin take part in?

15 What might cause a client to get a pressure sore?

16 Name three types of muscle in the human body.

17 Give an example of a smooth muscle.

18 How can posture show the state of a person's muscles?

19 Give an example of an antagonistic muscle system which moves a joint in the body.

20 What are the main causes of back problems?

Assignment A5.1
The human body systems

1 Produce a booklet of diagrams and simple explanatory notes on the human body systems. Include simple accounts of the structure and functions of the major organs.

2 Select one body system and prepare a presentation for the rest of your group

Include a full account of the structure and functions of the chosen system, and show how the system you have chosen relates to another organ system.

Advice
- Research widely using a variety of books and other resources related to human biology.
- For your presentation consider using the appropriate visual aids, overhead projector, flip charts, etc.
- Make a plan and discuss it with your tutor before your presentation.

Assignment A5.2
Observation and measurement

1 a Explain the routine observations made on **one** of the following:
  - elderly clients in residential care
  - 3-year-olds in a nursery setting.
  b Produce a file of information which you have collected on the client group you chose for **a**.
  c Choose two individuals from the group you chose and compare their heights, weights and eating habits.

Intermediate Health and Social Care

2 a Many organisations including Help the Aged, local authorities, and gas and electricity companies give help and advice on the prevention of hypothermia in elderly people.

Collect as much information as you can from the various sources available in your locality and write a concise report of your findings.

b How could you ensure that a 9-month-old baby was:
- kept warm in a very cold winter?
- kept cool during a hot humid summer?

Assignment A5.3
The application of science: moving and handling

1 Find out as much as you can about equipment to assist with moving and handling clients. Write to manufacturers and suppliers for information. Visit local suppliers, if you can.

2 Describe three pieces of equipment in detail. Explain how each one works.

Read Chapter 8, pages 293–312, for some ideas to get you started.

CHAPTER 6

Meeting the needs of individuals in different care settings

Element 6.1:	Examine methods used to assess individual care needs
Element 6.2:	Explore the way individual needs are met in care setting
Element 6.3:	Investigate factors which influence the delivery of care in different settings

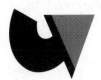

What is covered in this chapter

- Methods for assessing individual care needs
- How individual needs are met in care settings
- Factors which influence the delivery of care

These are the resources you will need for your Meeting the Needs of Individuals in Different Care Settings file:
- booklets explaining the health and social services offered to clients
- copies of job descriptions of the role and functions of carers in different settings
- a copy of your local authority annual Community Care Plan
- a copy of the Patient's Charter and the complaints procedure relating to local authority services and health services
- information collected on aids and adaptations
- your written answers to the activities in this chapter
- your written answers to the review questions at the end of this chapter
- your completed assignments: A6.1, A6.2 and A6.3.

Introduction

This chapter builds on what you have read in Chapter 4, Health and Social Care Services, and looks at the needs of individuals and how they may be met in differing care environments. Chapter 4 explained how services are provided by various statutory, private and voluntary agencies. This chapter focuses on care settings available within the community and on how these settings may meet the care needs of individuals.

Methods for assessing individual care needs

What is assessment?

Assessment is a process involving the client, carers and health and social care agencies. Its aim is to determine a client's care needs. The health and social

care worker gathers information in order to:
- understand the client's situation
- consider how the client might use a particular service or aid to daily living to improve their quality of life.

Assessment can range from the examination of a patient by a doctor upon admission to hospital for treatment to the more complex process involved in care planning under the National Health Service and Community Care Act (see page 230). A health and social care assessment covers the client's:
- physical environment
- health
- abilities
- financial needs
- formal and informal networks
- culture
- language
- religion
- emotional and psychological needs
- their personal perceptions and wishes.

The assessment process also involves the client in the identification of his or her own needs to ensure that any services provided are designed specifically to meet those needs. It is important that the client's own interpretation of their problems and needs is identified and recorded. Remember that carers and families should be involved in the process too, if possible.

The principles of assessment

Health and social care workers base assessments on the following principles:
- Assessment should be carried out **for** and **with** clients, not to them.
- The process of assessment should be as simple as possible. The basis of any decision-making should be described to the client clearly.
- As many people as appropriate should be involved in the assessment process, so that the outcome is enhanced.
- Assessment should be holistic – it should take account of the client's emotional, physical and practical needs.
- Care workers should have up-to-the-minute knowledge of the services which are currently available.
- Carers and clients should be aware of their rights as set out in any charter (see pages 118 and 230). There should also be a clear complaints procedures for both carers and clients.

Activity 6.1

Visit the head office or local area office of your social services department and obtain a copy of the latest annual Community Care Plan.

Make notes on the information the plan contains about:
- the assessment procedure
- the complaints procedure.

The needs of individuals

Before we examine the process of assessment, we need to consider some basic principles. An assessment carried out by a social worker, nurse or care worker is primarily an assessment of a person, their abilities, expectations and aspirations. To do this, the following areas of **need** should be examined:

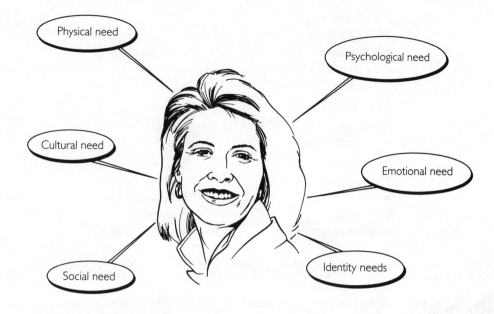

There are two ways of looking at needs that you may come across at work:
● Maslow's hierarchy of needs
● the activities of daily living.

Maslow's hierarchy of needs

This is a useful starting point when trying to understand human needs. According to Maslow, human needs are arranged in a series of five levels reflecting a hierarchy of importance (see the diagram on page 135). The needs at the bottom of the pyramid are the basic, essential requirements for life. The needs in the middle of the pyramid only come into play when many of the basic needs have been met. The theory implies a thinning out of needs as people progress up the hierarchy. Maslow assumes that for an individual to be functioning at their highest potential than all the needs shown should be considered and provided for.

Basic/physiological needs
These include such needs as:
● satisfaction of hunger and thirst
● the need for oxygen
● maintenance of temperature regulation
● the need for sleep
● sensory pleasures
● maternal behaviour
● sexual desire.

People who are denied any of these needs may spend periods of time looking for them. For example, if water or food is not readily available, a person's energies may well be directed to obtaining a supply. It would be pointless to try to teach a child about algebra when he or she was extremely hungry or desperate to go to the toilet.

Safety needs
These include:
● safety and security
● freedom from pain
● threat of physical attack
● protection from danger or deprivation
● the needs for predictability and orderliness.

Social/love needs
These include:
- affection
- sense of belonging
- social activities
- friendships
- the giving and receiving of love.

Esteem needs
Self-esteem, or self-respect, involves the desire for:
- confidence
- strength
- independence
- freedom and achievement.

The esteem of others involves:
- reputation
- prestige
- status
- recognition
- attention
- appreciation.

Activity 6.2

a List as many situations as you can think of in a residential setting where self-esteem needs might not be recognised.

b Discuss how self-esteem needs may be met in a residential home or a hospital ward.

Self-actualisation/self-fulfilment needs
This means the development and realisation of one's full potential. To be able to function at this level then all the needs identified in four lower levels should have been considered and provided for.

Activity 6.3

Look at the photograph opposite. What needs of this person do you think are being met?

The activities of daily living

This is another assessment method that you may see used. It looks at client needs by an examination of the normal activities that people (need to) carry out every day. Various areas of functioning are examined and strategies for helping the client either stay independent or become more independent are put forward for discussion and agreement.

Safe environment
- Is the client in a safe environment?
- Are they free from pain?

Body functions
- Is the client breathing comfortably?
- Is the client passing urine and faeces regularly?
- Is the client maintaining body temperature, etc.?

Nutrition
- Is the client eating a healthy diet?
- Has the client the ability to eat and take in suitable fluids.

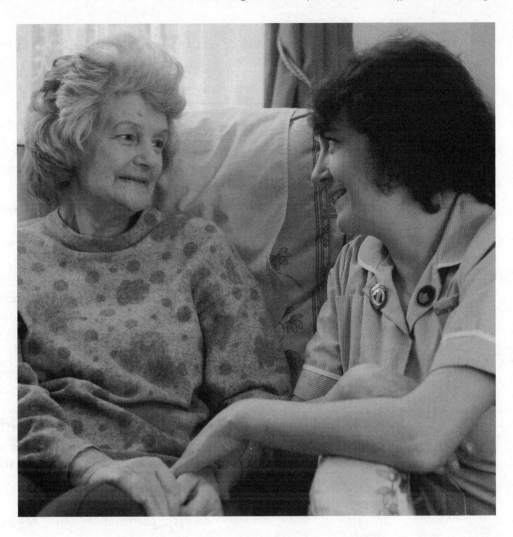

Personal cleaning and dressing
This includes care of the mouth, teeth, eyes, ears, skin, the wearing of appropriate clothing, ability to dress and undress.

Mobility
Is the client able to get out of bed or exercise?

Sleep
● What is the client's sleep pattern?
● Does the client wake during the night or sleep during the day?

Leisure and work
What recreation and rehabilitation needs does the client have?

Sexuality
Has the client the ability to express feelings and the ability to enter into meaningful sexual relationships?

Religion
● What are the cultural needs of the client?
● Have they the freedom to worship?

Communication
Has the client the ability to communicate verbally, express emotions, use smell, touch, hearing, etc.?

Activity 6.4

Identify a client that you have been supporting in your work placement. Observe their behaviour over a period of time and, using the information given in this section, list the needs that you think are being met and those not being met. Explain your observations.

Client participation: empowerment of the client

In the past, power resided with the providers of a service. Doctors, nurses and social workers have traditionally controlled services and made decisions about how they are delivered. Clients can be **empowered** (given control of their situation) by involving them in negotiating their own assessment and care plan.

By giving a client information and advice, they can be encouraged to make appropriate informed choices and decisions about services and take responsibility for their own lives. This approach assumes that they will be able to take risks to maintain their freedom and independence.

Services provided for clients should be delivered in a manner that respects the dignity and value of the client, and should be appropriate to the client's situation, culture and lifestyle.

Information
In order to make informed choices, clients must have adequate information about:
● services which are available to them
● their rights
● the complaints procedures.

The National Health Service and Community Care Act 1990 requires social service departments to provide information accessible to all potential service users and carers, including those with any communication difficulty or difference in language or culture. The information should set out:
● the types of community care services available
● the criteria for provision and services
● the assessment procedures to agree needs
● the ways of addressing those needs
● the standards by which the care management system will be measured.

This is done by publishing a Community Care Plan annually and also by setting up consultation procedures with clients and carers. Booklets and leaflets are also used to provide information.

Advocates
One way to help clients become involved can be though the use of advocates. Clients can be represented or accompanied by a person of their choice when meeting care staff. Such a person is known as an **advocate**. Advocates should

be available from the same racial or cultural background as the client. Voluntary organisations provide advocates for certain groups of clients. For example, Age Concern provides support of elderly people and MENCAP provides an advocacy service for people with learning difficulties.

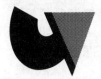

Activity 6.5

Obtain copies of information leaflets on various services and their availability. These will include particulars of elegibility criteria and assessment procedures. You should find the leaflets in your local library, GP's surgery, health centre or social services department.

We can empower clients by:
- not making assumptions about what a client needs
- recognising the differing interests of those involved in the assessment process: the client, family, agency
- recognising the need for negotiation between a client and a provider
- helping and supporting a client to regain control of their situation
- recognising a client's own abilities and experience
- giving accurate honest information to a client, their family and carers
- enabling choice for a client.

Activity 6.6

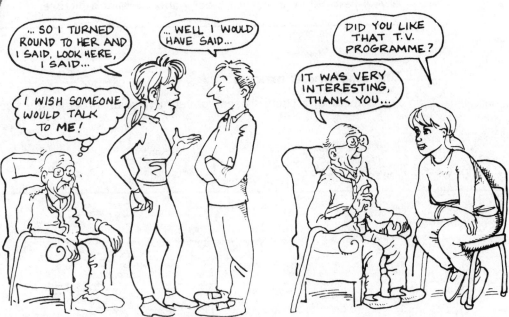

Which of these two situations illustrates the empowerment of the client? List the reasons for your answer.

Remember

● An assessment must be carried out with the explicit **consent of the client** and, if appropriate, those who care for the client. The client should understand the process and agree to the assessment unless there is a clear legal reason for intervention, for example under the Mental Health or Children Act.

● A care plan should be based on the views of all relevant carers and/or family. Any services offered should be based on **negotiated** agreement with all concerned. This includes statutory, voluntary and private sector services.

Activity 6.7

How might you help people help themselves in the following situations? Remember to think about your approach and take into consideration the feelings and wishes of the client.

How would you talk to or approach the client in each case?

a A 5-year-old child needs help tying their shoe laces.

b An 80-year-old woman is able to walk, but has difficulty when getting up from the sitting position.

c A person who is unsighted who is about to eat a meal in a strange environment.

d A fellow student who is confined to a wheelchair and wishes to use the lift.

e A 4-year-old in an infant school wants to paint a picture.

The assessment process

Assessment of a client's needs covers five main processes:

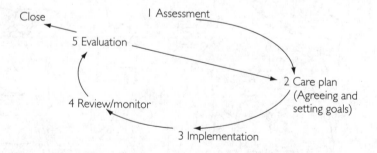

What information is necessary to carry out a first assessment?

When considering what information is necessary remember that only information that is **relevant** to the client's situation, illness or disability should be used.

Use the following headings as a guide to collecting information:
- **Basic details of the client** Date of birth, sex, marital status, ethnic origin, address, telephone number, household composition, next of kin and GP.
- **Abilities, attitudes and lifestyle** A person's ability to cope depends as much on their personal resources and motivation as on the extent of the disability. Two people with similar disabilities will manage differently and need different levels of support. How people have coped with similar situations is also very useful information in determining how the client may handle the present problem.
- **Race and culture** It is important that you take account and have an appreciation of racial and cultural differences, their differing perspectives and the impact of racism.
- **Contribution of formal and informal carers** Where a person is supported by, or is dependent upon, relatives or friends, you should be in a position to assess their contribution to any care. To achieve this you will needs to take account of the status of the carer and their relationship to the client, the care they provide and their other commitments.

Some needs are easy to define, for example, immediate needs, such as a health crisis needing the support of medical or nursing staff, and short-term needs, such as home care following discharge from hospital or respite care.

However, before the assessor prioritises needs with the client they should first discuss those needs of most concern to the client or family. What is perceived as important by the client should be addressed first unless there are conditions to the contrary. Giving clients full opportunity to make decisions about their own future can be time-consuming for those involved. Although certain needs may seem to the assessor as most important, it is essential to bear in mind those needs which the client is most motivated to address.

Activity 6.8

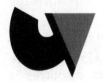

Mrs King is 82 years old. She lives alone in a small terraced house. She has a clear mind, a good sense of humour and keeps herself and her house in apple-pie order. She has difficulty preparing her meals. A month ago she had a slight stroke which left her with a tendency to dizzy spells. When she has a dizzy spell she simply falls down wherever she is and is unconscious for about 10 minutes.

Using the grid below, decide what solutions you might recommend to Mrs King.

Problems	Solutions
Unable to cook	
Fear of dizzy spells	

How much information should you collect?

To aid the assessment process a certain amount of personal information from the client is necessary. Simple needs, such as a request for meals-on-wheels will require less investigation than more complex request for support upon discharge from hospital after a serious accident.

When gathering information you should explain the reason for the interview to the client. What is the client's and carers' condition? What prevents them from functioning effectively? What aspects in their everyday life cause them most difficulty? How do they cope with dressing, cooking, cleaning, meals, walking and general household tasks?

Activity 6.9

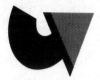

Mr Johnson has been referred to the social services by a neighbour because she thinks that he needs help with cleaning and getting into and out of bed. When the assessor arrives to see Mr Johnson, it is obvious that he could also be helped by the support of a community nurse.

Discuss what course of action you would take and why.

Facts about people are never straightforward. A client may say that they cannot cook for themselves, but there may be no physical reason for not doing so. They may be depressed or afraid that they might drop the cooking utensils. It is very important therefore to understand the client's perception of their situation. You need to ask yourself what can the client do for themselves? What support can family, friends, neighbours or carers give?

How can you ensure that the client participates in the process?

After the assessment has been carried the next step is to agree on the **care plan** to provide the support the client may need. If the client's needs are simple and can be met with a single service, such as a home help, then the care plan's goals may be quickly accomplished.

People like to feel in control of their lives as far as possible. This is achieved when people are enabled in making decisions for themselves. However, care planning which enables clients and carers to utilise their own resources is usually the most effective intervention.

What is an objective?

An objective, or goal, is a statement indicating what the client should be able to do after an agreed period of time.

For example, Mr Simmons is an elderly man who lives alone. He has family who live nearby. He has difficulty getting into and out of bed and is unable to wash himself. He also suffers from minor bedsores. An assessor might agree a care plan with the following goals for him:

How do you set goals?
● Goals should be kept as simple as possible and be understood by everyone. In this way they can be monitored and reviewed, and if necessary changed.

Problem	Help from	Goal
Domestic abilities:		
Cooking	Home Care	Provide meals
Cleaning	Home Care	Provision until bed sores heal
Self care:		
Get in/out of bed	Health Care Assistant	Until sister can do so
Bedsores	District Nurse	Heal bed sores

● Goals should reflect what the client can be expected to do. For example, 'Mary, who has just been discharged from hospital, will be able within six weeks to get herself out of bed in the morning without help from the health care assistant.' This simple goal can be monitored to see how Mary is progressing and at the end of six weeks the assessor can see if Mary can or cannot get out of bed unaided and re-adjust the care plan accordingly.

Activity 6.10

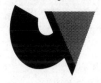

Ellen is an athlete. She is 23 years old. She has recently had an accident in which she injured her spine and she may be wheelchair-bound for some time. She is to be discharged from hospital to her flat where she lives alone. She has agreed to see an assessor with a view to obtaining services to enable her to live alone.

Copy the grid below and complete it.
What immediate problems do you think Ellen will experience?
What services would you offer her? What goals would you set?

Problem	Service	Goal

Reviewing the care plan

Care plan reviewing is the process by which the changing needs of the client are identified and support adapted accordingly. The review process will help determine whether the goals that were set have been achieved. Like the original assessment, the views and preferences of the client must be the focus of the review.

Normally the review will be undertaken through a meeting of all concerned parties. The review meeting is a formal one with a chairperson. A full record of the proceedings should be made. The client and carers should be clearly informed that they may be represented by an advocate or accompanied by a third party.

Purposes of the review:
- review the achievement of the care plan goals
- examine the reasons for success or failure
- evaluate the quality of care provided
- re-assess current needs
- reappraise eligibility for services
- revise the care plan goals
- redefine the service delivery requirements
- set a date for next review
- record the findings of the review and circulate to all parties.

Remember
- The focus of the review should not be on the services provided, but on the needs, views and preferences of the client and their carers.
- The outcome of the review should be an enhanced understanding of the needs of the client and their perceptions of the services provided. This should lead to a redefinition of the goals of future intervention and an allocation of responsibility for their achievement.

Activity 6.11

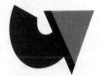

Mary is a very physically disabled, wheelchair-bound, 7-year-old girl, living with her father who has moved to this part of the country due to a change of job. Mary's mother lives many miles away. She still loves Mary and wishes to continue to have a say in her future. Mary's present accommodation is a large Victorian house in a suburb of a large city with good health and social care support services. The local education authority's policy is to integrate all children with a disability into mainstream education.

Planning

In implementing any care plan for Mary remember that the following principals of assessment should be adhered to:
- Assessment should be with the explicit consent of Mary.
- Mary must understand the assessment process. If there is a legal reason for intervention (non-school attendance, for example) this should be explained.
- The client should always understand when the assessment partnership is based on consent or on legal authority.
- Any intervention must be based on the views of all relevant carers and/or the family.
- Any services offered to Mary should be based on negotiated agreement with all agencies.
- Mary should have the greatest possible degree of choice in the services that are offered.

Assessment

1 Using a copy of the following grid, identify how you would attempt to meet Mary's needs.

Need	Possible support
Physical needs	
Social needs	
Cultural needs	
Emotional needs	

2 Using a copy of the following grid, set goals for Mary's care plan which can be monitored and reviewed by all the supporting agencies. Identify the agencies or individuals that Mary might obtain support from and the goal of such support

	Support from	Goal
Domestic abilities		
Self-care		
Social needs		
Intellectual needs		

3 What processes would you employ to help to empower Mary within the care planning process?

How can clients be involved in shaping their environment?

Clients can be involved in shaping their environment when they have been empowered — when they have **real** power.

'Real power results from knowledge and choice. Historically, care organisations met the requirements of groups in society other than clients themselves. The needs of those perceived to be more able, including families, neighbours, professionals and politicians, dictated policies in respect of those perceived to be less able. Care professionals often made decisions with reference to other professional groups first, and the client second. The problem had been compounded by the lack of choice in service provision, with particular services being offered by only one local provider, almost exclusively in the public sector. Clients had to accept what was offered, or have no service at all. Financial constraints on available provision has also been a major factor in limiting the choice of clients. All of these factors, over many years, developed into an institutionalised belief that care providers know better than clients what is needed, or wanted.

It is now apparent that such attitudes significantly contribute to the problems of those disadvantaged through health or social difficulties. The very process of health or social disadvantage results in a loss of power in society. A prime aim of health and social care is empowerment in respect to a client's rights and choice. Not only is such an aim morally correct, but it is also highly effective in terms of meeting the needs of those who require care services. By promoting and supporting individual rights and choice within service delivery, we may ultimately reduce a major source of difficulties that care workers themselves impose on clients.

Many social service and health authorities have set up consultative groups as one way in which clients can participate in developing and shaping services. A number of authorities have developed new initiatives to encourage users of services to become involved in the planning and management of services. The 'Margin to Mainstream' project, funded by the Rowntree Foundation, enables clients and carers to become involved in the organisation, management and delivery of services. This initiative gives people who use and provide services an opportunity to come together to distribute funds, meet those who provide services and organise workshops. The project supports a direct payment scheme which allows community care finance to be paid to users who can in turn purchase and manage the services they want. Other schemes under this project facilities users having an input into training schemes and developing ways in which clients can influence public policy.

Sheffield social services department has developed an Older People's Reference Group which meets every two months to consider day services, home care and residential care facilities. This group also plays a direct role in the preparation of strategic plans by being full members of such groups. This group is also developing a Direct Payment to Users Scheme for older people to enable them to purchase services which best meet their individual needs.'

Source: Sheffield's Community Care Plan 1994

How individual needs are met in care settings

Care settings in the community

Activity 6.12

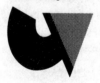

a Before we start to examine health and care settings, think about yourself for a moment and write down all the care settings you have had contact with during your lifetime.

b Write down those that your family may also have had contact with.

No doubt your lists were extensive and included settings like health centres, hospitals, nurseries, schools, dental surgeries, opticians, playgroups, possibly residential settings and lastly your own home.

Let's look at care setting in a more structured way and work through the services and resources offered in those settings from before birth through to old age.

Care services for babies and children

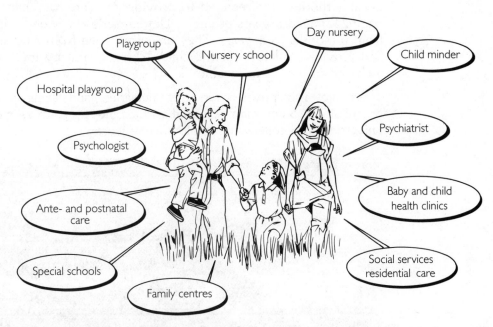

Services available to children and families

Antenatal and postnatal care

Once a woman is confirmed pregnant by her GP, she will receive regular checks by her GP and the local hospital. Arrangements will also be made for the delivery of the baby either at home or in hospital, depending on factors such as the mother's previous history, her present health or her wishes. The mother's home or the local hospital may be the care setting for the delivery of the baby.

If there are problems at birth then the baby may need the care of the special baby unit and the mother may need extra days in the hospital. If the labour and delivery are without complications then the family's home becomes the appropriate care setting. When mother and the baby arrive home there are various people whom the parents can call on for support and who will visit the home regularly, the health visitor, social worker or GP. The roles of these carers are dealt with more fully later in this chapter.

Baby and child health clinics

As the baby grows and develops, the parents may be assured through regular visits to baby clinics and child health clinics at the local health centre, where professional staff will monitor the child's development. Detection of disability can be very difficult with young babies. Sometimes there are concerns from the moment of birth, but it is often only when a child fails to follow normal patterns of development that a disability may become evident.

Children with difficulties may be referred to a specialist unit where experts from different disciplines or branches of medicine come together to assess the child. Audiologists (to assess hearing), physiotherapists, psychologists, speech therapists, orthoptist (vision) and doctors meet together after each has individually assessed the child. Many of the assessments are carried out through play. They make recommendations for services and help.

Day nurseries
Local authorities are required to provide day care for 'children in need' (see page 242) aged 5 years or under. Day nurseries provide facilities for children from 6 months to 5 years. They are often open from 8.00 a.m. to 6.00 p.m. and provide total care for the child. Nurseries run by local authorities make a charge according to income.

There are also privately-run day nurseries, and some run by voluntary organisations. Some may be linked with employers, such as the Midland Bank, universities and colleges or employment agencies.

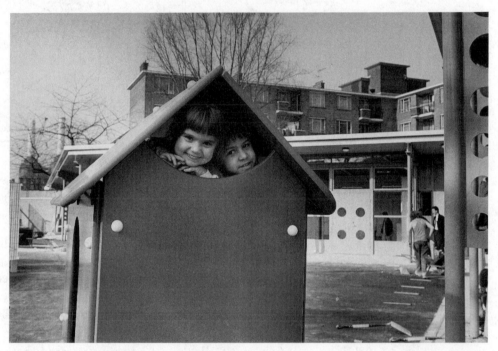

Children at the Patmore Centre in London (run by Save the Children), where community-based childcare services include a nursery, creches, parents and children's groups. The childcare services enable local women to take up training initiatives provided by the project

Activity 6.13

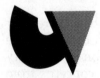

What day nursery provision exists in your community? Find out what provision is made by the local authority, private organisations and/or voluntary groups.

Nursery schools
Nursery schools and nursery classes are run by the local education authority and operate within school hours. Some places may be part-time, mornings or afternoons only. Children can attend nursery school from the age of 3.

In some local authority areas, children can attend 'Rising Fives' sessions at school two terms before they are due to start school. However, if a child takes a local authority nursery place then they cannot have a Rising Five place also. Local education authority nursery schools are provided free of charge.

There are also privately-run nursery schools which charge fees.

Child minders
Child minders are individual people who care for children in their own home. They must register and be approved by the local Social Services Department. A social worker can visit their home at any time to check numbers of children being cared for and the standard of safety measures being taken. Safety standards and the time a child can stay with a child minder are regulated under the Children Act. A local authority can cancel a child minder's registration if it is not happy with the standard of service offered.

Parent and toddler groups
These are usually run by volunteers using such premises as church halls or community centres. They provide a welcome break for people looking after young children. The children usually enjoy a different setting from home and fresh toys and friends to play with.

Playgroups
Playgroups must be approved and registered by local authority social services departments. They are usually run by volunteers who attend local authority training courses. Parents and carers of children often help on a rota basis. In some areas playgroups are the only structured pre-school provision within easy reach for families.

Some nurseries and playgroups have a policy of integration so that children with learning difficulties or special physical needs can work, learn and play alongside other children.

Activity 6.14

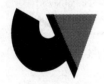

Arrange visits to different playgroups or toddler groups either as individuals or in pairs. Observe the requirements that the group has to comply with in order to register. Note the toys, activities and staff involved. Report back to your group and discuss.

Family centres
Family centres may be run by the local authorities or voluntary agencies, such as the Family Welfare Association. These centres offer day care to both the children and parents. They assist parents in the difficult job of bringing up children by providing discussion sessions, visiting speakers and encouragement to play with the children. Families may be referred to the centre by social workers possibly because of difficulties they are experiencing such as ill-health, poverty or bad housing.

The Children Act 1989
The Children Act places a duty on local authorities to:
- safeguard the welfare of all children in need in their area.
- identify those children in need

- publish information about services available so that those who need support will know about them
- keep a register of children with disabilities and provide services to minimise the effect of these disabilities so as to give children the opportunities to lead lives which are as normal as possible.

Services which may be provided include:
- advice, guidance and counselling
- occupational, social and cultural activities
- family centres
- home helps
- laundry facilities
- help with travelling to and from services
- assistance with holidays for the child and the family.

Children in need are defined in the 1989 Children Act as:
- those who are unlikely to achieve or maintain, or have the opportunity of achieving or maintaining, a reasonable standard of health or development without the provision of services
- those whose health or development is likely to be significantly impaired without the provision of such services
- those who are disabled, including physical, mental and sensory disability.

Care settings for adults with learning difficulties

The National Health Service and Community Care Act places emphasis on providing services to enable people with disabilities to have access to care settings such as:

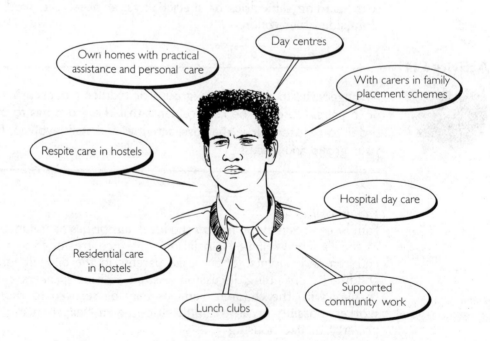

These services are provided through either statutory organisations, such as the social services or the health authorities, or voluntary organisations, such as United Response, Home Farm Trust or MENCAP.

Similar services are provided for people with mental health needs and involves voluntary organisations such as MIND or the National Schizophrenia Fellowship.

Residential homes and foster care homes are also significant care settings when ordinary family homes may not be able to provide the appropriate care.

Activity 6.15

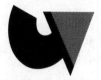

Find out what care settings exist in your community for people with visual and hearing impairment. For example, voluntary organisations such as the RNIB (Royal National Institute for the Blind) and RNID (Royal National Institute for the Deaf) provide facilities.

Care settings in the community for older people

For most older people the care they need can be provided in their own homes. For those with more dependent needs the following services provide support:

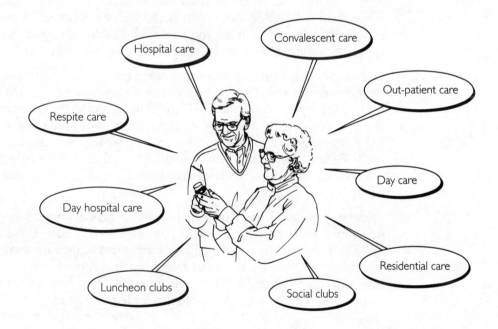

Within the community there may also be care settings for people with special difficulties concerning alcohol, drugs, domestic violence, HIV or other terminal illnesses.

The needs of individuals in care settings

As we have already seen, everyone has needs – think about yourself for a moment and write down what you think your needs are. No doubt most of you wrote about your basic needs like food, drink, rest, etc., but what about more difficult areas such as emotional needs and the need to realise your full potential?

Activity 6.16

Study the diagram on page 135 and discuss how far it applies to a care setting that you know well. For example, if you consider a playgroup, how are the basic physical needs of the children catered for? What happens in relation to safety?

Care settings appropriate for different individuals

Sometimes, people can still manage at home but they need extra support, practically, financially or emotionally – someone to talk to and help them cope.

If a child is born with a disability or a disability becomes evident as the child develops, then assessments may be carried out by multi-disciplinary teams. As part of the assessment, suggestions may be made in consultation with the parents to place the child in an appropriate care setting. Later, an educational psychologist will become involved and a 'statement' about the child will be drawn up in consultation with the parents and other professionals. The statement will make recommendations concerning appropriate care for the child.

Many parents and carers of disabled children take advantage of **respite care** – the child is based in their own home but stays for short periods in a home especially designed to meet the needs of disabled children. There are different types of respite care units to support different age groups.

Decisions concerning appropriate care settings for particular individuals are by no means easy. Even when decisions are reached, it may be difficult to find a vacancy in a particular residential or supportive setting. For most children the first care setting they encounter is their own home, but consider some of the reasons why a child's home may not be the best place for him or her to be. If there is a situation of potential or actual abuse or neglect, then the court may decide that the child is fostered or, if they are older, joins a family group home.

Older people may need residential care, practical and personal care at home or simply visits to help them to feel less lonely. Sometimes they may need links with education classes, clubs or activities which are available in the local community. This may be called **therapeutic support** – it is a form of therapy for them to go out and meet people, possibly learn how to cook for themselves if they are living alone. Many older people manage almost independently, but may visit a hospital day centre once a week so that nurses can help them bath and shave or shampoo their hair.

Activity 6.17

Read the case history on page 245 and decide which settings you think might be appropriate for Mrs Anderson. Make a note and give reasons for your decision. (Don't forget about domiciliary services which can enable people to use their own homes as the most appropriate care settings.)

Mrs Anderson has three children under 5 and her husband has been recently killed in an accident. Financially, she is reliant on state benefits. The shock of her husband's death has made her frequently depressed. She needs to grieve the loss before she can come to terms with it. The eldest child is very bewildered by his mother's lack of energy and involvement. The second child has developed some quite strong difficult behaviour because of lack of attention.

The role of care workers in meeting individual needs

Many of the roles and functions of particular personnel involved in social care are familiar to us if only through books and television images. It may be helpful to explain the roles of certain familiar personnel (see also Chapter 3).

The midwife

A midwife is a Registered General Nurse (RGN) who has gone on to further training to specialise in midwifery. The midwife assists a woman in labour and may deliver the baby in a home setting or a hospital. She (there are also a number of male midwives) cares for the mother and baby for ten days following the birth, both in hospital and at home. If there are problems she will refer them to the appropriate agency. She checks particularly that the baby is feeding well. After ten days the midwife hands over to the health visitor.

The health visitor

The health visitor is an RGN who has completed further training in social and preventative medicine. The health visitor deals with any early difficulties the parents may have. She also carries out various assessment checks to see that the child is developing properly. Some of her work may be carried out at the clinic or at the home. The fact that she or he picks up possible problems highlights the preventative aspect of their work.

The earlier any defect or disability is discovered the better the chance for help and treatment. The role of the health visitor may be significant in cases of abuse. Careful records of visits to families are made. They have no legal right of entry anyone's home, neither do they wear uniform. Some health visitors also visit elderly people in the community.

The district or community nurse

The district nurse may lead a team of nurses (usually based at a health centre or clinic). They are responsible for carrying out nursing care in the community. This may involve changing dressings on wounds, assisting a person who had a stroke to take a bath or checking a child after discharge from hospital.

The community psychiatric nurse (CPN)

The CPN is involved with people who have mental health difficulties in the community. They visit them in their homes or hostels, give them medication, arrange for therapeutic activities and generally support them to live as normal a life in the community as possible.

The psychiatrist

The psychiatrist is a qualified doctor who has also undergone training in psychiatry. They work with people with mental illness in a hospital or community setting, or as a member of a team, assessing people with learning disabilities.

The psychologist

The psychologist is not a medical doctor, but will have a postgraduate qualification in a specialist field such as clinical or educational psychology. They may work from a hospital base or be a member of the team assessing people with learning disabilities or physical disabilities such as brain damage. They are also involved in the treatment of patients.

Activity 6.18

Make an appointment with two of the above carers. Discuss their role, write down what they say they do and discuss it with the rest of your group.

The speech therapist/Communication therapist

The speech therapist may work with children with delayed speech development, children with learning difficulties, or people with speech problems after strokes.

The occupational therapist (OT)

The OT is concerned to increase an individual's ability to manage independently. They may work from hospitals or social service departments. They will devise ways to assist people to cope practically or psychologically with their everyday life.

The physiotherapist

The physiotherapist encourages clients, both young and old, to maximise their physical potential by exercises or other forms of movement.

The social worker

The social work role is complicated because it can vary so much, but basically the social worker is concerned to try to call in those services and helplines which can meet a client's needs. Some social workers are involved in residential settings, and here again their aim is to manage the setting so that the needs of the individuals are met in the best way possible.

Activity 6.19

Within your group, discuss how you could help and support clients in the situations described below.

a A client who is confused and dependent on the carer and who may:
- feel restricted by the routine of the establishment
- miss her home or family
- be upset at being unable to keep personal belongings
- be unused to the establishment's food
- feel she has lost friends, independence and freedom.

b A 3-year-old child leaving her mother to attend a nursery or creche for the first time and who may:
- miss her family
- be unable to express her needs or wishes to carers
- feel surrounded by strangers
- feel confused in an unfamiliar environment
- not fully appreciate what is happening to her.

Factors which influence the delivery of care

Care values

Inevitably, the caring role can give rise to difficult situations for both client and carer. Some of the more relevant situations are described below. Perhaps you can think of other issues which may arise?

Working with people is seldom an easy option. You may often feel:
- overworked and so feel you have not the energy to listen to clients
- that your personal problems are affecting your work and attitude towards clients
- tired and impatient
- immature and unable to understand a client's problem
- that you have difficulty in forming relationships with clients or colleagues
- worried because the demands of your job are excessive
- overwhelmed with paperwork
- not trained enough for the demands of the job.

Sometimes you may feel overwhelmed by the responsibilities and tasks you are expected to carry out. It is at times like this when you are under stress that it is most important that you remember and work with the **care values** in mind. Care values are principles, standards or qualities considered worthwhile or desirable by the care profession.

An individual's attitudes and values can be observed in their behaviour. Although it is difficult to change attitudes, and hence values, some vocations, such as health and social care, require a great deal of attention to be paid to them. In fact, the National Vocational Qualification (NVQ) in Care includes a Value Base unit.

The Value Base unit

This addresses five elements:
- **anti-discriminatory practice** Culture, race, religion, sexual identity, age, gender, health status, etc.
- **confidentiality** Clients have the right to say who should have access to personal data. Care workers are responsible for respecting the wishes of the client.
- **individual rights and choice** Clients' choice, preferences and wishes must be respected.
- **personal beliefs and identity** Each individual's own personal beliefs and preferences must be respected – religious, cultural, political, ethical and sexual.
- **effective communication** Listen to other individuals, promote effective communication in a variety of ways, consider language (verbal and non-verbal), understanding, environment, and social and cultural influences.

It is hoped that by stimulating thought and discussion, and exposing carers to a wide variety of situations, attitudes may be developed that are consistent with this value base.

Activity 6.20

Divide the class into five groups, each group taking one of the five elements that make up the Value Base unit. Discuss the contents of the element assigned with reference to professional practice in care settings. Make notes of your discussion and report back to the whole class.

The intention of the Value Base unit is to create equality for all individuals. Most professional carers are employed by agencies that have considerable power, and that also have responsibilities in law to others besides service users. While we emphasise the therapeutic, supportive and counselling roles of care workers, they are also responsible to the agency that they work for. A care worker may be better educated and therefore, by definition, possess more power through position, than their client. To counteract these processes the new Diploma in Social Work identifies values which are integral to competent social work practice. It states that social workers should:

- identify and question their own values and prejudices, and their implications for practice
- respect and value uniqueness and diversity, and recognise and build on strengths
- promote people's rights to choice, privacy, confidentiality and protection while recognising and addressing the complexities of competing rights and demands
- assist people to increase control of, and improve the quality of, their lives, while recognising that control of behaviour will be required at times in order to protect children and adults from harm
- identify, analyse and take action to counter discrimination, racism, disadvantage, inequality and injustice, using strategies appropriate to role and context
- practise in a manner that does not stigmatise or disadvantage either individuals, groups or communities.

The social or health problems of some clients may create real dependency. To be perceived as anything other than fit, able, and making a valuable contribution to society is to be stripped of power. Some care services inadvertently reinforce this problem in the way they provide their services. Those who provide care services are not immune from the attitudes of the society into which they themselves have been socialised. They may have attitudes which reinforce many of the prejudices that society has about people who are different, for whatever reason. Care settings may mirror the effects of power on vulnerable individuals in both public and private settings.

Activity 6.21

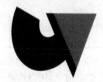

In a care setting (which may be a work placement), observe the behaviour of other care workers. Make a list of some of these behaviours, which may include things like assisting with bathing, eating or bedtimes. Decide for each of the behaviours that you listed whether the client is being empowered, or whether the care worker is exercising power over the client, and how.

Environmental factors and the care environment

A pleasant environment for people who are ill or in need of care is essential as it will make them feel better. Carers will also feel more motivated if their working conditions are agreeable.

Buildings and grounds in residential and day care establishments should be well-maintained and attractive. Decorations in buildings need careful planning so that certain areas look bright, cheerful and stimulating while others should encourage quiet and rest. In residential centres, a room where residents can entertain friends and family in private should be made available. Client's wishes must be considered and their views taken seriously. Wherever possible, clients should have their own rooms, a key to their room, and be offered choices in the furnishings and fittings.

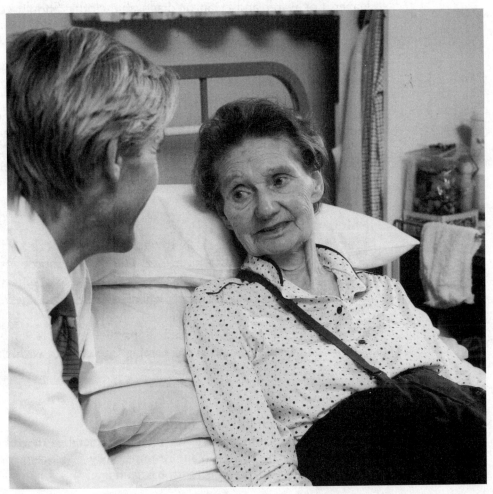

A patient receiving care in a Marie Curie Cancer Care hospice

Good hygienic practices will make for more pleasing environment and will reduce the risk of infections spreading. In your work placement, read the basic guidelines relating to hygiene and safety rules that must be enforced. These are explained in Chapter 1.

Ventilation
Adequate ventilation is very important to ensure that the air which is being breathed is stimulating and refreshing for clients and staff. No doubt we have all experienced rooms where conditions are less than perfect, where there is a stuffy atmosphere, making you feel tired and causing headaches and other minor ailments. Windows should be opened to allow cross-ventilation.

Household cleanliness
Much of this will be the responsibility of the domestic staff, but it is up to the carer to see that standards are maintained while the service is being offered. This will involve mopping up spills and wiping work surfaces, tables and chairs

as required. Proprietary cleaners in the correct dilution should be used. Special care will need to be taken with items which are upholstered, such as chairs and matresses.

Hand basins, baths, showers and bidets

These should be cleaned at least once every 24 hours using a proprietary cleaner, hot water and clean or disposable cloths. Should equipment become soiled, day or night, it is the carer's responsibility to see that it is clean and ready again for client's use.

Bed pans, potties and commodes

Scrupulous, routine cleaning is vital and all should be emptied immediately following use. You will find that different establishments use a variety of cleaning agents, including bleach solutions. Check the health and safety regulations in the workplace before you use these cleaning materials. Hospitals and some large establishments will use disposable bed pans and urinals. They may also require different forms of waste to be disposed of in separate containers.

Points to remember
- Always wear protective clothing when in contact with body fluids or waste.
- Always dispose of waste matter carefully, using appropriate containers.
- Always make sure you have instructions from your supervisor.
- Never leave cleaning materials where clients, especially small children, can reach them.
- Protect yourself by always reading instructions on labels of cleaning agents that you use and avoid coming into contact with them by using gloves and overalls or aprons.

Bedclothes and client's clothing

Most large establishments will have laundry facilities or will contract out any laundry work. The carer's main responsibility is to remove bedclothes and soiled clothing, and prepare them for laundry.

Points to remember
- Bedding and clothing must be changed as soon as soiling occurs.
- Remove any excreta which is on the bedding or clothing. Do not forget to use gloves. Place items in special coloured bags, as directed by your supervisor, before sending to the laundry.
- Small or delicate items should be hand-washed for individual clients. Sometimes relatives will do this for the client.

Food preparation areas

To avoid food poisoning, areas where food is prepared whether in a caring establishment or a client's home need to be kept scrupulously clean. In a residential establishment, this responsibility is shared between carers and domestic staff. All work surfaces must be wiped frequently. Bleach solutions are appropriate for this.

Play equipment, toys and games

Regular, thorough cleaning using household cleaners and sometimes weak solutions of bleach is essential for this type of equipment. Supervisors will give exact instructions.

Activity 6.22

a In your workplace, identify all domestic tasks which are shared between domestic staff and carers.

b In relation to domestic tasks, examine one area where domestic work is particularly important.

c Within your class or tutorial group, discuss the importance of co-operation between all members of staff within caring establishments.

Specialist aids, appliances and equipment

The aim of any care or treatment plan which has been devised with or for a patient or client is always to encourage them to be as independent as possible within the limits of the conditions from which they are suffering. Always allow clients to do as much as they can for themselves.

There are a wide variety ot aids which enable the person with mobility problems to move around, to get into and out of the bath, to feed themselves, to use the toilet, to dress and undress. Medical staff, occupational therapists and physiotherapists give advice as to the most appropriate aids and applicances.

Aids and appliances are described in detail in Chapter 8, pages 282–315.

Review questions

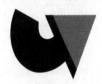

1 What does multi-disciplinary assessment mean?

2 What responsibilities does the Children Act 1989 place on local authorities?

3 List six care settings in the community for older people?

4 What is respite care?

5 What is the role of the midwife?

6 List six needs which should be examined during the assessment process.

7 List six ways that you as a care worker can empower clients.

8 What are the five main stages involved in assessment processes?

9 What are the four main categories of objective?

10 What aids are available to clients who have difficulty with eating or drinking?

Assignment A6.1
Assessing care needs

Mrs Pugh is 80 years old and lives alone. She has some family but they have lived in Australia for many years. She has difficulties getting into and out of bed. She is able to wash herself, but cannot get into or out of the bath. She would like to go out to the local bingo hall occasionally. However, she is very concerned about her dog which seems to suffering from some illness. She is so worried about the dog that she is not eating her food. Mrs Pugh wishes to get the dog to the vet immediately.

1 Copy the grid outlined below. How would you support Mrs Pugh so that she could continue to live in her own home?

Mrs Pugh	
Problems	**Solutions**
Unable to cook Cannot bath Unable to shop Wishes to go to bingo Dog ill	

2 What assessment methods would you use to assess Mrs Pugh's needs?

3 Explain to Mrs Pugh the stages of the care planning process.

4 How would you achieve the maximum involvement of Mrs Pugh in the assessment process?

Assignment A6.2
Meeting individual needs in care settings

David, aged 8, has broken his legs after falling down some stairs. He has been admitted to the local district general hospital

Mrs Malone, aged 90, has been admitted to a residential home for the elderly.

1 How can the staff of the two institutions meet the physical, social, emotional and intellectual needs of these two individuals? Give examples of how these care needs can be met in each individual's care.

2 Outline the general nature of the two care settings.

3 Explain the roles of the care workers in the district general hospital and the residential home in relation to David and Mrs Malone.

Assignment A6.3
Factors which influence the delivery of care

You have been asked to design a residential home for adolescents with physical disabilities.

I How would you do this, bearing in mind the care values (valuing individuals, client's ability to choose, dignity, confidentiality, independence and self-determination)?

2 How would you take into account environmental factors which might influence the care of the individual (location, physical environment)?

3 What staff would you appoint? What qualifications should they have?

4 What equipment would you need to meet the physical needs of the residents?

CHAPTER 7

Creative activities in care settings

Element 7.1: Examine the contribution of creative activities to the development of individuals

Element 7.2: Carry out a creative activity of value to individuals and client groups

Element 7.3: Investigate the contribution of creative activities to care settings

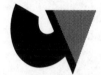

What is covered in this chapter

- Creative activities and the development of individuals
- Planning and carrying out creative activities
- The contribution of creative activities in care settings
- Ideas for creative activities

These are the resources you will need for your Creative Activities in Care Settings file:

- your written answers to the activities in this chapter
- your written answers to the review questions at the end of this chapter
- your completed assignments: A7.1, A7.2, A7.3.

Introduction

This chapter looks at the meaning of 'creative' activities, suggests a range of activities which can be described as creative and explains why they are of value to individuals. It outlines ways that carers can develop a client's creativity and also be more aware of their own creative potential.

The second focus of the chapter is on planning activities to meet the needs of individuals in particular client groups. It includes the way the activity may be presented and suggestions about approaching and motivating individuals when appropriate.

The final part explains the difference that creative activities can make in the care setting. It also highlights the resource implications of encouraging creative activities, in terms of staffing, family involvement, facilities, equipment and finance.

Creative activities and the development of individuals

What does being 'creative' mean? What are 'creative activities'?

To create means to make or to bring into being. When we are involved in creative work, we make or produce something. What we make or produce will vary according to the activity or task – it may be that we make a response to a film or some music, or we may produce a shirt by sewing, or a computer by engineering.

'Creative' is a broad term with a wide range of meanings, particularly in care settings. Generally, being creative involves some thought, even it if is combined with a natural or spontaneous action. Think of the differences being creative would mean for children with severe learning difficulties compared with lively, more able children and for elderly people with dementia, when compared with active, energetic elders. The response of each individual is valid and valuable to them. The processes each one has gone through will be of benefit, even if the results are very different.

> **Remember**
> Judgements about work should be made on the basis of the value to the individual client and not compared with the work of others.

Activity 7.1

In pairs, discuss your own creativity. Make a list of all the ways that you are creative and have been creative since early childhood.

You could include creative dress and hairstyles, and recreational pursuits, such as sports, which have value to you as a person. Don't confine your list to the things you are good at – think more broadly.

The value of creativity to an individual's development

It is important to remember that for any creative activity to be of value, individuals have to be allowed to try things for themselves and develop their own ideas.

If you are working with young children, for example, it is easy to stifle their creativity by continually telling them what to do – by being prescriptive. Often it is necessary to show how something is done, but it is important to avoid doing all the work yourself. The individual can be left feeling frustrated or with a sense of failure.

Creative activities will have little value for people if:
- the individual feels pressured into doing them
- they are badly presented
- they do not suit the ability of the individual (that is, if they affirm what is negative in the client), for example it is no use giving fine embroidery to someone who has poor eyesight and an unsteady hand.

The value of creative activities for babies and children
Babies and children who are denied creative activities or experiences may fail to develop as sociable human beings. For example, it was found in the past that children who had been abandoned (often because they were born outside marriage) and who were given just physical care, found it difficult to adjust to society, to make relationships, to play with other children, to eat in a socially acceptable way and to express themselves.

The choice of activity and its value to a child will depend on that child's:

- age
- stage of development
- needs (see page 135)
- personality.

It will also be affected by the number of children taking part in the activity and the setting you are in.

An activity can be valuable for a child in terms of its:

- **physical development** – by providing exercise and developing physical skills
- **intellectual development** – by providing opportunities for thinking, reasoning and problem-solving
- **social and emotional development** – by providing opportunities to mix with others, to learn to co-operate with them and develop relationships.

For example, when a baby learns to roll over it has developed physically by being able to change its position by itself. In doing so, it can see different objects from different viewpoints so providing intellectual stimulation. While the baby is learning to roll over, the carer will be encouraging it by talking, thus helping its language development, and strengthening the emotional bond between them.

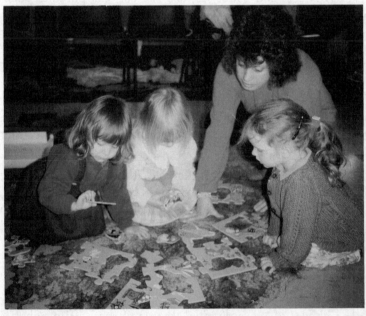
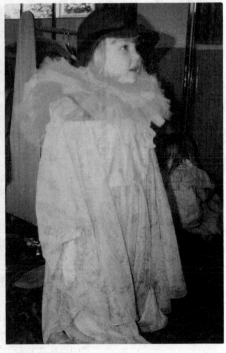

Puzzles aid a child's intellectual development, while dressing-up contributes to social development

Activity 7.2

Decide how a baby's development may be extended by each of the activities below. Draw up a table and put each activity under one (or more) of the following headings: Physical development, Intellectual development, Social and emotional development.

a Having brightly-coloured mobiles hanging in different positions
b Taking the baby out in the pram and pointing out different sights and sounds
c Massage
d Use of music and sounds – records, rattles, singing, musical instruments, household noises
e Talking
f Toys
g Simple exercises
h Splash sessions in toddler pools
i Songs and rhymes
j Books and reading

As the child grows . . .
k Playing with sand, water, dough and clay
l Pretend games
m Outings to parks, playgrounds, museums, shops, farms and the seaside

The value of creative activities for young people

Activity 7.3

Read the comments below. Describe the benefits each young person is gaining from his or her activities.

a 'I really enjoy playing tennis. Even though sometimes I feel a bit lethargic, I know when I start to warm up that I'll feel better. I seem to have more energy when I play than when I don't bother going down to the sessions.'
b 'When I've been working in the evening, I look forward to going to the coffee bar. It gives me a chance to catch up on the gossip, to relax and unwind with my friends.'
c 'I like the challenge of climbing, of pushing myself to the limit of taking a risk. Although I'm scared, it's still a thrilling experience.'
d 'I need to get out of the house a bit at weekends. That's why I like to meet up with my friends and go to a club. I need to talk to people of my own age. I notice when I've been away from home on outdoor pursuits weeks with the Duke of Edinburgh team, I appreciate home more. I think I need to have my own space – some independence.'
e 'I like going away on training weekends with St John's. It's interesting thinking about meeting new people and even more interesting when you might arrange to see someone again afterwards.'
f 'I'm not much good at art really, but I love painting, using colour. I feel really free when I settle down to paint, focussed but free – strange really.'
g 'I often spend time writing. Sometimes it helps to order my thoughts, sometimes it's just good to imagine situations and let the pen run. I like being by myself for a while too.'

h 'We have some really good discussions down at the youth group. The sessions really make me think about big issues like politics, religion and relationships.'

i 'When I'm at school, I feel I'm one of a huge number, but when I'm helping with the play scheme, I feel important, wanted and useful.'

How did you get on? Could you describe how the activities were of value to the young people? Did you think about how they might need physical challenges, company of people their own age, time to relax, chances to take risks, time to be away from parents, opportunities to meet people, chances to make friends with the opposite gender, time to be alone, space to concentrate, a forum to sort out what they really think, a way of raising self-esteem and self-identity?

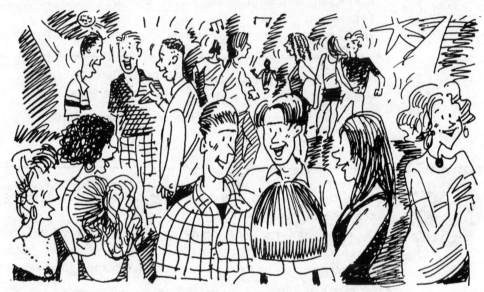

The company of people their own age is important for young people

The value of creative activities for people generally

Activity 7.4

Look at the list of possible values that may be gained from creative activities. Decide whether each benefit is physical, intellectual, emotional or social. In some cases there may be more than one benefit. You could do this by drawing up a table.

Creative activities can:
- stimulate a person's interest in something outside of their immediate problems
- encourage mobility, physical activity and improve general circulation and health
- encourage and build on interests people already have, providing a link with their past, reassurance and some security

- provide enjoyment
- provide a way of passing long days and breaking up boring routines
- provide an opportunity to meet others
- provide an opportunity for carers to get to know clients
- provide a way of satisfying more than basic needs (see page 227)
- provide a talking point for relatives and friends
- enhance a person's self-esteem and sense of self-worth
- in some situations, provide possible employment or remuneration
- put people in a situation of choice or decision-making which gives them a sense of their own autonomy or control over their own lives (empowerment, see page 231)
- be useful in terms of bring people together to form a closer group (group cohesion)
- be a way of relieving tension or anxiety in individuals or groups
- be a calming or soothing influence for an individual or a group
- be used for specific mental or physical treatment
- provide specific movement in a natural way (as in physiotherapy)
- increase dexterity or use of a non-dominant hand (if someone has had a stroke and has little use in their right hand, encouraging writing, baking, painting may assist dexterity in the affected hand)
- strengthen existing movements
- encourage better posture
- increase the range of movement in a stiffened joint
- improve concentration
- provide a counter-irritant to worry or sadness (a frustrated parent might go for a gruelling run after dealing with the tantrums of a 2-year-old)
- provide a client with a gift to give to a relative
- be used as an assessment of ability and motivation (as in occupational therapy)
- produce something for a resident to use themselves
- provide an opportunity for self-expression (possibly an autistic child will draw and paint, but not speak)
- provide an opportunity for someone to help someone else
- provide a chance for families to be together
- provide a chance for someone to express past experiences (as in reminiscence therapy)
- provide an opportunity for someone to gain order and be less confused (as in reality orientation, which seeks to assist people to join our present reality by reinforcing basic points such as the time, the day, the year. It is best carried out as a continual process, rather than a separate activity.).

The value of creative activities for disabled people

Activities may have to be adapted for people with disabilities, but the value or benefit from them may be just as fruitful. Some activities, such as those which concentrate on a particular sense, lend themselves more easily to disabled people.

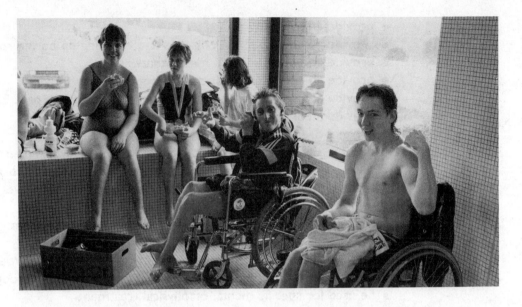

Negative aspects of creative activities

The list in Activity 7.4 demonstrates the positive aspects of creative activities, but some activities can be abused. For example:

- There may be pressure on people to produce items for financial gain. Work produced should always be considered in terms of physical, intellectual, social and emotional gains for the client, rather than what is it is worth commercially.
- If an activity is too demanding, it may cause distress and 'knock people back' emotionally.
- Some pursuits can inhibit social contact if they are taken too seriously.
- Some activities involve more risk-taking than others, and these need expert supervision and careful planning and preparation.

Opportunities for developing an individual's creative skills

When you are on work placement and have settled down in the establishment, it is a good idea to note possible times for creative activities.

Working with children

When working with young children, a lot of the day can be used creatively. Even routine tasks, such as washing and dressing, can be turned into game with language and singing, so that the child learns *and* achieves the task.

Toys such as Lego, Duplo, Sticklebricks, small figures, animals, road layouts and toy vehicles can all be used in creative ways, as obviously dough, clay, paints, crayons, glue and paper can too. Household items can be used to play shop, boxes and cartons for models, and of course there is always dressing-up.

Remember
Safety should be the watchword, whether you are taking children out or using scissors for cutting and sticking.

The timing of an activity is important. You cannot play creatively with a child if he or she is tired or hungry (see page 227). In addition, the choice of activity needs to link with the child's mood and personality. Obviously, if you are working with several children, you will need to choose a time when other help is available to assist you, or choose a very simple activity.

As children progress, creative activities tend to be timetabled in a more structured way. These slots need to be utilised to the full.

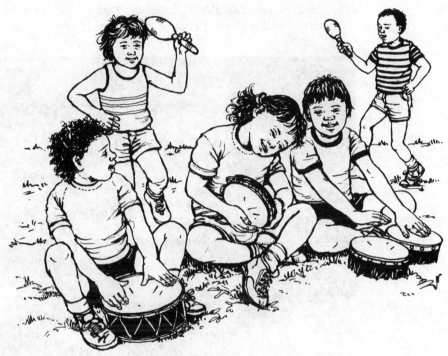

Making music is a valuable creative activity for children

Working with older people
Young people and adults have to consciously set aside time for recreational pursuits. It is easy to let spare time 'fritter' away. Some people's lives are so pressured that they seldom spend time in a creative way. It is not uncommon for people to have little opportunity to develop any creative skill in their entire working lives. It is not surprising, therefore, that they may be resistant to trying new skills when they go to a day centre or residential home in later life.

It may be less easy to identify opportunities for creative activities when working with older people. Apart from any personal lack of motivation and health problems they may have, the setting in which they live may not lend itself to such activities. Often staff are under extreme pressure simply to attend to people's immediate physical needs, without the added responsibilities of organising activities. Sometimes residents seem so confused that it is bewildering to think of suitable activities.

If you are working in a residential establishment with older individuals who are confused, you may be able to reinforce reality orientation messages while helping them with routines of washing and dressing by reminding them of the time, day and year. With those who are still mentally alert, you may be able to talk to them about their past, to find out about what they did, what they ate, what they wore in order to gain ideas for activities or reminiscence sessions later.

Some elderly people may feel brighter earlier in the day and this would be a good time for creative tasks. However, this may interfere with the physical routines that take place in the morning. The afternoons may be better, if the residents are not too sleepy.

Day centres are excellent places to carry out creative activities, both for individuals and groups, because creativity is one of their specific aims.

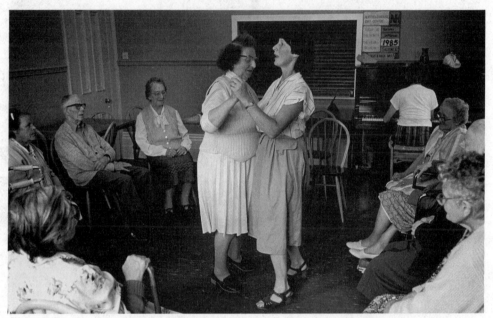

'I feel young again!' Note the reality orientation point on the wall

In all cases, you need the advice and support of experienced staff who know the individual or group, before preparing any structured activity. All plans and preparations need to be closely linked to the client and discussed fully with the staff concerned before any opportunity is taken.

Planning and carrying out creative activities

You will find ideas for creative activities on pages 276–9 . The most important thing is to select an activity that is appropriate for the group or individual.

When planning an activity, you will need to consider the following questions:
- Is the activity for an individual or a group?
- Is the activity self-contained, to be completed at one time, or is it on-going over several sessions?
- For whom is the activity aimed? Do they have any specific needs?
- Is the activity realistic and achievable for the individual or group? Think very carefull about this, especially if anyone has learning difficulties. You will need to take advice here.

- Is the activity relevant to the individual or group? Would they find it interesting, exciting, challenging, enjoyable, satisfying?
- What will the individual or group gain from the activity?
- Who is involved in running the activity?
- Where would the activity be held? Would this disrupt any long-standing routines or arrangements which might breed resentment?
- Is the room suitable in terms of space and furniture? Is it next to another room which is noisy?
- When would the activity be carried out (time of day, date)? Is this enough time for you to prepare? Do you to give notice to the individual or group? Is there enough time for them to prepare?
- Are you simply going to carry out the activity, or are you going to offer refreshments as an inducement? Who would be responsible for these? Who would pay for them? Prepare and serve them? Are the refreshments suitable? Has anyone any allergies, diabetes or special diet? Would the serving of such refreshments interfere with patterns in the establishment?
- What equipment do you need? Do you need to borrow materials and tools, or arrange transport?
- Have you considered the safety implications at every stage?
- What are the cost implications?
- Where will the money come from? Establishment? Fund-raising?

Once you have decided roughly who you are working with, a client or client group, a date and the type of activity, arrange an appointment to speak to the person in charge. Do not turn up without an appointment, because it is likely that the manager, supervisor or teacher will be busy. You need time to talk to him or her, with whoever is working with you, to discuss the issues thoroughly.

Be prepared to change your activity or plans on the advice of your tutor or manager in the workplace. Make notes during the discussion so that you have a clear record to plan from. When you are actually planning the activity, try to build in some way of gaining feedback from the individual or group to assist with your evaluation of the activity.

How creative activities meet the needs of different client groups

It is worth spending some time in the planning process trying to anticipate the needs of the group or individual, rather than being put 'on the spot' later. Think through the whole process of the intended activity to see how far it meets the needs of the group or individual physically, intellectually, emotionally and socially.

When you are thinking about meeting needs, consider:
- the need for company if a person is lonely
- the need to raise self-esteem – this is important for everyone (see Chapter 4)
- the need to reduce tension and anxiety if it is a new activity
- the need to link with the past
- the need to have a good time to allow a person to 'escape from themselves' for a while
- physical needs – can they cope with the length of the session or will they become tired or fidgety? Will anyone need food, drink, medication or to go to the toilet?
- Will they need quiet moments in the midst of a noisy session?

- Will they need particular chairs? Aids? Will they need to sit alongside particular people?
- Will they need to move physically from one room to another for the activity? Is help available for this?
- Is the activity suitable for their emotional needs? If you do a reminiscence session and people become upset, what can you do about this? If someone becomes angry because he or she loses a game, or feels frustrated by the activity, what alternatives can you offer?

Activity 7.5

Read the comments below. Decide what needs are being satisfied by each activity.

a 'When I practise yoga, I feel so completely relaxed that I sleep better and seem to be less harassed during the day.' *Mother of three young children*

b 'I was delighted when Phil was asked to swim for the school. He had been a bit low after that bullying incident.' *Father of a 10-year-old boy*

c 'Sometimes I think I won't go to the day centre when I feel in one of those "can't be bothered" moods. But then I urge myself to get going, have a wash and shave, change my shirt and make an effort. I always feel better for having made the effort. I need that motivation for a bit of self-discipline.' *Seventy-six-year-old man*

d 'I'm so glad I've mastered the eureka computer. It gives me chance to write my poems.' *Adolescent girl with very little sight*

e 'I look forward to playing a bit of snooker on Friday nights at the club. I can meet my friends and I'm improving – we have a laugh.' *Teenage boy*

f 'One thing about gardening, it's a good excuse to get out in the fresh air. It's an interest. I look forward to the spring, and in the winter I'm busy with seeds. All that bending and stretching, I don't need to go to keep fit – it's a pity I'm not so enthusiastic about housework!' *Older woman*

g 'I've always danced – I think I danced before I walked! I love to move and I feel I can interpret the music when I dance. The classes help me to improve.' *Seventeen-year-old boy*

h 'I can express myself through sculpture. I would like to spend a lot more on sculpture – working myself and seeing others work.' *Young woman in her early twenties*

i 'Sometimes the reminiscence sessions go really well. You can see the joy in the faces of some of the people when they are reminded of particular things. You can see them grow in self-worth as they link with their past and remember how they once were. I feel I learn a lot too – about them – I appreciate how their lives have changed and I find it easier to relate to them then.' *Occupational therapist in a nursing home*

j 'The simple games and armchair fitness exercises have really improved Mrs Brown's range of movement. She seems brighter in herself now.'
Physiotherapist in a day centre

k 'You can tell how restless the children become when they miss PE. Last week I took them out onto the field to play some games to release some energy and then we practised some ball skills.' *Infant school teacher*

l 'I enjoyed that quiz we did the other night on old Sheffield. I was really surprised how much they knew. It was fun checking out the answers beforehand. They seemed to chat on for ages afterwards.'
Care assistant in a residential home for the elderly

How did you get on? You should have been able to identify needs for relaxation, self-esteem, self-discipline, imagination, recreation, being sociable, physical fitness, self-expression, linking with the past, increasing self-worth, opportunities for getting to know people, and releasing energy.

Developing creative skills within the group

The introduction of any activity directly affects the way any skills are developed. To create an atmosphere in which skills may be developed, and therefore in which people will gain benefit from the activity, you will need to:
- encourage people to join in
- plan the timing of the activity
- encourage effective communication between the group members
- ensure all the necessary equipment is at hand.

People need to feel safe before they embark on a creative activity. They quickly sense tension, particularly if they have had a difficult time and feel vulnerable already. Everyone fears failure and making a fool of themselves. However straightforward the activity seems to you, you must never put anyone down who doesn't quite understand what to do.

Encouraging people to join in
In some situations people may be very apathetic (not interested or motivated). You may have to spend some time discussing ways people may be encouraged to join in, such as:
- the inducement of refreshments
- their friends are there
- they'll enjoy themselves – it's nothing heavy
- you would appreciate them joining in – it's special to you if they come
- the group will miss them.

Look at the comments below. Which do you think are the most positive? How do you think the person being asked may reply?
- 'What would you like to do?'
- 'Would you like to make a tea cosy?'
- 'Which of these would you like to have a go at?'

- 'I've brought this ... to try. Have a go and if it's no good, we'll have a go at something else.'

Children pounce on any sort of uncertainty:
- *Parent to child*: 'I wondered about going swimming today. Would you like to? I know it's a bit cold.'
- *Parent to child*: 'Let's go swimming today. It'll be fun – the water at Upperthorpe Pool is always warm.'

Can you see the difference in the two approaches? The point is that you have to be enthusiastic about the activity yourself before you can inspire anyone else.

If people are unsure what the activity involves, they are likely to 'vote with their feet' and say no or stay away. So it's important to be as clear and as simple as possible with the introductory explanation.

Being clear and simple does not mean being bossy or patronising. You must always work with the person and not talk down to them (see Chapter 4). Show that you are sensitive to their needs by paying attention to your tone of voice, language and non-verbal messages.

There may be people who simply don't want to participate whatever the activity or the inducements, or however skilful you are at persuasion. If that is their decision, you must respect it. Never force people to join in or reach a confrontation stage.

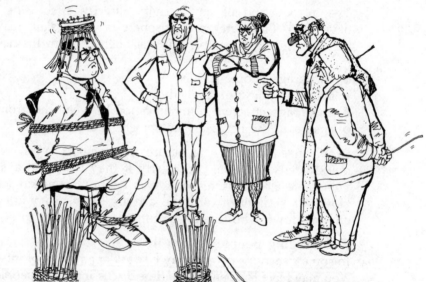

'They told me they didn't want to do it! Why didn't I listen?'

If a person refuses to participate, use the experience to learn. Ask yourself why. Was it something in their past? Was the activity inappropriate? Was it just a bad time? Learn from the incident, but don't take it personally.

Timing
Timing needs to be well thought-out.
- Start on time, but not in a rush. You may have a cup of tea first to act as an ice-breaker. Once the cups are cleared, that may be a signal to start.
- It is better to run shorter, effective sessions rather than long, drawn-out affairs with too little to do.

- Sometimes it may be necessary to change the activity, if the task in hand is flagging.

Effective communication

- If the members of the group do not know one another, or if you have brought other helpers with you, spend some time introducing people and asking them by which name they like to be called. Think of ways to reinforce names. By repeating them, for example, when playing a ball game, you might say, 'Pass it to Mary'. This will help people to feel relaxed and more able to communicate with other members of the group.
- If you have several helpers, it is good to alternate the 'presenting' so that everyone has a opportunity to observe, assist and talk to individuals.
- Use open and closed questions where appropriate:
  - If you are using part of the time to learn about an individual, use lots of **open questions**, such as 'Tell me a bit about yourself . . .'.
  - When you need to gain specific answers, use direct, **closed questions**, such as 'Do you need more clay next week?' Only one of two answers is required, yes or no (see Chapter 4).
- Some sessions may be made more challenging by dominant or unusual individuals. You will need to think some tactics through in advance and ask more experienced members of staff how they might approach the situation. Some people may need encouragement to speak in the group. If it is a reminiscence session, ask them directly, 'Arthur, what do you think?' Others may say too much, say 'Fred, I want to hear from the others a bit.'

Equipment and materials

Development of creativity will be hampered if sessions are not well-prepared and if equipment or facilities are not available and in good working order.

This is something you need to consider carefully when planning an activity. It is tempting to be ambitious, but if you have few facilities and materials, it is better to be simple, effective and realistic than complicated and unsuccessful, and to reinforce failure.

An example of planning a creative activity

It was decided to organise an afternoon of creative activities for a group of 6-year-olds. The students decided to work as a team rather than individually.

They were asked to present the stages of their planning as a series of meetings and then to decide on a time-scale for the planning process.

Group meeting 1
- Brainstorm contacts
- Brainstorm possible activities
- Allocate one person to record ideas and decisions made
- Reach a decision on which client group and activity, so that, in this case, the teacher can be approached and work can begin on preparation.

Group meeting 2
- Draw up a draft plan for the activities afternoon
- Make arrangements to see class teacher to discuss plans and introduce helpers
- Prepare list of questions for teacher (see 268)

The students used a contact from one student's work experience. This meant that one team member knew the level and needs of the group and situation. The place for the activity was fairly accessible for most of the team.

Draft plan (to be modified on class teacher's advice)
1.30 Introduction
1.40 Explanation of activities
2.00 Music and movement in hall using music from 'The Snowman'
2.20 Small group work – creative writing theme of snow, cold, excitement of seeing new snow, building, playing
2.40 Break time – squash and snowmen cakes (prepared by group member)
2.50 Small group work – art/craft creation of large frieze (pre-prepared)
3.25 Clear up, wind down, ask for feedback
3.35 Home

Questions for class teacher
1 Is suggested afternoon OK?
2 Do we also need to check with headteacher?
3 How many children will there be?
4 Could we have a list of names
5 Is there anything we need to know about individual children?
6 Are the proposed activities suitable?
7 Equipment – Can we use paint, glue, scissors, lolly sticks? We will bring pre-prepared background frieze from college – it will roll up to bring on the bus.
8 Where can we mount the frieze? Can we use a staple gun? Blutack won't work.
9 Can we arrive at lunch time to set up?
10 Is it OK to let the children eat and drink in the classroom?
11 Will you stay around and give us feedback?
12 Timing – Is break-time at 2.40 as Sarah said?
13 Can we use the hall and tape recorder for music and movement?

Group meeting 3
More detailed planning.
1 Check strengths of group. Allocate tasks of:
   a Introduction, explanation and wind down
   b Leading the music and movement
   c Each member to take a small group – time to get to know some children individually for writing and crafts. Half the groups could write and then alternate to reduce pressure on equipment.
   d Cake making, purchasing squash and paper cups
   e Everyone to clear up
   f Checking tape recorder and tape
   g Preparation of background frieze and craft ideas for children

2 Check timing – time of arrival to prepare

3 Costs – Shall we all chip in for squash and buns?

Group meeting 4

- Make a detailed plan of action for the day
- List the items to bring and allocate who is to bring them
- Exchange phone numbers for last minute details or hitches

Once the stages of planning had been drawn up and the students could see the amount of organisation that would be necessary, a timescale was decided. They had four weeks until the day of the activities afternoon. Meetings 1, 2 and 3 needed to be carried out by 30 November to give time for all the tasks to be completed.

Timescale

Meeting 1	16 November
Meeting 2	20 November
Meeting 3	30 November
Meeting 4	11 December
Activities afternoon	14 December

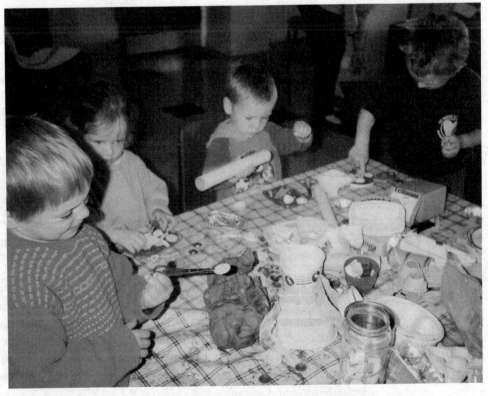

Children's creative activities can be fun – the messier the better!

> **Points to remember when planning an activity**
> - Know the group, take advice
> - Select the activity carefully
> - Plan the activity methodically
> - Check what resources are needed and what is available
> - Introduce the activity simply and enthusiastically
> - Try to get feedback from participants and other staff
> - Learn from each activity
> - Evaluate the activity thoroughly

Evaluation

Make use of any feedback you can get from participants in the activity and from members of staff, and also ask yourself:
- Was each part of the activity appropriate for the group and each individual?
- Was the setting right? Could it have been improved or would this have been too difficult to organise
- Was the helper/children ratio right?
- Were the materials and equipment appropriate and ready for use?
- Timing – Did you need longer than planned for certain activities? Did the time drag?
- Content of the activity – Did the activity interest, stimulate and challenge the children? Was it too difficult for some? Did it allow for individual creativity?
- What benefit did the children gain physically, intellectually, emotionally and socially?

The contribution of creative activities in care settings

We have already discussed the benefits creative activities may have for individual clients, groups of clients and for the helpers and carers themselves. What difference do creative activities make to particular care settings? Let us look at some examples.

> **The family home**
> Harry is a thoughtful carer. He looks after three children, aged 6, 4 and $2\frac{1}{2}$. The 6-year-old is at school. Harry knows he has to see to their physical needs, such as providing lunches, snacks and sleep times, but he also takes time to plan special outings, simple craft sessions, lively games, dressing-up sessions and stories to read aloud.
>
> The home is an interesting place where the children are happy to be. They enjoy seeing Harry and feel secure and occupied when he is around. Their parents feel assured that their children are developing rapidly, and admire the creative efforts of their children when they come home from work. The parents are very supportive of Harry in terms of costs, helping with transport when they can and encouraging contacts with other local children, groups, organisations and events.

Activity 7.6

Imagine life in the house without Harry's thoughtfulness and ideas. What tensions might there be among the children? With the parents?

Think of the general atmosphere in a home where the children are bored, where people don't call and the children don't get out much.

Family life can be enhanced by shared creative and recreational activities, such as walking, skiing, cycling, camping, paper crafts, reading, watching a film or video together, cooking, or just eating a meal together and talking. Often it is difficult to get everyone in the family to agree to do the same thing at the same time. So, 9-year-old Kate might spend time writing stories, but she feels she can go to the kitchen, where her Dad is preparing a curry, to read him the story she has just written. At the same time, 6-year-old Jamie may be making a rag rug, while his mum is working on the computer, but they are all available to each other.

The day centre: I
Jane looks forward to going to the day centre at the local home for elderly people. She has got to know the regulars now. If she notices anyone new, she quickly makes an effort to include them. That's why she enjoys the games — people join in, feel included — they have a laugh. It's good to have some occupation, a focus, a talking point. If they all just sat around, they would only discuss their aches and pains. They can think about those at home. Yes, creative activities help people to get to know one another in the day centre and provide a different setting from home.

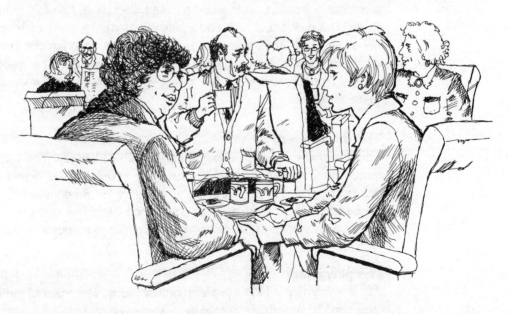

Day centres provide an opportunity for social contact for elderly people who live on their own as well as creative activities

271

The day centre: 2

Albert's day centre is very active. He says that he's learnt more since he retired from the steelworks, with all the trips, outings and speakers, than during all the time he spent at school.

The residential home: 1

Peggy was upset when she left her own home to go into residential care. 'Lovely home', her daughter said, 'spotlessly clean and curtains with tie backs.' She didn't mention the endless hours of boredom, waiting for someone to visit or for the next meal. Only the television blaring away. Peggy feels her life has altered for the worse since she left her home. The staff seem to be under pressure – they do what they have to and then go home.

The residential home: 2

Ruth feels just the opposite to Peggy. She was lonely at home on her own and glad to give up her house and go to Primrose View. The home really caters for people's needs. There is always something happening – people coming for keep fit, aromatherapy, to play music, to sing, to dance, to demonstrate crafts, not to mention the outings.

'I've never had it so good', says Ruth. The staff really seem to enjoy being around the home. They seem interested and glad to be part of a set-up where things are going on, where people are interacting and appreciative. Of course, some people don't want to join in things, but that's up to them – the staff do their best and understand.

The hospital

Joan was in hospital after a complicated operation. She felt awful lying there. She didn't feel well enough to do anything, until a friend brought her some small embroidery cards to complete. Joan felt she could get on with these and build up a store of greetings cards for her friends and family. The nurses noticed her improvement and how few demands she made on them.

The day nursery

There is always a bustle about Buchanan Day Nursery. You can sense it the minute you walk in. The children eagerly anticipate the events planned and the tasks prepared for them. It's a real asset to the community. Parents feel pleased that their children get such a good deal. The staff seem to act as a team because they do so much and the children respond well.

The playgroup

'My Tommy really likes his playgroup sessions. The main organiser really tries hard to encourage creativity. I always enjoy helping. I learn a lot myself and I'm always first to volunteer when they need extra help.'

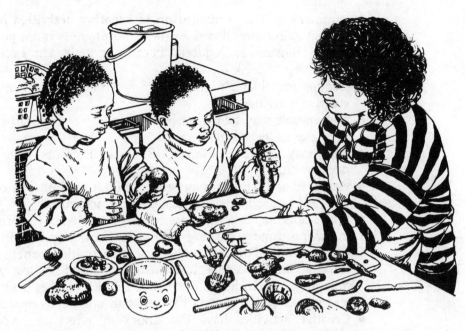

Playgroups offer a wider range of creative activities than children have access to at home

The special school

'I didn't want Karl to go away from home. He has little sight. I felt
almost bereaved when he started school. I worried myself sick. But now he
is always chatting on about what he has done, asking me to collect this and
that. I've noticed too that he can occupy himself more at home now
because of how they have encouraged his creative capacities in spite of his
poor eyesight. It seems to have given him confidence, made him more able.'

Did you make the connections?
- Harry's creative approach helps the children to develop, creates a happy home where parents and children feel at ease and fulfilled. Family relationships may benefit from working together on their own creative projects – home becomes a happy place to be.
- Jane's day centre isn't just a place for moaning people to share their ailments. They get on and do something.
- Albert's day centre has extended his education.
- Peggy's home only caters for the residents' physical needs. They have nothing to think about, look forward to, make them feel useful, empowered or able.
- Joan's hospital stay was brightened by creative work and it also reduced the pressure on staff.
- The Buchanan Day Nursery affects the community. Creative approaches are part of a positive atmosphere and it therefore provides an advantage in a disadvantaged area.
- Tommy's mother feels involved in the playgroup through creative work.
- Karl's mother can see the benefits that going to school has brought to Karl.

A summary of the contribution of creative activities in care settings
- Clients gain more, therefore the atmosphere is more positive.
- Group tension is reduced, because people are occupied. They have something to look forward to.
- Groups may blend together better if they have a common goal through creative activities.
- Staff morale may be higher because they are more satisfied seeing more of their clients' needs fulfilled.
- Staff may not be 'pestered' as much if clients have some meaningful occupation.
- Relatives and parents may sense an improved quality of life for clients in care settings which encourage creative activities.
- Staff teams may become more cohesive because of the organisation involved in having a more creative approach. They may be stimulated, challenged and encouraged themselves because the activities are new and interesting.
- Care settings become less 'institutionalised' – less clinical and more home-like. The inclusion of creative activities makes the place more dynamic and breaks down barriers beween staff and between staff and clients.
- Creative activities have the 'knock-on' effect of involving parents and relatives. The tasks gather momentum and people feel generally uplifted. The activities provide links between home and school, between care establishments and relatives.
- Clients may be able to use the creative skills and ideas they have learnt in their home settings.

Creative activities appropriate for different care settings

You will find a list of creative activities on pages 276–9. The main point to consider when choosing an activity is the level and capability of the client, as well as the facilities necessary. Consider the following questions:
- Is the client physically able to cope with the activity?
- On an intellectual level, is the task too simple, or too difficult? For example, would a child understand the rules?
- On an emotional level, what will the client gain from the activity? Enjoyment is a very valid emotion to gain!
- On a social level, will the client be encouraged? Even if the activity is solitary, such as reading, you may be able to organise discussions of particular authors, read stories aloud and discuss them, book swops, displays involving background information about an author or a particular book. (Note that these suggestions link with intellectual needs too.)

Sources of support for creative activities

People
One of the keys to successful creative activity sessions is not to be too independent. Do not forget the people who have a lot of emotional investment in clients: their family and friends. These people are often unstinting in their time and energy, because they are aware of the benefits and rewards such effort brings.
- Often family and friends help with fund-raising for equipment and materials.
- Family and friends may have talents and experiences that can be shared. For example, parents of children in a playgroup who are of Asian background may share their knowledge of cooking, crafts and textiles. Another parent

may enjoy photography and could take photographs of events to make displays.

- People who have recently retired may help with reminiscence sessions, or have photographs and objects of interest that they could show to small groups of children.
- People who have worked with disabled people may give you ideas and approaches to use with clients who have disabilities. Similarly, youth workers may help if you are unsure about activities for adolescents.
- Experienced, professional people, such as occupational therapists, physio-therapists, teachers, music therapists, dance therapists, art and drawing therapists, are all excellent sources of inspiration. Going to events, open days, performances and exhibitions yourself will also give you ideas that can be adapted.

Remember
- Don't be ambitious about what you can cope with on your own. Make sure you have enough helpers to assist, particularly when working with children and people with disabilities.
- Be aware of the health and safety regulations related to a particular situation

Environment
Many of the issues concerning facilities, equipment and materials are beyond your control. However, you may be able to put pressure on more senior members of staff so that rooms meet basic requirements in terms of size, temperature, cleanliness, safety, access, lighting, and signposting.

Sometimes posters, plants and displays give a room a pleasant, welcoming appearance. Check the layout of furniture in the room (remind yourself about barriers to communication in Chapter 4).

Materials, equipment and facilities
Materials may be purchased using a budget, through fund-raising and through the sale of items made. It is not a good idea, however, to put clients under pressure to produce items for sale (see page 260).
- Simple materials may be collected from home.
- Sometimes it is possible to gain usable scraps from factories and offices.
- Scout and Guide groups, and other organisations such as the RNID and RNIB, may be able to lend equipment and facilities.
- Use any local resources you can. For example, if you live in a flat area and your client group is able, think about cycle hire. If you live near an area like the Peak District, think about abseiling or climbing. If you use public sessions at local facilities, such as a swimming pool, inform the attendant of any individual that has a disability. In many pools, there are usually sessions for particular groups of people, such as parents and toddlers, or people with disabilities.

Ideas for creative activities

This list has not been arranged according to age, ability or gender, because many activities can be adapted for different abilities and there are few activities that cannot be enjoyed by either gender. Age does affect some activities involving thought processes, such as chess, but even in this some children are able to challenge older people. People with disabilities often surprise helpers with their abilities and talents, so do not deny them opportunities, but present them sensitively and work at the client's pace.

Arts and crafts

3D-work
Appliqué
Basketry
Batik
Brass rubbing
Candle making
Card making
Carving
Collage
Construction and model-making
Decorating objects, bottles, tins
Découpage
Drawing, sketching
Embroidery
Fabric printing
Feltwork
Finger/hand/toe/foot painting
Home furnishings/upholstery
Jewellery making
Knitting, crocheting
Locker hooking (using wool and canvas to make bags, rugs, etc.)
Marbling
Masks and puppets
Modelling – clay, plasticine, doughcraft, mod rock (using soft plaster and bandage-type material)
Painting – watercolours, oils, acrylics
Paper making
Papier maché
Pressed flowers
Printing with wood, leaves, vegetables, lino, loofah, sponges
Scupture
Sewing
Silhouettes
Stencils
Tracing
Wax patterns
Weaving

As with all creative activities, anticipate any safety hazards.

Look for ideas for stimulating activities in books, libraries, open days, exhibitions and galleries. Themes, festivals and celebrations from other cultures can provide exciting ideas. If possible, encourage clients to learn from others, 'the older masters' and the displays at the local infant school. Materials themselves can be inspiring. Leaves, pine cones, flowers, tree barks and wood are natural sources of ideas. There is also much potential in considering other media, such as plastic and man-made fabrics.

Outdoor activities

Abseiling
Bird watching
Bug hunting, or other wildlife
Butterfly spotting
Camping
Canoeing
Climbing
Cycling
Fishing
Gardening
Skiing
Sports
Traditional games
Walking

Movement

Armchair keep fit
Dancing
Jogging
Keep fit
Music and movement
Playground games
Ball skills (throwing, catching, kicking, goal scoring, batting, bouncing)
Running
Sports
Swimming
Team games
Using apparatus
Using weights and gym equipment
Walking

- Use movement to raise awareness of body parts, space, moving safely using the floor (Note how confident children roll easily on the floor, while timid, anxious children are afraid to let their weight go. Think how such exercises may be used with other client groups.)
- Movement using hoops, balls, ropes, partners, bean bags, skittles, hockey sticks

Indoor activities

Armchair keep fit
Baking
Board games
Card games
Computer activities
Construction play
Cooking
Flower arranging

Model railways
Music
Pot plants
Reading
Reminiscence sessions (see below)
Videos
Word/discussion games

Reminiscence sessions
Use music, photographs (use them as prompts, 'There's an open fire there — who was your coalman? How often did you have your chimney swept? Did you run out to see the brush at the top?'), smells (lavender, Vick, ginger, pear drops, aniseed — just a couple at a time, otherwise it is confusing), film clips, recordings of speeches, objects to be touched (scrubbing brush, toasting fork, flat iron). Be conscious of all your interpersonal skills with individuals and groups (see Chapter 4). If some clients are deaf, check whether there is a loop system.

Music

Exploring different themes in music (see below)
Exploring different types of music (see below)
Expressing feelings through music or sounds
Inviting people in to perform
Listening to records, tapes, CDs
Making music (see below)
Outings to concerts
Tune of the week (Hum that tune, Clap that rhythm, songs with actions)

Themes in music
- Animals: Rimskykorsakov, *The Flight of the Bumble Bee*; Walt Disney, *The Jungle Book, Dumbo*; Saint Saens, *Carnival of the Animals*
- Space: Holst, *The Planets Suite*; Dr Who theme
- Weather: Vivaldi, *The Four Seasons*; Stravinsky, *The Rite of Spring*

Types of music
- Music to alter mood
  - Quiet influences: Beethoven, *Symphony No. 6 Pastoral*, 2nd and 5th movements; Delius, *Summer Night on the River*
  - Strong, exciting movement: Tchaikovsky, *1812 Overture*
- Light dancing music: Tchaikovsky, *The Nutcracker Suite*
- Old time music: *The Lambeth Walk, We'll Meet Again, Pack Up Your Troubles, It's A Long Way To Tipperary*
- Look for other types: reggae, Indian music, rapping, big band music (e.g. Glen Miller), the Beatles, Chinese music, Elizabethan lute, folk music

Making music
Make music:
- through singing (groups or individually — group singing makes for a united group)
- through playing instruments and experimenting with them
- by making sounds with everyday items, such as a bicycle bell, milk bottles, shakers made from rice, bracelet with bells, maracas (made with Jif lemon

container, rice and dowelling), drums (layers of greaseproof paper and muslin glued together with wallpaper paste)

Drama

Drama with groups
Drama with toys
Local drama group performances
Making an audio-play
Mime
Theatre visits
Visits by travelling drama groups and dance groups

Drama can assist skill control, co-ordination, body awareness and oral skills. Disability need not be a bar to dramatic activities or dance performances. 'Can do Co.' are a group of disabled people who give stunning dance performances.

Review questions

1 List the factors that are important in selecting a creative activity for children.

2 List the factors that are important in selecting a creative activity for elders.

3 Explain the value of creative activities to the individual.

4 Explain the value of creative activities in the care setting.

5 Which organisations may help with lending equipment for outdoor use?

6 How can creative activities help to fulfil people's social needs?

7 Give an example of an activity which may meet several needs of an individual.

8 How can creative activities be therapeutic?

9 What does empowerment mean

10 How can creative activities empower people?

Assignment A7.1
Creative activities and individual development

For each client group, describe an opportunity you could use to develop an individual's creative skills. Choose a different skill in each case. Explain how the skill would benefit the individual.

Client groups:
- children
- adolescents
- older people
- people with learning difficulties
- people with physical disabilities.

Keep your descriptions brief. For example:

> **Client group: Children**
> **Setting: Playgroup for 3–4-year-olds**
> Often the children simply play with the toys that are available. Sometimes helpers set up a specific activity for those who want to join in. I could set up a dough table – I could make the playdough and let the children experiment with it first, then introduce cutters. I might make a baker's shop and talk to the children as they play.
>
> Value: manual dexterity, manipulative skills, hand-eye co-ordination, group skills, children may talk to each other depending on the level of concentration, may give me a chance to get to know the children.

Assignment A7.2
Carrying out creative activities

1 Select a client group and describe how creative skills may be developed with that group.

2 Organise a creative activity for your chosen client group. Produce a plan and carry out the activity.

Consider the following points when selecting a client group for a creative activity:

- Have you any contacts already? Knowledge of the client group is vitally important to the selection of the activity. Do you think the usual carers, or people responsible for the group, would be welcoming and supportive of students introducing an activity?
- Will you manage the whole group? Or will you make arrangements for part of the group to be occupied elsewhere?
- Are there any members of the group that you don't feel confident about coping with? Is it better to ask to some help with these members? Is it better for them to be excluded for the sake of the others, or will you include all those who wish to participate?
- Do you know the level, needs and interests of the group? Is there anyone who has a specific disability or health problem? Have you noticed anyone who seems particularly hard of hearing or slow to see (such problems may not even be diagnosed, if you are working with elderly people and they are deteriorating rapidly).

Assignment A7.3
The contribution of creative activities to care settings

Write a report describing two different creative activities which two different individuals have set about. You could use your experiences from your work placement for this. The client group and setting must be different in each case.

In each case, describe:
- the activities
- the setting
- what is available in terms of staff, materials, space and equipment.

In your conclusion, explain how the activities have benefited each individual and the differences that the activities made in each care setting.

CHAPTER 8

Practical caring skills

Element 8.1: Investigate the function of different care settings
Element 8.2: Describe methods used to support social and life skills
Element 8.3: Use the practical skills required to support physical needs

What is covered in this chapter

- The function of care settings
- Methods to support social and life skills
- Practical skills to support physical needs

These are the resources you will need for your Practical Caring Skills file:
- evidence of any caring tasks you carry out
- a record of any research you have done for activities
- your written answers to the activities in this chapter
- your written answers to the review questions at the end of this chapter
- your completed assignments: A8.1, A8.2, A8.3.

Introduction

You have most probably decided to follow this Intermediate GNVQ course in Health and Social Care because you have a caring personality and want a job in which you help people. Your caring attitude is an important asset in care work, but you will also need to know how to carry out practical tasks.

This chapter begins by describing the function of care settings. It then goes on to explain how to support social and life skills, and how to carry out the routine practical caring skills that are necessary when working in care settings, particularly in residential and nursing homes for elderly people.

The function of care settings

Types of care setting

As a care worker you may work with clients whose ages range from birth and late old age, who have a range of abilities – they may be able-bodied, ill, physically disabled, or have learning difficulties. The type of care setting that a client uses depends on the age, ability and **needs** of that client. Types of care setting include:
- residential homes for elderly people
- nursing homes for elderly people
- hospitals

- day centres
- clients' own homes
- nurseries
- creches
- playgroups
- primary schools

- schools for children with learning difficulties
- centres and residential homes for adults with learning difficulties and disabilities.

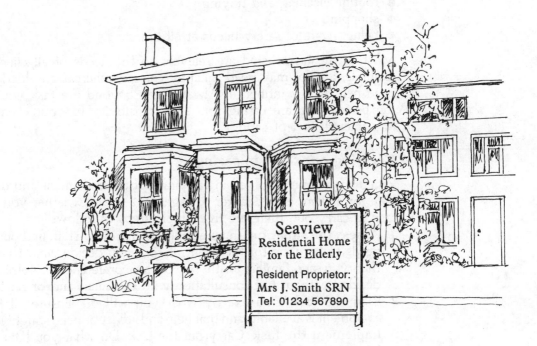

Seaview
Residential Home
for the Elderly

Resident Proprietor:
Mrs J. Smith SRN
Tel: 01234 567890

The purpose of care settings

The purpose (or aim) of any care setting is to provide for the specific needs that a client or client group may have. Needs cover four areas:

- physical needs
- intellectual needs
- social needs
- emotional needs.

Read Chapter 6, pages 226–30 to remind yourself about needs.

In this chapter, we will be concentrating on the practical skills needed when working with elderly people living in residential homes and nursing homes, where the focus is on residents' physical and emotional needs.

The functions of workers in care settings include:

- providing personal support
- assisting and encouraging clients to achieve
- encouraging clients to be as independent as possible
- taking part in the assessment of client needs, planning, implementing, monitoring and reviewing care.

When working with clients the tasks involved in these functions will include:

- attending to toilet needs
- attending to personal hygiene
- helping with dressing and undressing
- assisting with mobility
- attending to physical comfort

- using appropriate aids and appliances
- helping with meals and feeding
- organising and taking part in play activities and creative activities
- organising and taking part in educational activities
- organising outings, visits and social events
- setting up and clearing away equipment
- routine cleaning and tidying
- shopping
- being aware of safety needs at all times.

Most of the tasks listed are relevent to the needs of all client groups. For example, a baby may need a nappy change, whereas an elderly person may need help with continence. Always look beyond the task you are doing to the person you are caring for. Your sensitivity to your client's needs is a fundamental part of caring.

Carrying out tasks in caring

Whether you are involved in carrying out an assessment and devising a care plan for a client (see Chapter 6, pages 232–7), or whether you have a single task to carry out, there are five simple steps to follow:

1 **Assess the situation** In consultation with other staff, find out exactly what needs to be done for the client. Before you decide what to do, make sure that you are familiar with his or her preferences. Nothing should be decided without full consultation with the client and/or relatives.
2 **Plan the task** Plan exactly what you will do. Ensure all the necessary equipment is available, and that help and advice as been sought if necessary.
3 **Implement the task** Carry out the task. Do what you have planned.
4 **Monitor and review the task** Monitor what you are doing – what went well, and what didn't work so well.
5 **Evaluate the task** What lessons have you learned from the task? Could it have been done better?

Activity 8.1

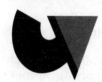

a Make a list of all the tasks you are involved in at your work placement.

b Describe one task in detail. Write an evaluation of what took place.

A caring attitude

As we have already mentioned, your caring personality is your most valuable asset as a care worker. It is also important that you appreciate how it feels to be dependent on others for even the simplest personal task. Try the next activity.

Activity 8.2

At your next family meal, ask someone to feed you using a spoon and bowl.

a How does it feel to be dependent on another person? Discuss your feelings as a group.

b Discuss situations when a client might find dependence upsetting.

Effective communication

To help your clients in a caring and sensitive manner, pay constant attention to the effectiveness of your communication skills. Be polite and respectful, speaking to clients and co-workers in a clear voice.

All caring work involves good interpersonal skills (see Chapter 4). Talk to your client about what you are doing and why to help them feel at ease. Always try to have a friendly, welcoming approach. Show interest and understanding of your clients' individual needs. Try to be helpful and supportive. Be ready to respond with conversation, a laugh, a smile or a word of comfort. Your clients will also derive comfort from a touch, so hold their hands, put an arm around their shoulders or give them a cuddle.

Aim to:
- Listen and respond to communications from clients and co-workers.
- Use good eye contact and keep smiling.
- Be sincere, sympathetic and understanding.
- Be kind, gentle and tactful.
- Be willing to assist, but always remember to allow your clients to do as much as possible for themselves. Encourage them to be as independent as possible.
- Respect your clients' right to confidentiality.

However caring you are, care work is not easy. You may encounter problems – some of them are listed in Chapter 6, page 247.

Legislation affecting care settings

There are a number of laws that relate to you as a care worker, to your clients and to the establishment where you work. The legislation covers five areas:
- registration of care settings
- residents' rights
- employment
- health and safety
- medicines.

Registration

The Registered Homes Act 1984
This Act governs the registration of residential care establishments by local authorities. Registration is required for establishments providing care for four or more residents.

The process of registration is concerned with:
- the suitability of the applicant to run the establishment – this includes details of previous employment, references (including a banker's reference), any previous criminal convictions
- the suitability of the premises, including:
  - planning consent for use as a residential home
  - building regulations – the premises should be suitable for use as a residential home (including construction and state of repair)
  - the premises have to be inspected and approved by the Fire Service
  - the premises have to be inspected and approved by the Environmental Health Service officer
  - the electrical installation has to be inspected

- the suitability of the accommodation, including:
  - bedrooms
  - lifts and stairs
  - dining and lounge areas
  - bathrooms and toilets
  - kitchen and food storage areas
  - laundry areas
  - emergency call system
  - security of valuables
  - heating, lighting and ventilation
  - furniture and furnishings
  - drug storage
- the staffing levels – the ratio of staff to residents is set depending upon the number and category of residents, and their level of dependency
- the suitability of the services and facilities – the appropriate range of services and facilities should be provided. Residents should have choice, privacy and be consulted about the running of the home.

Residents' rights

In Chapter 6 (page 230) you will have read about the rights that all clients (and everyone else too) have to anti-discriminatory practice, confidentiality, choice, personal beliefs and identity and effective communication. These rights are most often set out in charters (see the Patient's Charter on page 118).

Some rights are set out in laws – these too are rights that apply to everyone in our society. For example, the Race Relations Act of 1976 (see page 287), the Access to Personal Files Act and the Sex Discrimination Act (see page 287). You can probably think of others.

> **Remember**
> A care worker must always respect a resident's right to confidentiality. Information about a client must never be discussed with others. If information is to be passed on to another professional, the resident must be consulted and agree to it.

Employment

The Employment Protection Act 1978
Both the employer and the employee have rights and duties under this Act.

Employers' duties Employees have a right to expect that their employers will:
- remunerate them for work carried out
- provide work
- indemnify (compensate) them when necessary
- treat them with respect
- give them time off
- meet the safety requirements for the tasks they are expected to carry out
- provide a **contract of employment** for any employee who works for more than 16 hours a week. The contract could be in the form of a letter or form part of a staff handbook outlining the **conditions of employment**. This should state: the name of the employer, the name of the employee, the full job title, the rate of pay, the hours of work, holiday entitlement, period of

notice and details of any pension schemes. The employee must be made aware of any grievance or disciplinary procedures that exist.

Employees' duties Employers have a right to expect that their employees will:
- give personal service
- give careful service
- obey reasonable orders
- act in good faith
- be loyal
- share the benefit of any inventions
- not disclose confidential information
- abide by the terms of the contract and conditions of work. For example, arriving at work on time each day.

The Sex Discrimination Act 1975
It is illegal to discriminate or give less favourable treatment on the grounds of sex or marital status. The Act allows for positive discrimination in certain circumstances. For example, in a situation where two applicants (one male and one female) have identical qualifications and experience, the post can be offered to the woman. You may see job adverts which state 'We are committed to equal opportunities.'

The Act established the Equal Opportunities Commission to provide advice and deal with complaints.

The Equal Pay Act 1970
This Act states that men and women must be paid the same when they are doing the same job with the same level of responsibility.

The Race Relations Act 1976
This Act makes discrimination on the grounds of race, colour, nationality and ethnic origin illegal. Positive discrimination may be allowed (see above). You may see job adverts which state 'We are equal opportunities employers under the Race Relations Act and welcome enquiries and applications from all ethnic groups' or 'While all appointments are made on merit, disabled people and members of minority ethnic communities are under-represented in our company and are particularly encouraged to apply.'

The Act established the Commission for Racial Equality to provide information and advice, and to deal with complaints.

See Chapter 4, pages 156–8, for more about discrimination.

Health and safety

The Health and Safety at Work Act 1974
Under this Act, all staff have a responsibility for their own safety and the safety of others in the workplace. They should be aware of, and follow, the health and safety policy of their workplace.

Managers of care settings must provide a safe, healthy workplace. This covers hygiene, disposal of waste, ventilation, heating and lighting, safety of equipment, safe handling of materials such as drugs and chemicals.

They must also ensure that staff are properly trained for the tasks they are required to do, such as safe lifting techniques.

Control of Substances Hazardous to Health Regulations (COSHH) 1990
These state that employers must undertake to eliminate hazardous substances in the workplace. Employees must be informed of any risks associated with substances they are using.

Reporting of Injuries, Diseases and Dangerous Occurrence Regulations (Riddor) 1985
See Chapter 1, page 56. Responsibility for reporting lies with management, but employees should be aware of the regulations. Establishments usually keep their own accident books in addition to the information required under Riddor.

Fire Safety and Safety in Places of Sport Act 1987
The key duties of establishments are to provide:

- means of escape
- fire doors
- fire exit signs
- fire alarms
- fire drills
- fire fighting equipment
- emergency lighting
- fire resistant building materials and furnishings.

When an establishment applies for registration (see above), the registering authority has to satisfy itself that the fire precautions in the premises are adequate. Inspection is carried out by the Fire Service.

As an employee, you must ensure that fire precautions are carried out, such as keeping fire doors shut, signing in and out, and making sure any no smoking rules are followed.

Medicines
Sometimes medicines are referred to as drugs.

The Misuse of Drugs Act 1971 (modified 1985)
This sets out regulations concerning the ordering, custody and administration of habit-forming drugs, such as morphine. Persons allowed to administer drugs are medical personnel, registered nurses and specially-trained paramedics.

The Medicines (Prescription Only) Order 1977
This provides a list of medicines which must be prescribed by a doctor. It includes medicines which have powerful actions and side effects, such as tranquillisers.

The Medicines (General Sales List) Order 1977
This is a list of all the drugs which can be purchased at a chemist without a doctor's prescription, such as paracetomal or aspirin.

Handling medicines in care settings
There are some rules regarding the handling of medicines:

- Proprietors and managers of homes have a responsibility to see that staff are trained in the handling and administration of medicines. A senior care assistant may be trained to administer drugs.
- Medicines must not be given without a doctor's prescription.
- Medicines must only be administered by a responsible person authorised by the manager, such as a senior care assistant.
- Proper arrangements must be made for the safe keeping of medicines. Pharmacists visit establishments to check on the administration and storage of medicines.
- All medicines should be kept in their original containers and must be clearly labelled with the resident's name and the required dosage.
- If residents keep their own medicines, they must have a safe, lockable drawer or cupboard.

- If residents fail to take prescribed medicines or if any side effects occur, they must be reported to the doctor immediately.
- Do not give a medicine which is prescribed for one person to another person.
- If containers are difficult to open, pharmacists can supply alternative packings on request.
- If instructions are not clear, check with a pharmacist.
- Always store medicines as directed, for example 'a cool dry place', 'in a fridge', 'away from the light'.
- Always check the expiry dates on labels.
- Unwanted medicines should be returned to the pharmacy.
- Always make sure that the complete course of medicine is taken.
- Keep medicines out of the reach of children.

Remember
- Check the medicine to make sure it is the correct one.
- Give the exact amount.
- Give it to the correct resident.
- Give it at the exact time specified by the doctor.

Activity 8.3

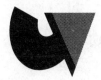

In your work placement:

a Find out about the implementation of fire precautions and write a short report of your findings.

b Find out who is responsible for giving medicines. Write a short report on the procedures followed.

Methods to support social and life skills

The maintenance of life skills

As we grow up and develop, we acquire the life skills we need to look after ourselves, such as:
- movement and mobility
- co-ordination
- manual dexterity, manipulative skills
- attending to personal hygiene, washing
- attending to toilet needs
- grooming, dressing and undressing
- maintaining a suitable body temperature
- living safely
- cleaning the home
- preparing and cooking food
- shopping
- arranging entertainment and outings.

A person's age, disability and state of health can all affect their ability to care for themselves adequately.

Age

Today, people's life expectancy (the age to which they may live) is greater than ever before. People are continuing to lead active, independent lives well into late old age (see page 115). However, there are some aspects of ageing that can affect a person's ability to maintain their life skills, such as:

- physical changes – deterioration of eyesight, hearing, teeth (making it difficult to eat), cardio-vascular system (leading to poor circulation, tiredness and breathelessness); slowing down of the digestion (causing constipation); incontinence; weak muscles, reduced bone mass making fractures more likely
- psychological (emotional) changes – difficulty in remembering, especially recent events; dislike of change (elderly people prefer well-established routines)
- social changes – retirement, family changes, loneliness, changing roles
- changes caused by disease – brain degeneration as a result of Alzheimer's disease or as a result of deterioration of the arteries supplying the brain; pain and immobility due to arthritis.

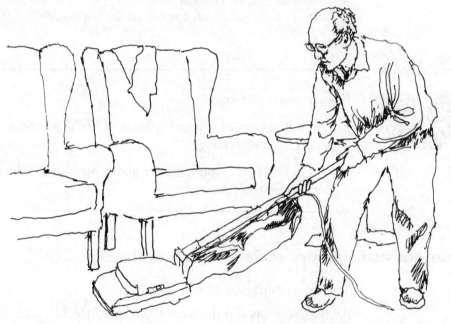

A married man may have to learn new skills after the death of his wife

Disability

A disability is a restriction on a person's ability to carry out an activity with the range considered 'normal'. For example, a person whose sight is impaired person may not be able to shop without assistance.

Preventing the spread of infection

The word 'infection' means the passing of disease from one source to another. This can occur in a number of ways:

- from droplets or dust in the air
- from skin and mucous membranes
- from wounds
- from food and drink
- from soil
- from animals
- from infected articles.

Infections are caused by **microbes** (small living organisms). The main groups of microbes involved in infection are bacteria, viruses, fungi and protozoa.

Activity 8.4

Find out about, and make lists of, diseases caused by:

a bacteria

b viruses

c fungi

d protozoa.

The body has its own defences which help to protect it against infection as shown below.

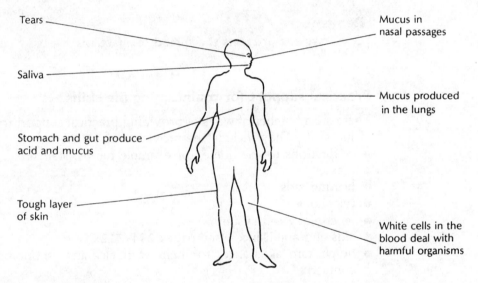

Tears

Saliva

Stomach and gut produce acid and mucus

Tough layer of skin

Mucus in nasal passages

Mucus produced in the lungs

White cells in the blood deal with harmful organisms

The body's defences

When working in a care setting, you should know how to prevent infection from spreading:
- by adopting high standards of personal hygiene
- by enforcing high standards of food hygiene
- by providing high standards of accommodation
- by adopting high standards of sanitation, including facilities for washing hands
- by disinfecting or burning articles used by infected persons
- by avoiding contact with infected people
- by ensuring good ventilation
- by reporting all infective illnesses immediately
- by making sure the establishment is clean throughout
- by educating everyone in the prevention of infection.

Activity 8.5

a In your work placement, find out the measures taken to prevent the spread of infection.

b Compare them with the list above.

Routines to prevent the spread of infection

- Avoiding contact with blood and body fluids. Always wear plastic gloves. Wash your hands thoroughly with soap and water after contact.
- Avoiding contact with cuts and abrasions. Cover open wounds with waterproof dressings. Blue plasters should always be provided for food handlers.
- Disinfecting. Wear plastic gloves and an apron when mopping up. Disinfect areas contaminated by blood and excreta with a bleach solution. Dispose of contaminated waste by using the appropriate bags and containers.

> **Remember**
> Good hygiene prevents the spread of infection.

Practical support for maintaining life skills

There are a number of ways of providing practical support for the maintenance of life skills. They include the provision of:

- adaptations to the home, for example ramps, stair lifts
- glasses
- hearing aids
- telephone
- emergency call system
- aids and applicances (see pages 294–312)
- home care assistance (for help with cleaning, shopping, cooking, social contact)
- visitors
- sheltered housing
- meals-on-wheels
- social worker to advise on services available (such as visits to a day centre), benefits, help with heating bills, etc.
- home visits by doctor, dentist, chiropodist, physiotherapist, community nurse, community psychiatric nurse.

Activity 8.6

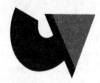

Produce a list of possible adaptations to an ordinary home to assist with mobility.

Avoiding danger in care settings

It is the responsibility of carers to ensure a safe environment for clients (see pages 46–56).

Activity 8.7

Write a checklist of criteria for the selection of safe furniture, furnishings and equipment for a residential home.

> **Remember**
> Encourage and help your clients do you as much as possible for themselves. They will feel much better (increased self-esteem).

Practical skills to support physical needs

In a residential home for elderly people, the most important physical needs of the residents are for:
- personal hygiene
- mobility
- comfort.

Practical skills to maintain personal hygiene

Washing and bathing a resident should always be carried out with tact and care. Always ask the resident whether he or she would prefer a bath, a shower or a strip wash. Sometimes, if a person is very frail or ill, a bed bath will be necessary.

How much help is required?
Remember to encourage the resident to be as independent as possible, but ensure that extra help is available if necessary. Hoists and other appliances should be used where appropriate.

Assisting with a bath
Always consider the physical, emotional and safety needs of residents when helping them to bath.

Physical needs
- Ensure the bathroom is clean and warm.
- Have all special equipment ready, such as lifting equipment, bath seat.
- Have all the toiletries ready:
  - towels (warm if possible)
  - bath mat
  - face cloth
  - body cloth
  - soap
  - talc
  - barrier cream
  - nail cutters
  - nail brush
  - clean clothes
  - laundry bag
  - bath thermometer.
- Ensure help is available if necessary.
- Allow the resident to use the toilet first.
- Attend to mouth, nail and hair care (see pages 296–7).
- Note any marks or rashes and report to the person in charge.

Emotional needs
- Explain clearly what you want the resident to do, so that he or she can co-operate with you.

293

- Ensure privacy so that the resident feels safe and secure by keeping the door closed.
- Keep the resident covered up until you help him or her into the bath.
- Allow the resident as much independence as possible to wash him or herself. In this way, they can retain their dignity.
- Maintain client confidentiality.
- Do not chatter constantly or talk to a colleague over the resident's head.
- Do not rush. Allow the resident time to relax in the bath.
- Leave the resident feeling comfortable and refreshed.

Safety needs
- Do not leave the client alone in the bathroom in case he or she slips or falls.
- Water temperature should be between 38–43°C. Always put the cold water in first. Check the temperature with your wrist or use a bath thermometer.
- Use equipment safely. Use lifting equipment and bath seats where necessary and available.
- Use non-slip mats.
- Do not lock the bathroom door.
- The bath and all equipment should be scrupulously clean before and after use.

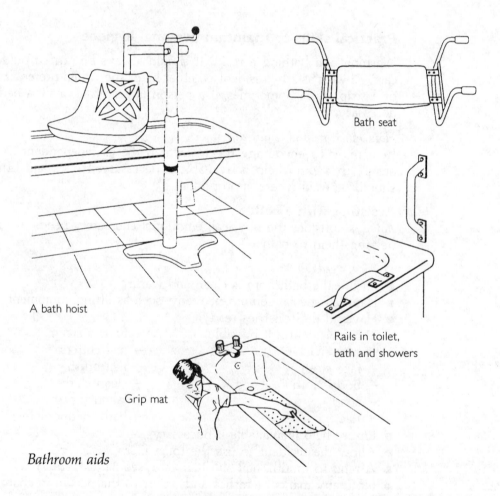

A bath hoist

Bath seat

Rails in toilet, bath and showers

Grip mat

Bathroom aids

Remember the techniques for lifting and moving clients – see pages 219–22.

Assisting with a shower

A shower requires less physical effort than a bath for elderly residents. However, if the resident has not been used to a shower at home he or she may well prefer a bath. Also, if the resident needs a lot of help it is quite difficult for a carer to assist without getting wet.

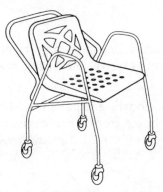

A mobile shower chair

> **Points to remember**
> ● Check the water temperature.
> ● Check the position of the resident – use a shower seat if necessary.
> ● Assist the resident with getting in and out and drying skin.
> ● Clear up, and clean shower. Make sure surrounding floor is dry.

Assisting with a strip wash

Many residents will have wash basins in their rooms. The strip wash can be carried out with the resident sitting beside the wash basin.

Help the resident as required with removing and replacing clothing, turning taps on and off and washing and drying. The resident should be left feeling comfortable and clean. Finish by cleaning the basin and clearing away equipment.

Giving a resident a bed bath

This is a way of giving a resident an all-over wash in a bed. It is usually carried out by two people and takes 15–20 minutes.

● Collect all the equipment required and place it at the bed side:
  - a bowl of water
  - soap
  - two flannels
  - towels
  - brush or comb
  - toiletries
  - mouth care equipment
  - nail scissors
  - barrier cream
  - tissues or wipes
  - clean nightwear
  - clean bedclothes
  - laundry bag.
● Explain the procedure to the resident.
● Ensure privacy – close doors and windows.
● Ask first if the resident would like to use the toilet, commode or bed pan.
● Remove top bed clothes and leave the resident covered with a large warm towel.
● Remove nightwear.
● Wash the resident methodically starting with the face and neck. Rinse and dry thoroughly.
● Use separate flannels for face and body.
● Wash or assist the resident to wash the genital area. Dry thoroughly.
● Use cream or talcum powder as required.

- Note the condition of the skin. Always report signs of redness or soreness to the supervisor.
- Help the resident to put on clean nightwear.
- Attend to mouth, teeth, hair and nails.
- Remake the bed using clean bed clothes.
- Leave the resident with everything within easy reach, feeling comfortable and refreshed.

Pressure area care
Pressure and friction can lead to sores on various parts of the body. Read Chapter 5 (page 178) for causes and ways of alleviating pressure.

Assisting with hair care
A visit to the hairdresser is a morale-boosting experience. Many elderly people enjoy a visit to a salon or a call at home from a professional hairdresser. Hair may also need to be washed between visits to the hairdresser.

Points to remember
- Frequent washing may cause excessive dryness.
- Mild shampoos and conditioners should be used.
- Hair should be thoroughly rinsed.
- Hair should be dried gently and styled according to the resident's wishes.
- Be gentle, older people often complain of tender scalps.
- Hair can be washed in bed if necessary.

Head lice
Head lice infestation is most common in school children, but it may also occur in older people. The head louse is very small, about 3 mm in size, greyish in colour and prefers to live in clean, short hair. Lice are transferred from person to person by close contact. They cannot jump or fly and do not survive away from the body for more than 24–48 hours. The eggs (nits) are firmly cemented to the hair. It takes about 18 days for an egg to mature. The mature adult louse lives about 10 days feeding on blood from the scalp of their host.

Treatment for lice involves washing the hair with insecticidal shampoo which kills both lice and eggs. Eggs which stick to the hair can be removed with a fine tooth comb.

Points to remember
- Ensure privacy.
- Be tactful and gentle.
- Staff can be infested in the same way as residents.

Assisting with mouth care
We all understand the importance of keeping our mouths and teeth clean. If we fail to do this effectively, particles of food will remain in the mouth and will decompose. Harmful microbes will multiply resulting in bad breath (halitosos), an unpleasant taste and tooth decay.

Elderly people should be encouraged and helped to:
- visit the dentist regularly
- avoid too many sugary foods
- eat a healthy diet
- drink adequate amounts of fluid
- brush teeth thoroughly at least twice a day
- change tooth brushes regularly.

Cleaning dentures
- Ask the resident to remove their dentures and place them in their own individual container. You may have to help them with this.
- Rinse the dentures under cold, running water.
- Brush the dentures with a special brush to remove food and debris.
- Use denture toothpaste to clean dentures. Rinse thoroughly.
- Help the resident to replace dentures.
- Any soreness or discomfort caused by the dentures should be reported to the person in charge.
- Dentures may be soaked in stain-removing solutions overnight.

Remember
Each resident should have their own labelled denture container which should be kept in their own room to avoid displacement of dentures.

More specialised mouth care
This will be necessary when a resident is helpless. The mouth can become dry and the tongue furred or discoloured. The breath will smell unpleasant. Special mouth care needs to be carried out regularly, before and after meals.
- Have all the equipment ready:
  - a tray
  - a towel
  - a small soft toothbrush
  - toothpaste
  - sodium bicarbonate solution – 1 teaspoon to 1 pint of water
  - mouth wash
  - a bowl to spit in
  - lip salve
  - tissues.
- Explain the procedure to the resident.
- Wash his or her hands.
- Place a towel under resident's chin.
- Using the toothbrush and the sodium bicarbonate solution, clean the teeth and mouth.
- Clean the teeth with toothpaste.
- Assist the resident to rinse mouth out with mouthwash.
- Apply lip salve to lips to prevent cracking and dryness.

Looking after children?
- Assist small children to clean their teeth.
- Encourage them to develop a teeth cleaning routine.
- Discourage the eating of sticky sweet foods.

Assisting with shaving

Sometimes men require assistance with shaving. If a man is in the habit of shaving regularly, he can feel very demoralised if he is left unshaven. Your placement supervisor will advise you precisely how to assist with shaving. You need to know the capabilities of the resident as well as the type of shave he prefers.

Shaving with an electric razor
- The face is shaved before washing.
- Some men like to use a pre-electric shave lotion.
- Shave the face in the direction usually followed otherwise pulling and tenderness will result.
- Hold the razor firmly and let it cut the stubble.
- Never scrub the razor across the face.
- Aftershave lotion may be used if the resident wishes.

Shaving with a safety razor
- Place a towel under the resident's chin.
- Lather his face using shaving soap (avoid the eyes).
- Shave his face in the direction he indicates.
- Use long firm strokes.
- Rinse the razor frequently.
- Rinse the face and dry gently.
- Apply aftershave lotion if the resident wishes.

Some older women have a considerable amount of facial hair which they might like removed by shaving or epilation.

Assisting with nail care

When you are assisting residents with washing and bathing, you will have the opportunity to observe the condition of their finger and toe nails.
- Nails should be kept clean and neatly manicured.
- A nail brush should be available for regular use.
- Never cut a resident's nails without consulting your supervisor. This is particularly important when elderly people are suffering from diabetes or circulatory disorders.
- Finger nails are filed or cut to the shape of the finger. Toe nails should be cut straight across.
- As people grow old, their nails can become very hard and horny. It is advisable to see a chiropodist if this happens.
- Female residents may well appreciate a manicure and an application of nail polish.
- It is important to sterilise scissors and metal files after use to prevent the spread of fungal or other infections.

Helping residents to manage continence

Much of the assistance you will give to residents concerning their toilet needs will be of a basic nature. It is always desirable for them to use the ordinary toilet and washing facilities even if considerable help is required from carers and the use of aids and appliances is necessary.

Taking a resident to the toilet
- Assess the resident's capabilities.
- Always respond promptly to requests to be taken to the toilet.

- Help the resident to get to the lavatory, either walking with him or using the wheelchair.
- Make sure the resident is seated or standing comfortably. Any aids he requires should be at hand.
- Allow privacy, if possible.
- Make sure lavatory paper is available. Assist if necessary.
- Make sure clean clothing, incontinence pads and pants (if necessary) are available.
- Make sure the resident is able to wash his hands before helping him back to his room.

Assisting with use of a commode

The commode is like a portable toilet which can be taken to the individual rooms.

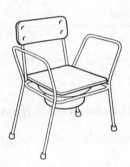

A commode

- Ensure privacy.
- Position the commode and remove the lid.
- Assist the resident to sit comfortably on the commode.
- If the resident is weak or unsteady, stay with him.
- If possible, allow the resident to manage on his own, making sure lavatory paper is to hand.
- Allow the resident to wash his hands and return him to his bed or chair.
- Empty and clean the commode.
- Wash your hands.

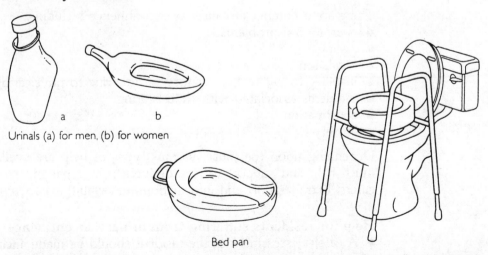

Urinals (a) for men, (b) for women

Bed pan

Other toilet aids

Raised toilet seat

You may find yourself looking after people who are unable to manage their own continence including babies and small children, mentally and physically disabled children and adults, and elderly people.

Continence and incontinence

The terms you may come across include:

● **Continent**, which literally means exercising self-restraint, in this context it means having control of both bladder and bowel

● **Incontinent** which in this context means lack of control of bladder and bowel

● **Incontinence of urine** which means that the resident wets himself with his water

● **Incontinence of faeces** which means the resident soils himself with his motions

● **Single incontinence** which means either urinary *or* faecel incontinence

● **Double incontinence** which means the resident soils and wets himself

---

Managing continence in older people

Most of us can readily accept that babies and small children do not have bowel and bladder control until a certain stage of development is reached. However, loss of bowel and bladder control can occur at any time in life, for a variety of reasons. Some of the disabled people you will be caring for may never achieve complete control and will need constant help and support from carers. The overall aim is to assist residents to have as much control as their abilities and circumstances allow.

Chapter 5 describes the urinary and digestive systems (pages 194 and 196).

There are a number of causes of incontinence including:
● neurological problems
● ageing
● confusion
● inability to get to the lavatory in time due to physical disability
● problems associated with child-bearing
● constipation
● anxiety.

Depending upon the cause, various types of help are available. In all cases, much help and support can be derived from a patient, kindly approach by carers. Extra support and information is available from Continence Advisers.

Help for residents suffering from urinary incontinence
● A careful assessment of the resident should be made, including how many episodes of incontinence occur, how long the resident remains dry, how much fluid is drunk and the physical and mental capabilities of the resident.

As a carer you may be involved in this process. Urine may have to be measured or visits to the lavatory recorded on a chart.

- Take the resident to the toilet at regular intervals instead of waiting for the resident to ask.
- Advise residents to drink regularly, to have a drink with every meal and not to drink too much late in the evening.
- Make sure that the skin is always kept dry and clean to prevent soreness. Barrier creams may be necessary for extra protection.
- In some cases physiotherapy may be offered to improve muscle control.
- As far as possible, normal clothing should be worn. However specially adapted designs are available. All clothing should be machine-washable.

When it is not possible to control urinary incontinence by the above measures, a wide variety of aids and appliances are available to assist the sufferer and the carer, including:

- A box style mattress cover made of waterproof material will protect the top and sides of the mattress. Cotton sheets should be placed on top to minimise sweating and discomfort.
- A waterproof draw sheet and a cotton draw sheet may be used. They can be changed without completely stripping the bed.
- Kylie sheets can be used in situations where there is severe urinary incontinence. The area next to the skin remains dry unless the sheet is completely saturated. Kylie sheets are machine-washable and can be tumble-dried.
- Incontinence pads and pants are useful for day and night wear. Many different sizes and styles, including unisex styles, are available from a range of manufacturers. The pads are disposable. Pants may be washable or disposable.

Look out for examples of these items in your work placement. Notice how they are used. If you see any interesting aids and appliances which are not mentioned in this text, report back to your tutor and your fellow students.

Help for residents suffering from faecal incontinence
The most common reason for faecal incontinence is constipation. This causes accumulation of faecal material in the bowel which begins to decompose and cause leakage of liquid from the rectum. Medical advice and treatment is required to deal with this. Once the blockage has been removed, a high fibre diet and plenty of fluids can usually keep the bowel functioning fairly well. In persistent cases or where mental or neurological disorder is contributory to faecal incontinence, incontinence pads and pants will have to be used. Changing the thorough cleansing immediately soiling occurs is of course essential.

The choice of incontinence aids is an important matter. Continence advisers, carers and clients need to consider the following factors:
- the type of incontinence – urine or faeces or both
- the amount of wetness or soiling
- day or night incontinence
- male or female
- mental and physical abilities
- condition of skin, pressure sores
- washing facilities
- availability of aids
- amount of help available.

Activity 8.8

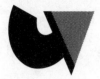

Your tutor will arrange a talk from a continence adviser. Write a short report on the talk.

Assisting people with mobility

Old people should be encouraged to be as active as possible, this can be achieved by:
- taking them for short walks round the establishment and garden or taking them shopping
- providing activities which involve active participation
- involving residents in gentle housework – dusting
- gentle exercises in groups.

Aids to mobility

Sometimes it is necessary to enhance mobility by using specialist equipment. You will come across a number of aids to mobility in your work.

The aim of any care plan is always to encourage the clients to be as independent as possible within the limits of the conditions from which they are suffering. Allow clients to do as much as they can for themselves.

There are a wide variety of aids which enable the client with mobility problems to move around. They range from an electronically-controlled wheelchair to a simple walking stick. Clients will have been advised by medical staff, occupational therapists and physiotherapists as to the most appropriate help for them.

Wheelchairs

These may be electronically-controlled, hand-propelled by the client or pushed by a helper. Various accessories are available including trays, soft seats, safety straps and spring lifter seats. The amount of help a wheelchair user will need will obviously depend on the ability of the client involved. Remember that the aim is to encourage mobility as far as possible. Never take over if a client wants to try to move unaided.

The steps which may be used when assisting clients in wheelchairs are as follows:
- Assess the situation and decide what is going to be required.
- Explain to the client what is going to happen.
- Look at the chair carefully to establish the position of the brake, the foot rests, the arm rests and any safety straps.
- Always ensure that the user is comfortably and, more importantly, safely seated.
- Make sure that arms and legs are positioned carefully in order to avoid knocks on doorways and other obstacles.
- When negotiating steps and kerbs, place your foot on the tripping lever, hold the chair firmly and tip it back to go up.
- Lower the chair down the kerb; the back wheels should touch the ground at the same time.
- If you are pushing a wheelchair, never go too quickly as this can be frightening for the client.

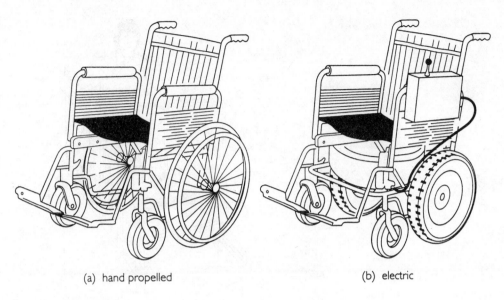

(a) hand propelled   (b) electric

Examples of wheelchairs

• When transferring clients to and from wheelchairs, make sure the brakes are firmly applied, foot rests are turned out of the way, small front wheels are turned inwards and the appropriate arm of the chair is removed.

Walking frames
The best known walking frame is the Zimmer frame. Frames give good support enabling clients to stand or walk safely.

Adjustable walkers with wheels
These aids to mobility are made from steel and usually have two fixed wheels at the front and two rubber feet at the back. They can be adjusted in height so that the user can rest their arms on the frame.

Activity 8.9

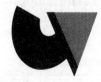

Within your group take turns to spend an hour in a wheelchair being pushed to classes and around the building.

Produce a written account of your feelings. Present your account to the rest of the group.

Hoists
These are devices which enable carers to move clients gently and safely from one place to another. Many different types are available; some are electrically-powered and some are manually-operated. Usually there is some kind of sling in which the client is supported, attached to the hoist by metal hooks. The client is then moved in the sling either mechanically or manually, depending upon the type of hoist. As a student you will only be allowed to observe the use of hoists.

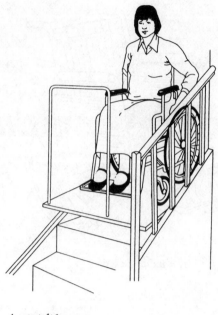

A stairlift

Lifts
Some homes for the elderly and disabled are fitted with stairlifts. These allow clients to move from different levels easily and safely, but carers should help and supervise their use.

Walking sticks
For people who need extra support when walking, a variety of sticks are available. They are usually made from aluminium and can be adjusted in length or folded. Variations include tripod and quadruped sticks which provide extra stability, and traditional, wooden sticks are still popular. Seat sticks are useful, being made of light-weight aluminium and can be turned into a seat when the user wants to rest for short periods.

Crutches
For people who are unable to bear their own weight or who need extra support when walking, a range of light-weight, aluminium elbow crutches are available.

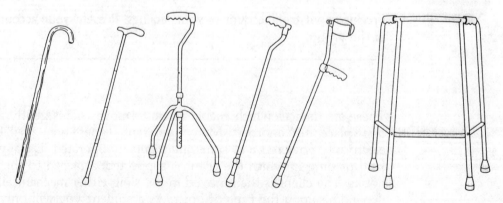

A selection of sticks, crutches and a zimmer frame

Their height can be adjusted to suit the individual. It is important that clients and carers should understand the correct way to use crutches and a physiotherapist will usually advise on this.

Making beds

The choice and care of bedding

Most of you will have had experience of bed-making in your own homes. You will be able to put this knowledge to good use if you have work experience with the elderly people.

Beds

If a resident spends considerable amounts of time in bed, it is essential that the bed is not only comfortable but functional too. An ideal bed has a firm mattress and firm base. It is also useful if the height of the bed is adjustable.

Bedding

- Sheets should be cotton where possible and in pleasing colours.
- If blankets are used, cotton cellular ones are very good as they are washable.
- Bedpsreads should preferably be made of a washable material.
- Duvets are now in common use in many establishments. The washable type are most convenient to use.
- A small bottom sheet called a draw sheet is sometimes used. This is helpful in cases of incontinence. If it is used with a small polythene sheet, it saves changing the large bottom sheet every time a resident wets the bed.
- Washable pillows are most useful. They can be protected with waterproof covers if necessary. Cotton pillow cases to match the sheets and duvet covers are desirable.

Making the bed

Methods will vary depending on where you are working and who you are working with. The method described below can be adapted to a variety of situations.

- It is easiest if two people are available to make the bed.
- Have all the equipment ready:
  - 3 pillows
  - 2 sheets
  - 1 draw sheet
  - 1 polythene draw sheet
  - 2 or 3 blankets
  - 1 bedspread.
- Make sure the mattress cover is in position.
- Place the bottom sheet in position. Make corners – hospital-type, if appropriate.
- Place the plastic draw sheet in position and cover with draw sheet which should be firmly tucked in. Check that there are no creases.
- Place top sheet in position. Do not tuck in too tightly at the bottom to allow for movement of the legs and feet.
- Place blankets in position. Make corners. Allow for movement. Leave some blanket at the top so that the client can adjust it for extra warmth and comfort.
- Arrange the bedspread neatly on top of the bed.

Stripping a bed

It is important that this is done in a tidy manner.

- Never put bed clothes on the floor. Use two chairs.
- Loosen the bed clothes first.
- Fold neatly and place on the chairs.
- Put any dirty items in the linen basket.
- Linen which is wet or soiled should be kept separately and dealt with in the appropriate manner.

Dealing with wet or soiled linen

In hospitals and homes for elderly people, there are usually special arrangements for dealing with soiled linen. If sheets are soiled with excreta, they will usually be placed in a special bag of a specific colour and will be dealt with separately.

In situations where laundry is dealt with by the care staff, follow these general rules.

- Urine soaked sheets should be sluiced immediately in cold running water. They may be left to soak in a bleach solution and then washed on a hot wash programme. They should be thoroughly dried and aired before using again. It is best if they can be dried outside.
- Bed linen which is contaminated with faeces must be thoroughly sluiced to remove all the excreta. The items should then be soaked in bleach solution, rinsed and washed using a hot wash programme. Sluicing can be done even if there is not a proper sluice by holding the items firmly in the lavatory bowl and flushing water on them repeatedly.

NB All linen which has been soiled with urine and faeces should be washed in a separate wash.

It is vital that residents should be changed as soon as wetness or soiling occurs – firstly for the client's comfort and secondly so that the establishment always smells clean.

It is always desirable to get residents out of bed when the bed is being made. This also applies when attending to the client's toilet and personal hygiene needs.

Making a bed when a resident cannot get up

In some situations, it is not possible or advisable to get the resident up when the bed is being made. Perhaps bed rest is necessary because of a medical condition, such as a stroke or a heart attack, or perhaps confinement to bed is necessary because of fractures.

This is a method for making the bed when it is not possible to get the resident up:

- Two carers are necessary.
- Make sure that you have all the equipment ready as you did when making an unoccupied bed. There may be additional items which you will need, such as incontinence pads.
- Make sure the resident understands what you are about to do.
- Ensure privacy.
- Offer the client a bed pan or urinal before you start. Make sure they are able to wash their hands and that the bed pan or urinal is removed immediately after use.
- Strip the bedclothes from the top of the bed leaving the resident covered with the top sheet.

- Position the resident carefully and roll them gently to one side of the bed where they should be firmly supported by one carer, remember to support the head with a pillow.
- Roll the dirty sheets up towards the client's back.
- Any incontinence is dealt with at this point. Thorough washing and drying of the affected area is very important to prevent skin sensitivity and pressure sores (see Chapter 5).
- Insert the clean bottom sheet and draw sheet and roll them close to the resident.
- Gently roll the resident to the opposite side of the bed, making sure they are well-supported and not unnecessarily exposed. Remove the dirty sheets and place them in the appropriate receptacles.
- Ease the clean sheets into position and tuck in firmly.
- Assist the resident into a comfortable position and make up the top of the bed.
- Clear away and anticipate and/or respond to any needs of the resident.

If you are working with residents who are confined to bed for any length of time you will probably notice that their positions are changed frequently. This is important to improve circulation and to prevent continuous pressure on one part of the body which would lead to pressure sores. See Chapter 5.

Similarly, if residents are spending a lot of time sitting in a chair because of impaired mobility, they will require frequent changes of position.

Activity 8.10

a With a partner practise making a bed and stripping it.

b In a group of three, practise making a bed where it is not possible for the resident to get up.

Take it in turns to be the resident. How did you feel? Tell the others in the group so they can improve their bed-making skills.

Aids to bed comfort
Although residents are encouraged to get up and to be as mobile as possible there will always be situations where they spend considerable periods of time in bed or sitting in a chair. Comfort can be improved (see below) by using:
- pillows to give extra support (triangular-shaped pillows are often used)
- back rests to give support when sitting upright in bed
- bed cradles to protect or take the weight of bed clothes
- rings and cushions to sit on
- fleecy pads to protect buttocks, elbows and heels
- ladder hoists which consist of a simple arrangement allowing clients to pull themselves into a sitting position when in bed or in the bath
- trapeze lifts to help residents to move in bed or in the bath.

Remember that as a learner you would not use any of these items without help and advice from your supervisor.

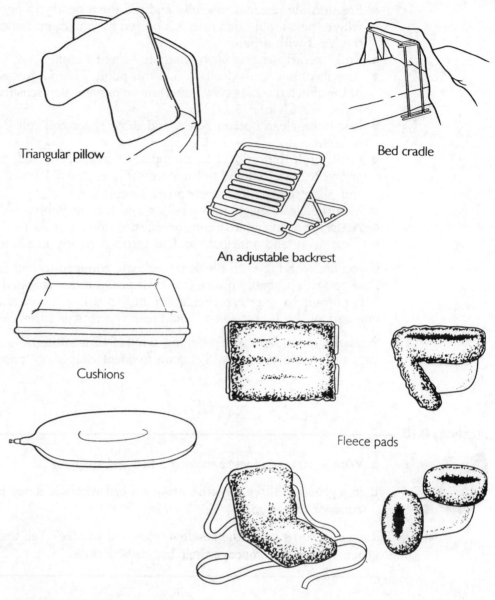

Triangular pillow

Bed cradle

An adjustable backrest

Cushions

Fleece pads

Aids to provide bed comfort

Assisting residents with eating and drinking

To survive we all need to eat a balanced diet – that is, a diet which contains all the nutrients in the correct proportions for our age and activity levels. This is discussed in Chapter 1.

In your work placements whether you are working with children, disabled or elderly people, you will probably have noticed that preparing and serving meals takes up a considerable part of the day. Meals are a very important social aspect of the day, especially when people are elderly and/or disabled and mobility is restricted.

The nutritional needs of elderly people
- Fewer calories are required because the body metabolism slows down and many older people become less active.
- Plenty of fluids are needed − about 2 litres or 8 cup-sized drinks daily.
- A little alcohol may be enjoyed.
- Small frequent meals are best.
- Traditional dishes are often preferred.
- Lifelong eating habits should be tolerated even if they are bad habits.
- Having ensured that a nutritious diet will be served, it is essential that food preparation, serving and storage are carried out under strict hygienic conditions.

Tasks involved
Some of the tasks you may be asked to help with in your work placement include the following:
- communicating effectively with residents while offering food and drinks
- collecting dishes and trays
- stacking, washing, drying and putting away dishes
- operating a dishwasher
- keeping the food preparation and serving areas clean and tidy
- setting meal tables and trays
- assisting residents with personal hygiene before and after meals
- helping residents to the table or to sit comfortably so that a meal can be enjoyed
- assisting the cook with food preparation
- helping to serve food
- selecting appropriate eating and drinking aids
- helping residents to feed themselves
- feeding helpless residents.

There are some important points to consider when carrying out the above tasks. These involve:
- the setting of tables and trays
- serving food
- knowledge of residents' cultural and religious dietary
- knowledge of special dietary requirements.

The setting of tables and meal trays
Clean table cloths and tray cloths should always be provided. Each resident should have a table napkin or bib. Paper products are best as they can be thrown away afterwards.

Serving food
Different foods should be separate on the plate. Ideally individuals should be helped to food from a serving dish. Amounts given should not be too large. Dishes of food should be kept hot so that residents are able to request another helping.

Cultural and religious dietary requirements
It is essential to know the religious beliefs of residents as some foods are not consumed by certain groups because of religious laws. For example, Orthodox Jews do not eat pork. Other religious groups observe fasts. For example, Muslims fast until sunset during Ramadan. Individual likes and disliked are also very important.

Activity 8.11

a From the area where you live compile a list of all the different religious and cultural groups. Select five of the major groups.

b Prepare a leaflet which sets out clearly the dietary laws and requirements specific to each of the groups you have selected. Compare your findings with those of your colleagues.

Special dietary requirements

Sometimes medical problems make it necessary for a resident to be given a special diet. Examples of special diets include:

- light diet (small, nourishing meals of easily digestible food)
- high-fibre diet
- fluid diet
- diabetic diet
- high protein diet
- low calorie diet
- low fat diet
- low salt diet
- gluten-free diet.

It is essential that carers assist residents to observe the restrictions of any special diets which they are following.

Activity 8.12

Research the requirements of the diets which are listed above. Prepare an advice sheet for each diet. Ask your tutor to check the information and retain it for future reference.

Providing assistance with eating and drinking

The following groups of residents will require some degree of assistance with eating and drinking:

- mentally and physically disabled adults and children
- residents who have varying degrees of paralysis
- confused residents
- residents with serious injuries, such as two broken arms
- residents who are very weak and perhaps dying.

Activity 8.13

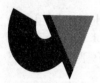

Apply the guidelines on page 284 to the following task.

You are asked to prepare and serve mid-morning drinks to 15 people who live in a home for elderly people.

Using the headings, Assess, Plan, Implement and Evaluate, explain precisely how you would carry out the task. Be prepared to present your ideas to the rest of your class.

Note: You will need a lot of information in order to do this effectively.

Hints for feeding helpless residents

- The resident must be comfortable, having had toilet needs attended to and hands washed.
- Have ready any specialist eating aids which may be required.
- Explain what you are about to do and describe the food. The sight and smell of food will enhance the resident's appetite.
- Salt and pepper should be available if permitted.
- A drink should be ready.
- The food should be at the appropriate temperature.
- A clean napkin or bib should be used to protect clothing.
- Place small amounts of food on the fork or spoon and gently introduce into the mouth. Support the head if necessary.
- Give plenty of time to chew and swallow the food.
- Offer drinks during the course of the meal.
- Try to respond to requests about the order of eating the food. Many people do not care for various foods to be mixed up together.
- The meal should be an enjoyable experience.
- Report any problems to your supervisor. For example, you may feel the resident has eaten or drunk insufficient amounts.

Safety factors
- Be aware of a resident's ability to chew and swallow. Choking is a particular hazard when these abilities are impaired. You must know the First Aid measures relating to choking (see Chapter 1, page 59).
- The temperature of food and drink should always be checked. Residents should not be left without assistance when hot drinks are offered.
- Strict hygiene measures must always be employed to prevent cases of food poisoning.

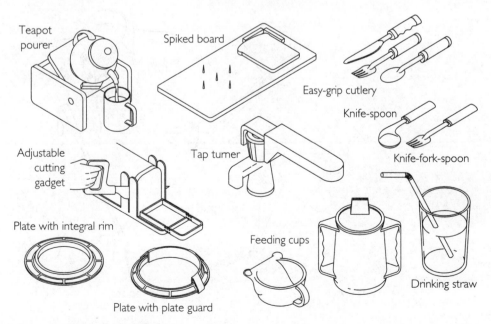

Teapot pourer

Spiked board

Easy-grip cutlery

Knife-spoon

Knife-fork-spoon

Adjustable cutting gadget

Tap turner

Plate with integral rim

Feeding cups

Drinking straw

Plate with plate guard

Aids to eating and drinking

Helping clients with dressing and undressing

In your work, you may have to help residents to dress and undress. This may sound straightforward, but the type of clothes we wear and the reasons we wear them can be very significant.

We wear clothes for warmth, protection and to look good, or to denote religious or cultural groups or professional identity. Some people may find it a disturbing experience if they are unable to follow their usual style of dressing.

In order to maintain both physical and psychological comfort, you should aim to dress a resident as closely to his or her normal style as possible. Before your start look at the following checklist of questions to consider:
- What can I learn about the resident from his or her clothes?
- Are there any specific religious observances that I need to know about?
- What age is the resident?
- Does he or she follow fashion trends closely?
- What are their special likes and dislikes?
- Will frequent changes of clothing be necessary?
- Is special clothing necessary in cases of incontinence?
- Is the client able to cope with fastenings?
- What time of year is it?
- Is protective clothing required to allow the resident to indulge in various activities?

Try to encourage residents to do as much as they can for themselves. It makes them feel better and encourages independence.

When helping a disabled person to dress it is best to start by putting the sleeve or trouser leg on the most affected limbs. Reverse this process when removing garments.

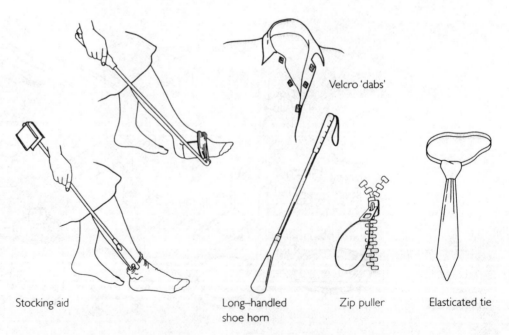

Stocking aid

Velcro 'dabs'

Long–handled shoe horn

Zip puller

Elasticated tie

Aids to dressing and undressing

Ensuring that residents have a good night's sleep

The home should be quiet, with the lights turned down. Noisy machines should not be left on at night. Carers should work quietly and be prepared to talk to and comfort residents as required.

The resident should have:
- attended to toilet needs and, if desired, have a commode, bed pan or urinal where it can be reached during the night
- had a good wash or relaxing bath
- a warm comfortable bed
- a warm well-ventilated room
- had a drink and possibly a small snack
- a book, music or relaxation tapes
- a bell or buzzer to call for assistance.

Unfortunately the sight of residents sitting gazing blankly at a TV screen from morning to night has been all too common in some residential homes. If residents are ignored and no stimulating activities are provided they will become introspective and spend time worrying about real or imagined ailments.

Good residential homes will make sure that carers know what the hobbies and interests of residents are and provide facilities for them to be followed. In addition homes will endeavour to be part of the local community and involve residents in activities outside the home. Recreational and creative activities are discussed in Chapter 7.

Review questions

1 List four care settings where a carer might be working.

2 State four physical needs of residents in a care home.

3 List four tasks that a care assistant may carry out when working with elderly people.

4 Define residential care.

5 List three residents' rights.

6 What is COSHH?

7 What is the Medicines General Sales List?

8 Who is responsible for staff training relating to medicines in care homes?

9 How are food areas kept clean?

10 List four appliances which assist residents with mobility.

11 List four aids which assist residents with eating and drinking.

12 What is the function of a zimmer frame?

13 List four aids to bed comfort.

14 List three aids which make dressing easier.

15 Why is mouth care important for elderly residents?

16 How much fluid should an elderly resident drink in 24 hours?

17 State three hints for shaving a man's face.

18 Why is it important to sterilise nail care equipment?

19 How do the nutritional needs of elderly people differ from those of young people?

20 Suggest ways of helping an elderly resident to sleep.

Assignment A8.1
The function of care settings

1 You have been asked to carry out a survey of the care establishments for elderly people in your local area and to report on your findings.
  a Carry out your research using directories and any additional information you can obtain from your local social services department.
    You might find it useful to collect any brochures that are available about each establishment.
  b On a map of your local area, mark the position of each establishment. Use a key to identify them. You might decide, for example, to a different colour to indicate the different types of establishement.
  c Explain the function of each type of establishment you have marked on the map.
  d Find out whether the establishments are statutory (run by the local authority), private or voluntary.

2 Describe the main legal factors which influence the registering and running of a residential home or nursing home for elderly people.

3 Visit your local pharmacy. Make lists of:
  a ten general sales medicines
  b five prescription only medicines
  c five controlled drugs.

Assignment A8.2
Supporting social and life skills

You are a care assistant in a residential home for elderly people. Mrs Simpson, an 86-year-old woman with limited mobility, has been offered a room in the house. You have been asked to help her to make recommendations to the manager of the home about decorations and furnishings in her room.

1 Explain how advancing age, disability and illness can alter a person's ability to carry out tasks associated with daily living. Give examples.

2 Describe the practical support which can be obtained to enable individuals to retain their independence and live as full a life as possible.

3 a Draw a plan of the room offered to Mrs Simpson. Include in it the position and dimensions of doors, windows and sanitary applicances.
   b Choose paint and wallpaper for the room. Work out the costs of decorating the room, excluding the cost of labour.
   c Select curtains and carpets, and work out the costs.
   d Select furniture (bed, chair, table, etc.) and cost them.
   e Write a full explanation to justify your choices. Include samples of materials and wallpapers if possible, and colour charts clearly showing your choices.

4 Consider the adaptations that would be necessary to an ordinary home to accommodate a person in each of the following situations:
   a a teenage wheelchair user
   b an old person who walks with the help of a zimmer frame.

5 Describe the full range of help and physical support available for an elderly man who is living alone in a two-storey house and who is unable to go out unless he is taken by car.

6 Write a short report on the safety factors involved in the planning of accommodation and provision of equipment for people with various disabilities.

7 Hypothermia and pyrexia are discussed in Chapter 5.
   a Prepare a leaflet which gives advice to old people on keeping warm and preventing hypothermia.
   b Give reasons why a person may have a raised body temperature. Explain the measures which could be taken to reduce body temperature.

8 In your local area, visit the following:
   a a cinema
   b a football ground
   c a department store
   d a place to eat
   e a leisure centre.

For each venue, produce a report on access and facilities for different client groups.

9 In your local area there is probably a supplier of aids and applicances for disabled people. Either visit the showroom or ask for a product catalogue to be sent to you.

Choose **one** of the following situations:
   ● a young man who is paralysed and confined to a wheelchair
   ● an elderly person who is deaf and only able to walk with assistance
   ● an elderly woman who suffers from arthritis in her hands and has difficulty with manipulative skills

- an 8-year-old child who is very overweight and is unable to stand or walk without assistance.

a Make a list of all the aids and appliances which would assist the person you have chosen.

b Explain carefully the function of each appliance you have listed.

c Find out the cost of each item and then work out the total cost of all the items you have listed.

d Find out what financial assistance is available for people who need to purchase items to support them in everyday situations.

Assignment A8.3
Practical skills

1 Keep a diary of what you do at your work placement. Include accounts of any practical experiences you have, such as serving meals, bathing, hair care, etc.

2 Your tutor will arrange a series of demonstrations and opportunities for you to practise caring skills in some or all of the following situations:
- assisting clients with using mobility appliances
- moving and handling techniques
- minimising the effects of pressure
- assisting with personal cleanliness
- assisting with eating and drinking
- assisting with clients' toilet needs
- assisting with clients' need for rest
- assisting with bed-making.

a Make notes of all the knowledge you gain.

b Take part in the assessment of your skills. (Your tutor will be able to provide you with an assessment sheet.)

In future you may wish to take a full NVQ assessment in your workplace.

Human development

Age	Physical factors	Intellectual factors	Emotional factors	Social factors
At birth The newborn baby	An average newborn baby weighs about 3.5 kg and is 50 cm long. Compared with other newborn animals, at birth a human baby is a helpless creature and its growth is very slow. Certain **primitive reflexes** are present, and these usually disappear by the time the baby is 3 months old and is beginning to make conscious movements on his or her own: • sucking reflex • swallowing reflex • rooting reflex – if one side of a baby's cheek or mouth is touched gently, the head will turn in the direction of the touch • grasping reflex – the fist clenches if an object is placed in the palm • Moro reflex – arms and legs are flung out and then drawn inwards in response to being startled • stepping reflex – if the front of a leg is brought into contact with the edge of a table, the baby will raise a leg as if to 'step' up • walking reflex – if held upright, with the soles of the feet on a flat surface, and is moved foward, the baby will respond by making 'walking' steps.			
1 month The infant	Holds head erect for a few seconds. Eyes follow a moving light.	Interested in sounds.	Cries in response to pain, hunger and thirst.	May sleep up to 20 hours in a 24-hour period. Stops crying when picked up and spoken to.
3 months	Eyes follow a person moving. Kicks vigorously.	Recognises carer's face. Shows excitement. Listens, smiles, holds rattle.	Enjoys being cuddled and played with. Misses carer and cries for him/her to return.	Responds happily to carer. Becomes excited at prospect of a feed or bath.
6 months	Able to lift head and chest up supported by wrists. Turns to a person who is speaking.	Responds to speech. Vocalises. Uses eyes a lot. Holds toys. Explores using hands. Listens to sound.	Can be anxious in presence of strangers. Can show anger and frustration. Shows a clear preference for mother's company.	Puts everything in mouth. Plays with hands and feet. Tries to hold bottle when feeding.

Age	Physical factors	Intellectual factors	Emotional factors	Social factors
9 months	Stands when supported. May crawl. Gazes at self in mirror. Tries to hold drinking cup. Sits without support.	Tries to talk, babbling. May say 'Mama' and 'Dada'. Shouts for attention. Understands 'No'.	Can recognise individuals – mother, father, siblings. Still anxious about strangers. Sometimes irritable if routine is altered.	Plays 'Peek-a-boo'. Imitates hand clapping. Puts hands round cup when feeding
12 months The toddler	Pulls self up to standing position. Uses pincer grip. Feeds self using fingers. May walk without assistance.	Knows own name. Obeys simple instructions. Says about three words.	Shows affection. Gives kisses and cuddles. Likes to see familiar faces but less worried by strangers.	Drinks from a cup without assistance. Holds a spoon but cannot feed him/herself. Plays 'Pat-a-Cake'. Quickly finds hidden toys.
1.5 years	Walks well, feet apart. Runs carefully. Pushes and pulls large toys. Walks upstairs. Creeps backwards downstairs.	Uses 6–20 recognisable words. Repeats last word of short sentences. Enjoys and tries to join in with nursery rhymes. Picks up named toys. Enjoying looking at simple picture books. Builds a tower of 3–4 bricks. Scribbles and makes dots. Preference for right or left hand shown.	Affectionate, but may still be reserved with strangers. Likes to see familiar faces.	Able to hold spoon and to get food into mouth. Holds drinking cup and hands it back when finished. Can take off shoes and socks. Bowel control may have been achieved. Remembers where objects belong.

Age	Physical/Motor	Language/Intellectual	Emotional/Social	Self-care
2 years	Runs on whole foot. Squats steadily. Climbs on furniture. Throws a small ball. Sits on a small tricycle and moves vehicle with feet.	Uses 50 or more recognisable words; understands many more words; puts two or three words together to form simple sentences. Refers to self by name. Asks names of objects and people. Scribbles in circles. Can build a tower of six or seven cubes. Hand preference is obvious.	Can display negative behaviour and resistance. May have temper tantrums if thwarted. Plays contentedly beside other children but not with them. Constantly demands mother's attention.	Asks for food and drink. Spoon feeds without spilling. Puts on shoes.
2.5 years	All locomotive skills now improving. Runs and climbs. Able to jump from a low step with feet together. Kicks a large ball.	May use 200 or more words. Knows full name. Continually asking questions, likes stories and recognises details in picture books. Recognises self in photographs. Builds a tower of seven or more cubes.	Usually active and restless. Emotionally still very dependent on adults. Tends not to want to share playthings.	Eats skilfully with a spoon and may sometimes use a fork. Active and restless. Often dry through the day.
3 years	Sits with feet crossed at ankles. Walks upstairs using alternating feet.	Able to state full name, sex and sometimes age. Carries on simple conversations and constantly questioning. Demands favourite story over and over again. Begins to understand sharing. Can count to 10 by rote. Can thread wooden beads on string. Can copy a circle and a cross. Names colours. Cuts with scissors. Paints with a large brush.	Becomes less prone to temper tantrums. Affectionate and confiding, showing affection for younger siblings.	Eats with a fork and spoon. May be dry through the night.

Age	Physical factors	Intellectual factors	Emotional factors	Social factors
3 to 5 years The pre-school child	Continues to perfect physical skills, including running, walking, climbing, riding a tricycle, sitting cross-legged, moving in time to music, playing ball games.	Begins to speak grammatically, recounts recent events accurately, enjoys jokes. Starting to gain control in writing and drawing. A recognisable person may be drawn, or a house with windows and a roof. Pictures are coloured neatly. Begins to understand rules of games and idea of fair play.	Needs companionship of other children. Begins to develop personal relationships. Gradually becoming more independent from parents. Play with other children and by self. Will comfort playmates, choose friends.	Can dress and undress self. Make-believe play.
5 to 10 years The school child	Taller and slimmer. Features have more adult look. Movements well co-ordinated. Physical skills increase. Growth rate steady, but slower. Girls tend to develop more quickly than boys.	Improved ability to concentrate on one task and finish it. Starts school – structured activities to help child gain knowledge and skills.	Beginning to develop self-image and sense of identity. Growth of feelings about others. Special friendships start to develop. Some may be excluded.	Range of contacts grows when school starts. Influences now include teacher and other children. A child who is used to a lot of individual attention, may find it difficult to adjust to school.
11 to 18 years The adolescent	Start of puberty – physical changes as a result of increased production of sex hormones (oestrogen in girls; testosterone in boys). Growth spurt. In girls, breast development, pubic and armpit hair, broadening of hips, redistribution of fat, menstruation. In boys, deepening of voice, pubic, chest and armpit hair, enlargement of penis, scrotum and testes, broadening of shoulders, ability to ejaculate. Possible spots.	Thinking more about self and what others think of them. Begins to compare real world with the ideal world, in terms of family, politics, religion. Starting to think about future – job, career, further education.	Mood swings and feelings of ambivalence. Difficult time for adolescents and parents. May seem to be rebelling, but by challenging ways of behaving, they are testing and developing their ideas of what is right and wrong.	Starting to take an interest in the opposite sex. Problems of shyness, embarrassment prevent socialising and inhibit the forming of new relationships.

Age	Physical	Intellectual	Emotional	Social
18 to 64 years — Adulthood	Physical development complete at about 20 – at physical peak. 30+: changes occur slowly and become more apparent in old age (see below). Main period of reproduction for women around 20–40 years. Menopause can start at any time after mid-30s. Ill-health more common as get older.	18–25: may still be in full-time education or starting work, learning new skills. 25–40: possibly for career progression – new challenges	Coming to terms with new role in work, as married person or partner, as a parent, or as carer of older parents. May experience problems with loss of grown-up children, dissatisfaction with work/redundancy/early retirement	Starting new relationships at work, and college, possibly settling down as a couple. Relationships with children and later grandchildren. Social activities probably less when bringing up family and increase again later.
65+ — Old age	Changes which occur throughout adulthood become more obvious: skin becomes dry and wrinkled; hair growth slows, may thin, turns grey; longsightedness may develop, side vision narrower, cataracts and glaucoma possible; hearing, smell and taste less acute; gum disease and tooth decay; lungs, heart, digestion, urinary system less efficient; high blood pressure; muscles less flexible; poor mobility due to arthritic disease; reproduction no longer possible in women, but still possible in men. Body more subject to degenerative disease, e.g. atheroma, osteo-arthritis, brain degeneration, cancer.	Ability to learn new things slows down, does not imply less intelligence. Memory may be less reliable. Relieved of employment may take up creative activities.	Problems may occur as a result of loss of status after retirement, loss of work relationships, loss of partner due to bereavement, change of role as grandchildren born, possible loneliness, isolation, role reversal as may become dependent on others, reduced income.	

Index

ABC 52, 56
abdominal cavity 181–2
access 106–7
accidents 46–51
accidents in the home 47
activities of daily
    living 228–30
adolescents 257–8
age 160, 290
Agpar score 203
AIDS 35, 39–41
aids and appliances 251,
    294, 295, 299, 302–4,
    307–8, 311, 312
airways 52, 58–9
alcohol 27–34
amputations 64
androgyny 78
ante-natal care 239
assessment 225–6, 232–6

basic nutrients 5–9, 11
bleeding 62–5
blood vessels 193–4
body language 144
body measurements 202–6
body temperature 209–12
breathing 52

calcium 6, 8
carbohydrates 6, 8
cardio-vascular
    systems 182, 191–4
cardiopulmonary resuscitation
    (CPR) 60–2
care plan 234, 235–6
care settings 238–44,
    270–4, 282–3
carers 109
cells 179–80
central nervous system 182,
    188–9
change 80–4, 86
chest compressions 60, 61,
    62
child minders 241

Children Act 1989 241–2
children 114–15, 125, 255–6
chiropodists 125
Chronically Sick and
    Disabled Persons Act
    1970 167
circulation 52
circulatory system 182
closed questions 142, 267
communication 129–52,
    267, 285
communication
    skills 133–52
community care 104
community health 44
community psychiatric nurses
    (CPNs) 123, 245
compulsory referral 107
confidentiality 170
connective tissue 180
continence 298–301
Control of Substances
    Hazardous to Health
    Regulations 1990 287
cranial cavity 181, 184
creative activities 254–79

day centre 271–2
day nurseries 125, 240, 272
defence mechanisms 83,
    112–13
deficit model 96
diabetics 11
diet 4–12
digestive system 182, 194–6
direct discrimination 158
disability 110–14, 116–17,
    160, 165, 290
Disabled Persons Act 1986
    167
discriminatory
    behaviour 152–68
District Health
    Authority 102, 103
district nurses 122
doctors 102, 121–2

dressing and undressing 312
drug abuse 34–7

eating and drinking 308–11
elderly people 115–18
emotional development 71,
    256
empathy 137
Employment Medical
    Advisory Service
    (EMAS) 56
Employment Protection Act
    1975 167
    1978 167, 286–7
empowerment 230, 237–8
endocrine system 182,
    198–9
energy 12, 214–17
environment 248–50, 275
epithelial tissue 180
Equal Pay Act 1970 167, 287
ethical issues 173–4
evaluation 270
excreta 207–8
exercise 2–3, 12–17
eye contact 138–9

facial expressions 138
families 85, 88–91, 108–10,
    131–2
Family Health Service
    Authorities 103
family centres 241
fat 7–8, 178
feet 43
Fire Safety and Safety in
    Places of Sport Act
    1987 288
first aid 54–5
fluorine 6, 9
food chains 215
food web 216
foreign bodies 64
fund-holding GPs 104

gender stereotyping 159

323

general practitioners
    (GPs)   102, 104, 121–2
gestures   139–40
grief   113–14
group interaction   147–50
group membership   147
group pressure   146
groups   144–52

haemorrhage   62–5
hair   42, 296
head circumference   206
Health and Safety (First Aid)
    Regulations 1981   54
Health and Safety at Work
    Act 1974   287
Health and Safety Executive
    (HSE)   56
health and safety   287–8
health and social care
    services   100–28
health and well-being   1–99
health emergencies   52–66
health promotion   45
health visitors   122, 245
heart   191–3
height   204–5
HIV   29–41, 54
home care assistants   120
hormones   182, 198–9
hospitals   100–1, 105, 272
housing   95
hygiene   41–4, 53–4
hypothermia   209, 211

income   94
indirect discrimination   158
infection   290–2
intellectual
    development   71, 256
interpersonal
    relationships   84–8
iodine   6, 9
iron   6, 8

joints   186

language   157–8
levers in the body   218–19
life events   81–4
lifestyle   2, 96
listening   135–6

loss   113
lung inflations   60, 61

making beds   305–7
Maslow   134, 135, 227
meals-on-wheels   121
medicines   288–9
Medicines (General Sales
    List) Order 1977   288
Medicines (Prescription
    Only) Order 1977   288
midwives   123, 245
minerals   6, 8–9
Misuse of Drugs Act
    1971   188
mitosis   180
mobility   302–5
mouth care   296–7
mouth-to-mouth
    resuscitation   60, 61
mouth-to-mouth-and-nose
    resuscitation   62
moving and
    handling   219–21
multi-disciplinary
    teams   102, 105
muscles   178, 180, 182,
    186–8, 218–19
muscular system   182, 186–8

nails   43, 298
National Health Service
    (NHS)   101–5
National Health Service Act
    1973   102
National Health Service Act
    1977   167
National Health Service and
    Community Care Act
    1990   103–4
National Vocational
    Qualifications
    (NVQs)   125
needs   134–5, 225–30,
    293–4
nervous tissue   180
non-verbal
    communication
    137–44
nose bleeds   65
nursery schools   240–1
nurses   121, 122, 123

observation   135, 201–2,
    206, 208
occupational therapists
    (OTs)   124–5, 246
open questions   142, 267
organs   181–2

parent and toddler
    groups   241
passive smoking   24–5
Patient's Charter   118–19
pelvic cavity   181, 182
people with
    disabilities   110–14,
    259
personal bias   155, 165–6
personal hygiene   41–44,
    293–301
phosphorus   6, 8
physical development   70,
    256
physiotherapists   124, 246
planning meals   11
playground accidents   49–50
playgroup   272
post-natal care   239–40
posture   139
potassium   6, 8
poverty   117
practical skills   293–313
practice nurses   122
prejudice   155, 165–6
pressure sores   217–218, 296
primary groups   145
protein   5–6
providers   103
psychiatrist   245
psychologist   246
pulse   16, 58, 212
purchasers   103
pyrexia   209, 212

questioning   142–3

Race Relations Act 1976
    166, 287
racial discrimination   162–3
radiographers   123
recovery position   57–8
recreation   2
referral through a
    professional   107

Registered Homes Act 1984 285–6
registration 285–6
relaxation 4
Reporting of Injuries, Diseases and Dangerous Occurrences Regulations 1985 (Riddor) 56, 288
reproductive system 182, 197–8
residential homes 272
residents' rights 286
respiration 213
respiratory system 182, 189–91
road accidents 48
roles 91–3

school nurse 123
secondary groups 146
self-concept 74–5
self-esteem 75, 228, 263
self-fulfilling prophesy 77
self-referral 107

Sex Discrimation Act 1975 167, 287
sexual behaviour 38–41
sexual discrimination 163–4
sexually transmitted diseases 38
shaving 298
shock 65–6
skeleton 178, 182–6
skeletal system 182–6
skin 42, 182, 200–1
sleep 3, 313
smoking 23–7
social and life skills 289–93
social class 93–4
social development 71, 256
social services 105–6, 107
social workers 119, 246
socialisation 75, 132
sodium 6, 8
solvents 37
space 141
special school 273
speech therapists 125, 246

stages of human development 72–4
stereotyping 153–4
stress 3, 17–23

teeth 43
thoracic cavity 181, 186
tissues 180
touch 141
transition times 86
trusts 103

unconsciousness 57
urinary system 182, 196

values 155, 247–8
varicose veins 65
vitamins 6–7, 9

weight 203–4
work 95

zinc 6, 9